Clinical Homoeopathic Organotherapy

Theory & Practice of Homoeopathy

Dr. Jakir Hossain Laskar, PhD

Homoeopathic Pharmacy

Organon of Medicine
& Homoeopathic Philosophy

Clinical Repertory & Materia Medica

Mother Tinctures & Biochemic Remedies

Practice of Psychiatry

Rare Medication

Note from the Publisher: Any information given in this book is not intended to be taken as a replacement for medical advice. Any person with a condition requiring medical attention should consult a qualified homoeopathic practitioner or theraputist.

"Homeopathy is a classical science which knows the art of curing both for somatic and psychic illness without side effects. We care the physical constitution and mental disposition of the patients, we cure both acute and chronic diseases and we help regain immunity and vital force of the patient." — ***Dr. Jakir Hossain Laskar, PhD,(Indian Homoeopath and Medical Author).***

CLINICAL HOMOEOPATHIC ORGANOTHERAPY

Dr. Jakir Hossain Laskar, PhD

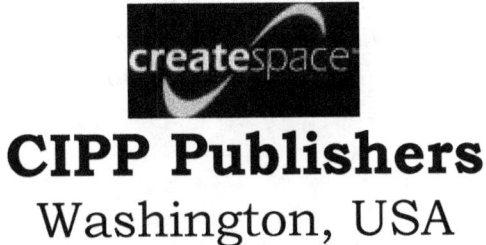

CIPP Publishers
Washington, USA

First Edition
September, 2017 (Clinical Homoeopathic Organotherapy)

Copyright
@ Reserved with the Author

Published by
CreateSpace Independent Publishing Platform
Seattle, Washington, USA

Marketed & Distributed by
Amazon USA, Amazon UK, Amazon Europe,
Amazon India, Amazon Worldwide, CreateSpace eStore

Book Cover Designed by
CreateSpace Cover Creator
Seattle, Washington, USA

[All rights reserved. No part of this book may be reproduced, stored in a retrieval system, or transmitted in any form or by any means, electronic, mechanical, photocopying, recording or otherwise, without the prior permission of the author and publisher. Any person who does any unauthorized act in relation to this publication will be liable to legal prosecution and civil claims for damages. Disputes if any are subject to Kolkata jurisdiction only. - **Author**]

Price : 9.50 USD

Preface

There is no royal road to perfect understanding of art of curing. This book is virtually meant for giving the Homoeopaths an out-and-out knowledge about Pharmacy, Materia Medica, Repertory, Organon of Medicine and Homoeopathic Philosophy.

I have incorporated Mother Tinctures, Biochemic Remedies, Indian Drugs, Specific Medicines, Group Remedies, Definite Medicines, Bedside Medicines, Drug Manuals in Materia Medica part of this book, considering the numerous practical difficulties encountered by most of the practitioners. Every possible attempt has been made for perfect choice of the similimum, amidst complicated symptomatology, from both the phermaceutical and philosophical point if view. I will find my humble endeavour fruitful if the purpose of the Homoeopathic professions could be fulfilled.

This unique book of its type has been written with great endeavour and sincerity with the purpose of acquainting our Homoeopathic Practitioners with infallible drugs.

We frequently use the word 'rare' for some drugs in the vocabulary of our homoeopathic literature - though when a medicine is prescribed frequently to the patients for curing the indicated disease, it then may not be called a 'rare' medicine. However, we are accustomed to use the word 'rare' against some drugs those have definite indications.

The book comprises more than 800 rare drugs with their cardinal therapeutic indications, doses and potency. All the new, old and forgotten remedies and essentials of published clinical experience have been incorporated. The busy doctor of to-day has no time for guess-work or theorizing. He simply wants to know what remedy is radically curative for his patient. I will find my endeavour fruitful and will be amply rewarded if the members of the homoeopathic profession become successful for treating most of the complicated cases by prescribing these specifically indicated drugs.

Lastly, I will only be happy to receive any constructive criticism or suggestion from professors, practitioners and students about this book and the method or style of presenting a drug, so that they may be duly incorporated if found worthwhile in subsequent editions.

18-th September, 2017
Kolkata, India

Author
Dr. Jakir Hossain Laskar, PhD

Dedicated...

To my beloved Mother

who helped me to become an Ethical Homoeopathic Practitioner.

Contents

1. The Preparation of Remedies and Scales of Dilution
2. Medicinal Vehicles
3. External Applications
4. Prescription Writing
5. Cardinal Principles of Homoeopathy
6. Regional Quick Prescriber
7. Bedside Medicine
8. Definite Medicines
9. Clinical Repertory
10. Combined Remedies
11. Master Guide
12. Specific Medicine
13. Internal Definite Prescription
14. External Definite Prescription
15. Biochemic Medicine
16. Psychiatry : Theory and Practice
17. Mental Philosophy
18. Bedside Prescriber (Potency)
19. Bedside Prescriber (Tincture)
20. Bedside Prescriber (Biochemic Remedies)
21. First-Aid Medicine
22. Compound Remedy
23. Drug Index
24. Drug Manual
25. Rare Medication with Therapeutic Index

Clinical Homoeopathic Organotherapy

Dr. Jakir Hossain Laskar, PhD

HOMOEOPATHIC PHARMACY

Chapter - 1
The Preparation of Remedies and Scales of Dilution

There are two main classes of original substance from the pharmaceutical point of view: (i) Soluble (ii) Insoluble.

Mother tinctures (the symbol ø is used to denote the mother tincture) prepared from alcohol-water extraction of the plant material are used in the class of soluble substances. Rhythmical violent agitations at each stage are carried out and the process is known as 'Succussion'. 'Trituration' is a prolonged circular grinding with mortar and pestle taking 'Lactose' as the diluent for the preparation of the natural insoluble substances. When the trituration has obtained 6x or $1/10^6$, this will be dispersed into alcohol-water diluent and afterwards it may be treated as a soluble substance. It is now fit to be converted into liquid potency.

Decimal scale involves a serial trituration 1/10, whereas centesimal involves a serial dilution 1/100. 'X' is denoted for decimal scale and the 'C' is for centesimal.

Three scales are used for the preparations of the homoeopathic potencies of liquid drug substances, i.e. (a) Centesimal, (b) Millesimal and (c) Decimal.

Two scales are in use : (i) Centesimal and (ii) Decimal, to prepare potencies from solid drug substances.

The Centesimal Scale : Introduced by Hahnemann himself. In this scale the 1st potency contains 1/100th part of the original drug and the 2nd potency will contain 1/100th part of the 1st potency and so on. Available centesimal potencies are: 1,3,6,12,30,200,1M, 10M, 50M, CM etc.

The Fifty Millesimal Scale : Introduced as per Organon of Medicine, 6th edition, Aphorism 270 (published 78 years after Hahnemann's death). In this scale the 1st potency contains 1/50,000th part of the original drug, the 2nd potency will contain 1/50,000th part of the 1st potency and so on. Potency available in this scale is denoted by 0/1,0/2,0/3,0/4 up to 0/30.

The Decimal Scale : Introduced by Dr. Constantine Herring. In this scale the 1st potency contains 1/10th part of the original drug, the 2nd potency will contain 1/10th part of the 1st potency and so on. Potencies available in this scale 1x, 2x, 3x, 6x, 12x, 30x 200x etc.

In practice, first centesimal (1 or 1C) potency is equivalent to second decimal (2x) potency and the first Fifty millesimal (0/1) potency is equal to second centesimal (2C) potency. So, 0/1=2C=4x.

Chapter - 2
Medicinal Vehicles

In Homoeopathy, vehicle is an inert substance, having no medicinal property of its own with chemically neutral in medicinal effects, in which medicines are prepared or mixed and given for their internal administrations either by oral or olfaction method and external application for medications.

Uses of Vehicle

1. Used in the preparation of mother tinctures, mother solutions and mother powders from crude drug materials.
2. It is used for dispensing medicines according to the prescriptions.
3. Used for further trituration and increased potentization.
4. For the preservation of certain medicines.
5. Used as 'Placebo' or 'Phytum' in cases of chronic diseases and where long acting remedies are used in between the administrations of the two dosed of remedies. 'Placebo' is the second best medicine in our Materia Medica, which is given to the patient to please.
6. As bases for preparing external applications of medicines.

Forms of Vehicles

There are three forms of vehicles: (i) Solid (ii) Liquid and (iii) Semi-solid.

Solid Vehicles

Saccharum Lactis or Sugar of Milk

White fine powder prepared from goat's milk.

Globules : Are made from pure cane sugar. These are round in shape, white in colour, odorless, easily soluble in water but insoluble in alcohol having sweetish taste with the size of 10,20,30,40 etc.

Pilules : These are characteristically same with globules but the sizes of pilules vary from 40 to 80, designated by numbers, e.g., 40, 60, 70, 80 etc.

Tablets : They are white looking round but flat, prepared from pure refined milk sugar by compression or moulding.

Liquid Vehicles

Distilled Water : is a good solvent, having a physiological inertness.

Alcohol - (a) Absolute alcohol.

(b) Strong alcohol - Used to prepare of absolutealcohol, mother tinctures, dilute alcohol, dispensing alcohol etc.

(c) Dilute alcohol - For preparation of potencies particularly under decimal scale.

(d) Dispensing alcohol - Used for preparing most of the dilutions, because it is readily absorbed by sugar of milk or globules or tablets.

Glycerine - Mainly used in external applications..

Olive oil - Used in external applications.

Almond oil - Also used in external applications.

Sesame oil - Used in the preparation of the hair oil.

Semi-solid Vehicles

Vaseline - (i) White soft paraffin - Used in the preparation of medicinal ointments and is applied on wounds or ulcers in dressing.

(ii) Yellow soft paraffin - same as described in white soft paraffin.

Lanolin - Extensively used in ointments as because it has penetrating power within the skin.

Chapter - 3
External Applications

The principles of homoeopathy do not allow external applications. It mainly advocates internal administration of medicines alone on symptoms similarity for the treatment of both the acute and chronic diseases. But in aphorisms 284-285 in his Organon of Medicine, 6th Edition, Hahnemann has given an exceptional allowance for external applications.

So, when the curative remedy should be continued internally, the same medicine may only be applied externally as a liniment, ointment, lotion etc. The external applications are prescribed in various cases like burns, injuries, lacerations, accidental cases, to relieve muscle tension and antiseptic dressings.

Ointments - One part by weight or volume of the required mother tincture is mixed thoroughly with 9 parts by volume or weight of white soft paraffin to prepare this therapeutic cream.

Liniments - It is prepared by one part of the required mother tincture mixed with four parts of Olive oil.

Lotions - These liquid suspensions are prepared by one part of the requisite mother tincture mixing thoroughly with 9 parts purified water.

Glyceroles – Theses are mixtures of solutions of one part of required mother tincture and 9 part of glycerine.

Chapter - 4
Prescription Writing

Prescription means a written direction for preparing a remedy by a physician for his patient, which is most appropriate as considered by the attending physician.

The body of the prescription is divided in the following 4 parts:

1. Superscription - It is the heading consisting of the symbol which means 'to take'. In this part the name, address and age of the patient, along with the word 'For' before his name, may be included.

2. Inscription - This part is the main trunk of a prescription which contains the name of the remedy, potency, its quantity, also the vehicle with its required quantity.

3. Subscription - It contains the directions or instructions to a compounder or dispenser as to how he should dispense the remedy.

4. Signature - This part of the prescription contains the directions to the patients, as to how he will take the remedy, alone with the signature of the physician with his registration number and date.

EXAMPLE OF PRESCRIPTION WRITING

For,
     Ranita Balmiki (Miss)
     97/A, Kazi Nazrul Islam Road
     Ranikuthi, Kolkata - 700032.
Rx, ...Superscription
Puls. Nig. 200 (One drum in 30 no globules) ....Inscription
    4 globules to be taken thrice daily for 7 days.......Subscription
               ....

Signature
...........Regd. No.
.... Date ....

In a printed pad of the physician
Mode of writing Abbreviations

Abbreviations - Full form

A.C. / a.c. – Before meals / Before food
Ad us. exter. – For external use
Aq. dist. – Distilled water
B.D. – Twice daily
Cap – Let him / her take
C.M. – To be taken tomorrow morning
C.N. – tomorrow night
C.V. – tomorrow evening
D. – A dose
Dieb att – On alternat day; every other day
Ft. – Let it be made
f.m. – Make a mixture
Gr. – A grain
Gt. – Drop
Gtt. – Drops
H. – An hour
H.S. – At bedtime
M. – Mix
Mist – A mixture
M. et.N. – Morning and night
O.M. – Every Morning
O.N. – Every night
O.H. – Every hour
O.d. – Every day
P.C. – After food
P.r.n. – When required
Pulv. – Powder
Q.L. – Four times a day
Sig. – Mark., Level
S.O.S. – If necessary
Stat. – Immediately
T.D. – Thrice a day
Tr. – Tincture
Uncia – An ounce
Ut. Dict. – As directed
Vac. Ven. – In empty stomach

ORGANON OF MEDICINE

Chapter - 5
Cardinal Principles of Homoeopathy

1. Law of Similia
'Similia similibus curantur' which means 'like cures like'. The selection of the medicine is fundamentally based on the principle that the medicine must have the capability of producing most similar symptoms of the disease to be cured in healthy persons.

2. Law of Minimum
According to this principle, we give medicine to the patients in very minute dose to avoid unwanted aggravation.

3. Law of Simplex
As because the homoeopathic remedies were proved singly, we use just one remedy at a time.

4. Theory of Chronic disease
The chronic diseases are caused by three chronic miasms, i.e., Prora, Syphilis, and Sycosis.

5. Doctrine of Drug Proving
Proving of drug is a systematic investigation of disease-producing power of medicine on the healthy human being of different ages, both sexes and of various constitutions.

6. Theory of Vital Force
"The material organism without the vital force is capable of no sensation, no function, no self preservation; it derives all sensations, and performs all the functions of life solely by means of the immaterial being (the vital force) which animates the material organism.

7. Doctrine of Drug Dynamization
Homoeopathic dynamizations are processes by which the medicinal properties which are latent in natural substances while in their crude state, become awakened and developed into activity to an incredible degree.

Considerations for Selection of the Potency of Drugs

There are five-fold considerations for choosing the potency of a homoeopathic drug :

1. The susceptibility of the patient
Susceptibility is greatest in children and young vigorous persons and diminishes with age.

Higher potencies are best adopted to sensitive persons of the nervous, sanguine, or choleric temperament; to intelligent and intellectual persons, quick to act and react. Lower potencies and larger and more frequent doses correspond better to torpid and phlegmatic individuals, dull of comprehension and slow to act.

Persons who have already taken many crude drugs often require high potencies.

2. The seat of the disease
Certain malignant and rapidly fatal diseases may require material doses or low potencies of a drug.

3. The nature and intensity of the disease.
Diseases characterized by diminished vital reaction require the lower potencies; while diseases characterized by increased vital reaction respond better to higher potencies.

4. The stage and duration of the disease
At one stage of the disease when the vital reaction is low, the patient may need a low potency and frequent repetition at another a high potency.

5. The previous treatment of the disease
Cease all medication for a few days and carefully regulate the diet and regimen if the patient seems to have lost all susceptibility for the time being due to abuse of too many drugs in crude doses.

Repetition of Remedies

Three following rules are to be observed for not changing a remedy.

A. Never repeat a remedy when the patient himself is improving.

B. Never change a remedy when symptoms are following Herring's Law of Cure, i.e., from within outward from above downward and symptoms appearing in the reverse order of the sequence of symptoms.

C. Never change your remedy when a discharge or eruption follows the administration of a remedy.

Medicinal Aggravation and their Interpretations

If the aggravation is long, with a decline of the patient's strength - the case is incurable and can only be palliated.

If the aggravation is long, with a slow improvement - the case is just taken up before it was too late; all will be well if the remedy is not too soon repeated.

If the aggravation is short and violent-the patient has enough vitality and their best result will follow.

If the quality and quantity of the remedy administered are in exact progression to the quality and quantity of the disease force-there will be ideal cure, i.e., cure without aggravation.

If there is an immediate amelioration, followed soon by aggravation-it is a failure, the case is incurable.

If too short an amelioration follows a pronounced aggravation-it will prove incurable.

If a full time amelioration of symptoms occurs without any increase in the patient strength - he will prove too weak for a respiration to health.

If the patient develops symptoms of the remedy given without improvement in his disease symptoms - the case is a hard one to treat as he is very sensitive to all remedies like a prover.

If the old symptoms appear with the aggravation.-One has to wait and need study no more; the most suitable remedy has been selected.

Second Prescription

Repetition : If the original symptoms come back with the same generals and particulars as formerly.

Complementary : Selected first medicine is an acute one and for the completion of cure, it is to be complemented with the help of the constitutional medicine.

Antidote : When the patient experience a lot of new symptoms after the administration of the first prescription not belonging to the pathogenesis of the medicine, not even the old symptoms.

Cognate : Medicines closely related to each other are known as cognates.

Remedy changed : (i) If the symptoms are changed, but the patient is improving, no need to change the remedy.

(ii) When the patient is not improving with the changed symptoms administer a new remedy.

(iii) Turning up of striking new group of symptoms leading to an entire change of base of the symptoms.

(iv) Shun that remedy after testing more doses without effect.

Changed Plan of Treatment : If the symptoms of another miasm comes up prominently with disappearance of symptoms of previous miasm treated.

HOMOEOPATHIC MATERIA MEDICA

Chapter - 6
REGIONAL QUICK PRESCRIBER

STOMACH

Sour belching and vomiting of pregnancy – Acetic Acid, Lactic Acid.
Indigestion of teething children, can't bear milk, vomiting – Aethusa Cyn., Mag. Mur.
Gastric upset – Ant. Crude, Arg. Nit., Sulph.
Belching accompaies most gastric ailments, flatulence – Aloe. Soc., Arg. Nit.
Vomiting – Bismuth, Fer. Met., Kreos., Lac.Def., Tab.
Abnormal appetite for chalk and indigestable things – Cic. Vir., Alumina., Psor.
Nausea or vomiting from riding in carriage, boat or railroad car – Cacculus, Arn., Nux. V., Sanicula.
Smell painfully acute; nausea and faintness from the odro of cooking food – Colch., Ars., Sepia.
Regurgitation and eructation of food in mouthfuls (Alumina), without nausea. – Phos.
Empty eructations from morning to night, as if every particle of food was turned into air. – Iod., Kali Carb.
Round ulcer of stomach. – Kali Bich., Gym.
Malignant affections of stomach. – Kreos.
Extreme nausea and vomiting with profuse sweat. – Lobelia.
Spasmodic affections of stomach and intestine. – Colo., Mag. Carb., Mag. Phos.
Heartburn, of pregnancy. – Mag. Carb.
Colic. – Colo., Dios. Vill., Mag. Carb., Mag. Phos.
Weakness of old age; dyspepsia of old people. – Nux. Mos.
Pain and distress in stomach while eating, or immediately after. – Kali Bich., Nux. Mos.
Eructations : sour, nausea, vomiting every morning after eating, pyrosis. – Nux. Vom.
Morning sickness of pregnancy; the sight of food sicknes (Nux. Vom.); the smell of cooking food nauseates. (Ars.) – Sepia.
Chronic heartburn. – Acid Sulph.
Nausea. – Ipec., Tab.

ABDOMEN

Piles. – Aes. Hip., Aloe. Soc., Ars., Acid Mur., Acid Nit., Thuja Occ., Wyethia.
Constipation. – Aes. Hip., Alum., Bryo., Calc. C., Can. Sat., Am. Mur., Arn., Caust., Opium.

Dysentry with lower abdominal colic. –Aloe. Soc., Colch., Canth., Ipec.
Haemorrhoids : like a bunch of grapes, itching. – Acid Mur., Aloe Soc., Hamamalis.
Piles. – Am. Mur., Sulph., Baryta Carb., Ign., Colinsonia, Lach., Sulph., Thuja.
Mucous Piles. – Ant. Crude.
Cholera with vomiting. – Ant. Tart., Camphor., Cuprum Met.
Dysentry of old people. –Bapt. Tinc.
Colic from gall-stone. – Berb. Vulg.
Anal fistula. – Berb. Vulg., Calc. Phos., Sil.
Diarrhoea : of teething childrenm. – Chamo.
Constipation. – Plumb., Chelid., Lach., Caust., Acid Nit., Plat. Met.
Gall-stone. – Chelid. (Terrible attacks of gall-stone colic. – Card. Mar.)
Grinding of teeth. – Cina., Cic. V., Mer. V., Spig.
Flatulence. – China, Carbo. Veg.
Umbilical hernia.– Cocculus., Nux. Vom.
Abdomen distended with gas. – Colchicum.
Jaundice, gall-stone. – Cholesterin., Fel. Touri.
Peptic ulcer. – Uran. Nit.
Abdominal colic : (> by pressure). – Colcynth (> by heat. – Mag. Phos.), Dios., Ipec., Lyco., Plumb., Ver. Alb.
Diarrhoea. – Crot. Tig., Fer. Met., Phos., Psor., Ver. Alb.
Constipation. – Fer. Met., Lac. Def., Lyco., Mag. Mur., Am. Carb., Nat. Mur., Psor., Pyrozen., Melilotus Alb.
Rectal prolapse and itching of anus. – Fer. Met., Stann. Met.
Prolapsus ani from moderate straining at stool. – Ign., Ac. Nit., Podo., Ruta G.
Cholera Infantum. – Kali Brom., Podo.
Flatulence; good appetite but a few mouthfuls fill up to the throat. > (– Lower abdomen – Lyco.); (–Upper abdomen – Carbo. Veg.); (– Entire abdomen – China).
Hernia, right-sided. – Lyco. (Umbilical hernia – Nux Vom. Cocculus).
Hepatomegally. – Mag. Mur.
Constipation; can only pass stool by learning very far back. – Medo.
Bloody dysentry. – Merc. Sol., Merc. Cor.
Ulceration with fungus-like growths and pseudo-like membranous deposits of intestional tract. – Acid Mur.
Aversion from milk; diarrhoea from it. – Nat. Carb.
Stool : involuntary, knows not wheather flatus or feaces escape. – Aloe. Soe., Iod., Acid Mur., Nat. Mur., Podo.
Diarrhoea : much flatus, on first rising and standing on the feet. – Nat. Sulph.
Fissure of rectum, pain during stool. – Ac. Nit., Alumina, Nat. M., Ratanhia, Syphil.
Haemorrhage : from bowels in typhoid. – Acid Nit., Crot., Ac. Mur.
Abdomen distended after every meal. – Nux. Mos.
Diarrhoea : from, boiled milk, cold drinks. – Nux. Mos.
Alternate constipation and diarrhoea. – Nux. V., Sulph., Ver. Alb.
Constipation : of children; of corpulent, good-natured woman. – Opium.
Involuntary stool, from paralysis of sphinter. – Opium.
Painless cholera morbus; cholera infantum. – Podo., Sec. Cor.
Prolapse of rectum, before or with stool. – Podo., Syphil., Tab.

Intussusception with colic and faecal vomiting; strangulated hernia, femoral, inguinal or umbilical. – Plumb. Met.

Diarrhoea : driving out of bed early in the morning. – Aloe Soc., Psor., Sulph.

Constipation. – Chelid., Plumb., Opium., Pyrozen., Thuja., Sulph., Tab., Syphil., Ver. Alb.

Jaundice : the eyes, skin and urine yellow, dark-brown, liver spots. – Plumb.

Sour child : colic with sour stool. – Rheum.

Early morning diarrhoea. – Aloe Soc., Nat. Sulph., Rumex., Podo., Sulph., Thuja Occ.

Worm affections of children. – Cina, Sabad., Sil., Spigalia.

Diarrhoea : painless, involuntary, anus wide open. – Apis Mel., Sec. Cor., Phos.

Constipation : requires mechanical aids. – Aloe. Soc., Calc. C., Selen., Sil., Sepia, Sanic.

Pot-belliedness of mother. – Sepia.

Pot-belliedness of children.– Sulph.

Constipation : during pregnancy. – Alumina, Sepia.

Constipation : before and during menses. – Sil.

Diarrhoea : before and during menses. – Am. Carb., Bovista.

Fistula in ano alternating with chest symptoms. – Berb. Vulg., Sil., Calc. Phos.

Appendicitis. – Iris. Tenax.

Anal fissure with warts or condylomata. – Thuja Occ., Myristica.

Scrofulous children affected with ascarides and lumbrici. – Cina, Spig., Stann, Terebin., TMV., Santon.

URINARY

Diabetes. – Acetic Acid., Ars. Brom., Colchicum., Lyssin., Insulin, Merc. Sol., Helonias., Uran. Nit.

Incontinence of urine, scalds severely, painful, bloody. – Apis., Canth., Thuja., Kreos., Berb. Vulg., Equisetum Hy., Sarsa.

Urine passes unconciously day and night. – Arg. Nit., Caust.

Involuntary faces and urine. – Arn., Lil. Tig., Sanic.

Retention or incontinence of urine after labor. – Arn. Mont.

Nocturnal eneruesis. – Ac. Benz., Caust., Medo., Psor., Mag. Phos., Equisetum Hy.

Dribbling of urine of old men with enlarged prostate. – Acid Benz.

Pain at urethra. – Can. Sat., Canth., Equiset. Hy.

Urine involuntary : when coughing sneezing, blowing the nose. – Caust., Puls., Nat. Mur., Ver. Alb.

Urine : turbid, milky, involuntary. – Cina.

Urine : dark, scanty or suppressed; in drops, with white sediment; bloody; contains clots of putrid decomposed blood, albumin, sugar.– Colchicum.

Urine : catarrhal is churia in grown-up children, with milky urine; from wading with bare feet in cold water; involuntary. – Dulc.

Strangury : retention of urine. – Tereb.

Ranal colic. – Calc. Renalis.

Constant desire to urinate; large quantity urine passes. – Equisetum Hy. (scanty, few drops. – Apis., Canth.)

Painful tenesmus of bladder and bowels when urinating. – Medo.

Tenesmus of bladder, burning in urethra; urine scanty in drops with pain, bloody; albuminus. – Merc. Cor.

Urine passes slowly; bladder weak, must wait a long time. – Acid Mur., Heper. S., Nat. Mur.

Urine : scanty, strong-smelling. – Acid Nit.

Urine : retention, with bladder full, paralysis of bladder. – Opium.

Nephritis. – Plumb. Met.

Urine : involuntary with coughing. – Rumex. C., Sil., Caust., Puls.

Pressure on the bladder as if constantly full; can hardly retain urine on account of urging, involuntary. –Ruta G.

Severe unbearable pain at conclusion of urination. – Berb. Vulg., Equisetum Hy., Medo., Sarsa., Thuja.

Passage of gravel or small calculi, renal colic; stone in bladder; bloody urine. – Sarsa.

Painful distention and tenderness in bladder; urine dribbles while sitting; standing passes freely; air passes from urethra. – Sarsa.

Sand in urine or on diaper; child screams before and while passing it. – Borax., Lyco., Sarsa.

Urine : scanty, coffee-ground sediment; suppressed in brain troubles and dropsy; albuminus. – Heleborus.

Urine : flow inpeded, voided slowly, without force; is oblized to wait awhile before it passes; bladder weak, is unable to finish, seems as if some urine always remains. – Heper., Alum., Sil.

Paralysis of bladder : after labor, with retention or incontinence of urine; no desire to urinate in lying-in-women. – Arn. Mont., Hyos., Opium.

Smarting and burning during and after micturation. – Kreo., Sulph.

Red sand in urine, on child's diaper. – Lyco., Phos.

Child cries before urinating. – Borax., Lyco.

Pain in back > by urinating; renal colic, right side. – Lyco. (left side. – Berberis).

Weakness of bladder. – Mag. Mur., Staph.

Constant desire to urinate on seeing running water. – Lyssin., Canth., Sulph.

Eneuresis : nocturnal; after cathaterization. – Mag. Phos.

Severe back pain in renal region > by profuse urination; renal colic, with sensation of passing of calculus. – Medo.

Neuralgia or renal colic; excruciating pains from right kidney downwards. – Lyco., Sarsa.

Eneuresis : of old people, bloody. – Sec. Cor.

Urine : involuntary dribbling while walking. – Selen.

Eneuresis : bed is wet almost as soon as the child goes to sleep; always during the first sleep. – Kreos., Sepia.

Urging to urinate, has to sit at urinal for hours. – Staphis.

Urging and pain after urinating in prostatic troubles of old men. – Staphis.

Urine : painful to parts over which it passes. – Sulph.

Renal colic. – Tab.

Violent burning and drawing pains in kidney, bladder and urethre, bloody urine. – Berb. V., Canth., Terebin.

MALE SEXUAL

Complete impotence : no sexual power. – Agnus. C., Arg. Nit., Calad., Lyco., Selen.

Gleet, gonorrhoea. – Agnus., Can. Sat., Medo., Sepia, Merc. Cor., Kali Iod., Nat. Sulph., Psor.

Crushed pain in the testicles. – Arg. Met., Rhodo.

Semenal emissions : after onanism; almost every night; without erecion. – Arg. Met., Canth.

Induration of prostate and testis. – Baryta Carb.

Sexual desire increased, of both sexes. – Canth.

Emissions during sleep; vivid dreams of women at night. – Dios. Vill., Staphis.

Decided aversion to coition. – Graph.

Sexual desire absent in fleshy people. – Kali Bich.

Nocturnal emissions stained with blood. – Led. P., Merc. Sol., Sarsa.

Acute affections of prostate. – Merc. Dulcis.

Gonorrhoea and syphilis. – Merc. Solubilis.

Seminal emission : soon after coition; impotences, paralysis after sexual excess. –Nat. Mur.

Onanism : when patient is greatly distressed by the culpability of the act. – Acid Phos.

Priapism, with spinal disease, erection violent, long-lasting; profuse seminal emissions, satyriasis. – Acid Picric., Canth., Phos.

Orchitis. – Rhodo.

Bloody seminal emissions. – Ledum., Merc. Sol., Sarsa.

Priapism; glands drawn up. – Selen., Berb. Vulg. (drawn down – Canth.)

Testictes swollen, spermatic cord swollen, bruised, painful. – Spong.

Onanism : persistently dwelling on sexual subjects; constantly thinking of sexual pleasures. – Staphis.

Spermatorrhoea : atrophy of sexual organ. – Staph.

CIRCULOTORY

Heart troubles, palpitatoin. – Actea Rece., Digitalis., Lil. Tig., Iod., Lith. Carb., Calc. Ars., Cactus G.

Hypertrophy of heart. – Bromium.

Dropsy from cardiac disease. – Colinsonia.

Apoplexy. – Crot. Hor., Lach.

Weak heart, pulse slow; sensation as if heart would stop beating if she moved. – Digitalis.

Fears that unless on the move heart will cease beating. – Gels.

Fatty degenaration of heart. – Kali Carb., Phos., Lach.

Pulse slow. – Kalmia.

Rapid pulse (–150 to 170 /m) – Lil. Tig., Pyrozen.

Sensation as if heart would stand still; deep seated pain at base. – Lob. Inf.

Sensation as if heart was grasped in a vise.– Cactus., Lil Tig.

Palpiatition and cardiac pains, while sitting, < by moving about. – Mag. Mur., Spig.

Hypertrophy of heart, vulvular lesions, paralysis of heart, pain in the region of heart. – Naja. T.

Fluttering of heart; with a weak faint feeling < lying down. – Lach., Nat. Mur.

The heart's pulsations shake the body. – Nat. Mur., Spigelia.

Pains : neuralgic, myalgic, or rheumatic pains in walls of the chest.– Ran. Bulb.

Chest complaints of stonecutters with total loss of strength.– Sil.
Rheumatic affection of heart. – Kalmia Lat., Ledum., Naja., Spig.
Great weakness in chest; < from talking, laughing, reading aloud, singing; so weak, unable to talk. – Stann.
Heart : pain from base to apex. – Syphil.
Heart : pain from apex to base. – Medo.
Heart : pain from base to clavicle. – Spig.

FEMALE SEXUAL

Amenorrhoea in plethoric youngh girls. – Acon., Apoc., Euphresia.
Pregnancy : abortion at third month. – Act. Race., Sabina.
If given during last month of pregnancy, shortens labor. – Act. Race., Caulo., Puls.
Uterine prolapse. – Aes. Hip., Agar., Arg. Met., Aurum. Met., Kali Bich., Lyssin. Podo.
Leucorrhoea, yellowish. – Agnus. C. (whitish – Borax.)
Deficient secretion or suppression of milk in nursing women. – Agnus., Lac. Can., Lac. Def.
Profuse leucorrhoea. – Alum., Syphil., Psor.
Discharge of blood between periods, at every little accident – a long walk, after every hard stool. – Ambra Grisea.
Cholera-like symptoms at the commencement of menses. – Am. Carb., Bovista., Am. Mur., Ver. Alb.
Leucorrhoea : like white of egg, after every urination. – Am. Mur.
Amenorrhoea in young girls. – Apoc., Acon. Nap.
Coition : painful in both sexes; followed by bleeding from vagina. – Arg. Nit., Acid Nit.
Threatened abortion esp. at 3rd month. – Sec. Cor., Sabina.
Suppression of milk; the breast do not properly fill. –Sec. Cor.
Violent stitches upward in the vagina; lancinating pains from the uterus to the umbilicus. – Sepia.
Irregular menses of nearly every form – early, late, scanty, profuse, amenorrhoea, memorrhagia. – Sepia.
Vulva sensitive, can scarcely wear a napkin.– Plat. M., Staphis., Thuja Occ.
Menorrhagia : has not been well since her last miscarriage.– Sulph.
Uterine colic, uterine cancer. – T.B.P.
Menses, every 15 days. – TBP., Trillium.
Mamary cancer. – Bufo Rana., Carcinocin, Ars. Iod., Ast. Rub.
Bruised plevis. – Bellis P.
Uterine fibroid. – Thyroid.
Emenagogue. – Gossipium.
Metrorrhagia : in sterility. – Arg. Nit.
Sexual desire increased. – Ast. Rubens., Lit. Tig., Murex., Lac. Can., Plat. Met.
Membranous dysmenorrhoea. – Bromium, Collinsonia, Medo., Tub., Puls., Mag. Carb., Crocus Sat., Sabina, Ver. Alb.
Mammy : Stony hard. – Bryo., Phyto.
Pruritus vagina. – Calad., Kreos., Zinc. Met.

Any ailments during pregnancy, parturition, lactation. – Caulo.
Leucorrhoea in little girls.– Calc. Carb., Caulo., Mill.
Habitual abortion from uterine debility.– Caulo.
Haemorrhage after abortion.– Caulo., Sec. Cor., TBP.
Milk runs out in nursing women (runs out after weaning–Con.) – Chamo.
Leucorrhoea : in place of menses; like the washing of meat. – Cocculus.
Breasts sore, hard and painful before and during menstruation. – Con., Lac. Con., Kali Carb., Merc. Sol.
Menses : of short duration. – Baryta Carb., Con., Euphrasia.
Leucorrhoea. – Borax., Con., Bovista.
Malignant disease of uterus. – Crot. Hor.
Leucorrhoea : before and after. – Graph. (before – Sep.; after – Kreos.)
Hard cicatrices remaining after mamary abscess, retarding the flow of milk; cancer of breast. – Graph.
Decided aversion of coition. – Graph., Kali Bich.
For the bad affects of abortions and miscarriages. – Helon. Dioica.
Leucorrhoea : pruritus. – Hydrastis.
Leucorrhoea : most abandant at time of menses. – Iod.
Cancerous degeneration of the cervix. – Iod.
Threatened abortion. – Kali Brom., Kali Carb.
Weak before menses; backache, before and during. – Kali Carb.
Post climacteric diseases of women. – Kreos.
Severe headache : before and during menses. – Kreos.
Menses : flow intermittent, at time almost ceasing, then commencing again. – Kreos., Sulph.
Leucorrhoea : < between periods. – Borax., Bov., Kreos., Mag. Mur.
Violent corrosive itching of pudenda and vagina.– Kreos., Medo., Plat., Taran.
Climacteric ailments : haemorrhoids, haemorrhages, burning vertex, headache. – Lach., Sang., Sulph.
Serviceable in almost all cases when it is required to dry up milk.– Lac. Can., Asaf. (to bring back or increase it. – Lac. Def.)
Bearning down sensation : as though all organs would escape. – Lil. Tig., Lac. Can., Murex., Sep., Sanic., Nat. Mur., Nat Carb.
Weak and atonic condition of ovaries, uterus and pelvic tissues, resulting in antiversion, retroversion, sub-involution. – Helon. Dioica, Lil. Tig., Sepia.
Dryness of vagina; buring in, during and after coition. – Lyco., Lyssin.
Physometra. – Lyco., Lac. Can., Nux. Mos.
Vaginismus. – Mag. Phos.
Chronic ovaritis, salpingitis, pelvic cellulitis, fibroids, cysts and other morbid growth of the uterus and overies. – Medo.
Breast and nipple, sore and sensetive to touch. –Medo.
Leucorrhoea : with pruritus; < from contact of urine. – Merc. Sol., Sulph.
Painless drainage, from uterus; after labor or abortion; after miscarriage. – Mill.
Sore pain in uterus. – Helon., Murex., Lys., Taran.
Nymphomania, violent excitement in sexual organs, and excessive desire for an embrace. – Murex., Plat. Met., Taran.

Discharge of mucus from vagina after an embrace, causing sterility.– Nat. Carb.
Nausea and vomiting before, during and after menses. – Nat. Mur.
Haemorrhage : after miscarriage or post-partum.– Acid Nit.
Leucorrhoea : in place of menses. – Cocculus., Nux Mos.
Pain, nausea, vomiting during pregnancy. – Nux. Mos.
Menses, every two weeks. – Nux Vom.
Suppressed menses of young girls. – Podo., Puls. Nig., Tub.
Mammae, full of hard, painful nodusites; mammary abscess, nipple fissured (Graph).– Phyto.
Vomiting in pregnancy. – Psor.
Metrorrhagia : flow in black clots. – Plat. Met.
Threatening abortion : feels a lack of room for foetus in uterus; inability of uterus to expand.– Plumb. Met.
Fissures of nipples in nursing woman. – Ratan.
Tendency to miscarriage esp. at 3rd month.– Sabina.
Ailments : following abortion; pain from sacrum to pubis, in nearly all diseases.– Sabina.
Promotes expulsion of moles or foreign bodies from uterus.– Canth., Sabina.
Menorrhagia : during climacteric; with early 1st menses.– Sabina.
Leucorrhoea : with strong odor of fish-brine.–Sanic.
Retraction of nipples. – Sarsa., Sil.
Leucorrhoea : green, brown, offensive.– Sec. Cor.
Climacteric ailments : flushes of heat and leucorrhoea, burning of palms and soles, painful enlargement of breast; when Lach. and Sulph. fails.–Sang. Can.
Menses : labor-like pains in abdomen; continuous discharge of watery blood until next period. – Sec. Cor.

MENTAL

Great fear and anxiety of mind, with nervous excitability; afraid to go into a crowd where there is excitement.– Acon. Nit. Ac.
Idiocy in children : incapacity to think. – Aethusa Cyn.
Loss of memory.– Anacard., Baryta Carb., Can. Ind., Lac. Can., Con., Carbo Veg., Medo., Kali Brom., Lyco., Nux. Vom., Plumb. M., Syphil.
Bad effects of disappointed affection.– Ant. Crude, Calc. Phos.
Constantly dwelling on suicide. – Aurum Met., Naja. T. (But is afraid to die.– Nux. Vom.)
Full of ideas; no sleep on this account. – Coff. Cruda.
Cannot bear contradiction; easily offended; every triffle makes him angry; speaks hastly. – Cocculus, Anacard.
Bad effects of angar, grief or disappointed love. – Ign., Calc. Phos., Hyos., Aurum Met., Acid Phos., Lach.
Great loquacity; wants to talk all the time.– Agar., Lach., Stramo.
Indifferent : even to one's family; to one's occupation (Ac. Flour., Ac. Phos.); to those whom she loves best.– Sepia.
Night walking; gets up while asleep, walks about and lies down again. – Kali Brom., Sil.
Low-spirited, indifferent, weak memory from sexual abuses.– Anac., Aur. Met., Phos., Acid., Staphis.

Nocturnal halucinations. – Tuber.

The countenance is expressive of fear; the life is rendered miserable by fear; is sure his disease will prove fatal; predicts the day he will die; fear of death during pregnancy.– Acon. Nap.

Mental anxiety, worry, fear accompanies the most trivial ailment.- Acon. Nap.

Music is unbearable, makes her sad. (Sab.– during menses, Nat. Carb.) – Acon. Nap.

Puerperal mania; thinks she is going crazy tries to injure herself. – Actea Rece.

Sensation as if a heavy, black cloud had settled all over her
and enveloped her head so that all is darkness and confusion.– Actea Rece.

Illusion of a mouse running from under her chair. (Lac. Can., Aetrh Cyn.) – Actea Rece.

Absent-minded, reduced power of insight; cannot recollect; has to read a sentence twice before he can comprehend. (Lyc., Acid Phos., Sep.)– Agnus C.

Sudden loss of memory; everething seems to be in a dream; patient is greatly troubled about his forgetfulness; confused, unfit for business.– Anac. Orien.

Disposed to be malicious, seems bent on wickedness. Lack of confidence in himself and others.– Anac. Orien.

Irresistible desire to curse and swear (Lac. C., Lil. Tig., Ac. Nit.– wants to pray continually, stramo.) – Anac. Orien.

Feels as though he had two wills, one commanding him to do what the other forbids. When walking, is anxious, as if someone were pursuing him; suspects everything around him.– Anac. Orien.

Mentally restless; anxious fear of death; thinks it useless to take medicine, is incurable, is surely going to die; dread of death, when alone, or, going to bed.– Ars. Album.

Profound melancholy : feels hateful and quarrelsome; desire to commit suicide; life is a constant burden.– Aurum Met.

Perfect indifference, don't care to do anything, inability to fix the mind on work.– Bapt. Tinc.

Memory deficient; forgetful, inattentive; child cannot be taught for it cannot remember; threatened idiocy.– Baryta Carb.

Imagines he sees ghost, hideous faces, and various insects (stramo.); black animals, dogs, wolves. Fear of imaginary things, wants to run away from them; hallucinations. – Bell.

Violent delirium; disposition to bite, spite, strike and tear things; breaks into fits of laughter and gnashes the teeth; wants to bite and strike the attendants (stramo.); tries to escape (Hell.).– Bell.

Whole body feels as if caged, each wire being twisted tighter and tighter.– Cactus Grand.

Very forgetful : forgets his last words and ideas; begins a sentence, forgets what he intends to speak; inability to recall any thought or event on account of other thoughts crowding his brain. (Anac., Lac. Can.)– Can. Ind.

Constantly theorizing. Laughs immoderately at every trifling word spoken to him.– Can. Ind.

Great apprehension of approaching death. Delirium tremens; excessive loquacity; exageration of time and distance.– Can. Ind.

Hysteria, chorea or epilepsy at puberty, during establishment of menstrual function. (Actea.)– Caulo.

Full of ideas; quick to act, no sleep on this account. Weeping from delight; alternate laughing and weeping.– Coffea Cruda.

Hysteria with great hilarity, singing and dancing (Tar.); alternating with melancholy and rage.– Crocus Sat.

Fear of death (Ars.); utter lack of courage. The anticipation of any unusual ordeal, preparing for church, theatre, or to meet an engagement, brings on diarrhoea; state fright, nervous dread of appearing in public (Arg. Nit.)– Gels.

Hysteria or delirium tremens; with restlessness, jumps our of bed, tries to escape; makes irrelevant answers; thinks he is in the wrong place; talks of imaginary doings, but has no wants and makes no complaints.– Hyos. Nig.

Lascivious mania : immodesty, will not be covered, kicks off the clothes, expose the person; sings obscene songs; lies naked in bed and chatters. – Hyos. Nig.

Mental conditions rapidly change from joy to sorrow, from laughing to weeping; moody, exhausted by long-concentrated grief.– Ign.

Night terrors of children (Kali. P.); grinding teeth in sleep, horrible dreams. Somnambulism.– Kali Brom.

Mental excitability; ecstasy with almost prophetic perceptions; with a vivid imagination; great loquacity (Agar. Stramo.); wants to talk all the time; jumps from one idea to another; one word often leads into another story.– Lachesis.

Very forgetful, absent-minded; makes purchases and walks away without them. – Lac. Can.

Cannot concentrate the mind to read or study; very nervous. In writting, uses too many words or not the right ones; omits final letter or letters in a word. – Lac. Can.

Constantly loses the thread of conversation. Cannot speak without weeping. Irritated at trifles; cross during the day, exhilarated at night.– Medo.

Intolerable melancholy and apprehension; is wholly occupied with sad thoughts. Attacks of anxiety and restlessness during a thunder storm (Phos.).– Nat. Carb.

Illusions : that he is sick; parts shrunken; that she is pregnant when merely distended from flatus.– Sabadilla.

Apathetic, indifferent, low-spirited, weak memory from sexual abuses. (Ac. Phos.).– Staphis.

Dilirium : loquacious, talks all the time, sings, makes verses, raves.– Stramo.

Hallucinations which terrify the patient. Imagines all sorts of things; that she is double, lying crosswise.– Stramo.

Everything looks pretty which the patient takes a fancy to; even rags seem beautiful.– Sulph.

Loss of memory; cannot remember names of books, persons or places; arithmetical calculation difficult.– Syphilinum.

Fixed ideas : as if a strange person were at his side; as if soul and body were separated; as if a living animal were in abdomen; of being under the influence of a superior power.– Thuja Occ.

Mania with desire to cut and tear everything, esp. clothes (Taran.); with lewd, lascivious talk, amorous or religious.– Verat. Alb.

LOCOMOTOR

Rheumatism and gout.– Abort., Act. Rece., Ac. Benz., Colch., Rhus. T., Formica Rufa., Chin Ars., Berb. V., Kal. Lat.

Severe lumbo-sacral backache. – Acs. Hip., Agar., Kali C., Lac. Can., Nux. V.

Offensive feet-sweat. – Am. Mur., Graph., Psor., Sanic., Baryta Carb., Calc. Carb., Sil.

Bruised feeling in pelvic region.– Arn. Mont.

Stony hard, scrofulous or tuberculous swelling of glands, esp. on lower jaw and throat.– Bromium.
Joint weak.– Carbo An., Ledum. P.
Rheumatism of women, esp. in small joints. – Caulo.
Rheumatic affections, with contraction of the flexors and stiffness of the joint; tension and shortening of muscles. – Am. Mur., Caust., Nat. Mur.
Burning of soles at night, puts feet out of bed. – Chamo., Puls., Medo., Sulph.
Constant pain under the lower and inner angle of right scapula.– Chelid., Kali C., Merc., Sol. (under the left.– Sang. Can.)
Every joint pain, periosteum, as if sprained, sore all over.– China, Acid Phos.
Arthritis, joints. – Colchicum.
Burning sore pain in heels. – Cyclamen., Agar., Caust., Phyto.
Bone pains, affecting back, head, chest, limbs, esp. the wrist, as if dislocated.– Eupat. Perf., Ipec.
Rheumatism or gout; begins in lower limbs and ascends. (descends – Kalmia)– Led. Pal.
Joints become the seat of nodosites and "gout stones" which are painful; acute and chronic arthritis.– Led. Pat., Lithium Carb.
Swelling : of feet, up to knees; of ankle with unbearable pain
when walking; ball of great toe swollen, painful; in heels as if bruised.– Ledum. P.
Sacrum : extreme sensitive. – Lobelia Inf.
Cramps : of extremities during pregnancy; writer's cramp, piano or violin players.– Mag. Phos.
Lumber, sacrum, coccyx, pain, hip to keen pain.– Medorrhinum.
Ankle turn easily when walking.– Led. Pal., Medo., Nat Carb.
Deformity of finger joints; puffy knuckles; swelling and painful stiffness of ankles; tenderness of heels and balls of feet; swelling of all joints. – Medo.
Pain in periosteum of long bones. Long bones inflamed, swollen, carries, exostoses, tumour soften from within out.– Mez.
Painful contractions of the hamstring. – Amon. Mur., Caust., Guiacum. Nat. Mur.
Cracking of the joints, on motion.– Acid Nit., Cocculus., Graph.
Backache, while riding in a carriage.– Nux. Mos.
Rheumatism of fibrous and periosteal tissue.– Phyto.
Backache, motion < pain. – Lac. Can., Merc. Sol., Phyto. (Mation > Pain. – Rhus. Tox.)
Intercostal rheumatism : chest sore.– Ran. Bulb.
Acute inflamatory swelling of joints; rheumatic limb pains; gout with fibrous deposit in great toe-joint. (Colch., Led.).– Rhodo.
Mascular rheumatism, sciatica. (Colo.)– Rhus. Tox.
Backahe > by lying on back.– Ruta. G.
Rheumatic pain in the right arm and shoulder.– Sang. Can. (left.– Fer. Met.)
Rheumatism, bone pains.– Sarsa.
Arthritic nodosites of joints, esp. fingers.– Caulo., Lyco., Colch., Staph.
Facilitates union of fractured bones.– Calc. Phos., Symph.
Rheumatism of shoulder joint.– Rhus. Tox., Syphil. (Rt. shoulder. – Sang. Lt. Shoulder. – Fer. Met.)
Torticolis, rheumatic affection of neck – Lachnanthis.

RESPIRATORY

Croupy cough, dry, hoarse, suffocating.– Acon., Caust., Ant. Tart., Spongia.
Stoping of nose, "snuffles" of infants.– Amon. Carb., Heper. S., Lyco., Nux. V., Sambucus.
Best remedy for emphysema.– Am. Carb.
Whooping cough.– Ant. Tert., Cuprum. Met., Drosera, Euphrasia. Ipec.
Coryza with sneezing.– Arg. Met.
Hoarseness; of professional singers, public speakers.– Arg. Met., Alum., Arum., Tri., Arg., Nit.
Asthma.– Ars., Can. Sat., Heper. S., Ipec., Kali Carb., Chin. Ars., Tab., Sang. Can., Psor., Medo., Lob. In.
Hoarseness and aphonia.– Carbo Veg., Caust., Phos., Cina., Acon., Nux., Mos., Spongia., Stan., Met.
Cough : dry with sneezing; returning spring and fall.– Cina.
Cough : in spasmodic paroxysms.– Actea Rece., Con.
Deep sound hoarse barking cough; whooping cough; sensation of feather in larynx; sore-throat. – Drosera.
Chronic cough, chest sore.– Bryo., Eupat. Pref., Nat Carb.
Lungs ulcer.– Kali Carb., Merc. Sol.
Croup : > by lying down.– Kali Bich. (< when lying down.– Aral., Lach.)
Catarrh : hawking much thick mucus from throat.– Nat. Carb.
Dyspnoea, humid asthma in children. – Nat. Sulph.
Soreness of chest, during cough, has to sit up in bed and hold the chest with hands.– Bryo., Nat. Sulph.
Chronic cough, pus-like.– Psor.
Plurisy or pneumonia.– Acon., Arn. M., Ran. Bulb.
Raw sensation in larynx and trachea when coughing. – Caust., Rumex.
Dyspnoea : must lie on right side or with head high. – Cactus., Spig., Spong., Sepia.
Dryness of mucous membrane of air passages, throat, larynx, trachia, bronchi; dry cough.– Spong. T.
Palpitation : violent with pain and gasping respiration.– Spong.
Cough : deep, hollow, three paroxysms.– Stann. Met. (two paroxysms. – Merc.)
Cough : excited by tobacco smoke. – Staphis., Spong.
Haemoptysis : cough with blood, phthesis.– Trillium.
Takes cold easily without knowing how or where. – Heper. S., Tub.
Early stage of tuberculosis.– Ars. Iod.

FEVER

Fever with burning thirst.– Acon., Nux. Vom., Bell., Ac. Mur.
Typhoid : with delirium. – Agar Mas., Bapt. T., Carbo. Veg., Pyrozen.
Intermittent fever.– Apis., Cactus G., China., Eupat. P., Nat. Mur.

Typhoid or malerial fever.– Crot. Hor., Lach., Rhus. Tox.
Influenza.– Eupat. Perf.
Fever : scarlatina, rapidly becomes typhoid; involuntary stool and urine. – Hyos. Nig.
Pneumonia.– Lyco., Nat. Sulph.
Cerebral typhoid.– Ac. Phos.
Hay fever.– Psor.
Septic fever.– Pyrozen.
Weakness, after typhoid.– Selen.
Maleria.– Chin. Ars., Chin. Sulph.

SKIN

Chilblain, itching and burn.– Agar. M., Petrol., Zinc. Mat.
Panaritia.– Alliuim Cepa, Am. Carb., Dios. V., Sil., Graph, Myrist.
Itch appears each year, as winter approaches.– Aloe. Soc., Psor.
Dry, tettery, itching eruptions.– Alumina.
Warts on palms of hands.– Anacard., Nat. Mur.
Curbancle and malignant ulcer.– Anthracin.
Large horny corns on soles of feet. – Ant. Curde, Hypericum, Ran. Bulb.
Disposition to abnormal growths of the skin; finger-nails do not grow rapidly; crushed nails grow in splits like warts with horny spots.– Ant. Crude.
Acute exanthema : measles, scarlatina, urticaria.– Apis., Zinc. Met.
Oedema : bag-like puffy swelling under the eyes. – Apis. Mel. (over the eyes.– Kali Carb.)
Small painfull boil, one after another.– Arn. M., Sulph.
Tettery skin eruptions, dry and moist.– Bovista.
Acne, sty, boils.– Lappa. Major.
Eczema : no itching, exudation forms into a hard lemon-coloured crust. – Cic. Vir.
Pruritus in pregnancy with haemorrhoids.– Colinsonia.
Carbuncles or blood boils.– Anthracin., Bellis., Crot. Hor., Lach., Taran.
Acute eczema : over whole body.– Crot. Tig., Rhus. Tox.
Intense itching of genitals of both sexes.– Crot. T., Rhus. Tox.
Nail brittle. – Ant. C., Dios. V., Graph., Thuja Occ.
Rash before menses.– Dulc., Con. (during menses. – Bell., Graph.)
Urticaria. – Apis., Dulc., Calc. C., Nat. Mur., Heper. S., Sanic., Thuja Occ.
Thick brown-yellow crusts on scalp, face, forehead, temples, chin. – Dulc.
Warts, on face or back of hands and fingers.– Dulc.
Old cicatrices become red around edges and threaten to become open ulcers.– Acid Flour., Caust., Graph.
Varicose veins and ulcers.– Flour. Acid., Hamamelis.
Naevus flat.– Acid Flour.
Eczema, of lids.– Graph.
Corner of mouth ulcerated. – Heleborus.
Eruptions upon the ears, between fingers and toes and on various parts of body, from which oozes a watery, sticky fluid.– Graph.

Cracks or fissure in ends of fingers, nipples, labial commissures; of anus, between the toes.– Graph.

Herpes, surrounded by little pimples or pustules and spread by coalescing.– Heper. Sulph.

Acne.– Kali Brom., Carbo. An., Psor., Calc. Phos.

Violent itching.– Kreos., Merc. Solubilis. (itching without eruptions.– Dolicos.)

Punctured wounds by sharp-pointed instruments, as awls, nails, (Hypericum); rat bites, stings of insects, esp. mosquitoes.– Led. Pal.

Red pimples or turbercles on forehead and cheeks.– Ledum. P.

Ulcers of gum, tongue, throat, cheek.– Merc. Sol.

Furuncles and boils in external meatus, polyp.– Merc. Solubilis., Acid Pic.

Head covered with thick, leather-like crust, under which white pus collects. Hair is glued and matted together; pus offensive, breeds vermin. – Mez.

Vesicles appear around the ulcers, itch violently, burn like fire.– heper. Sulph., Mez.

Eczema : intolerable itching. – Mez., Staphis., Tub.

Freckles : eczema solaris. – Acid Mur.

Hangnails : skin around the nails dry and cracked.– Graph., Nat. Mur., Petrol.

Herpes about anus and on borders of hair at nape of the neck. (in bend of knees. – Hep., Graph.) – Nat. Mur.

Warts on palms of hands.– Nat. Mur., Nat. Carb., Ruta G.

Fever blister.– Nat. Mur., Acid Nit.

Eczema : esp. on edges of hair.– Nat. Mur.

Every spring, skin affections reappear.– Nat. Sulph., Psor.

Warts.– Ac. Nit., Staphis., Thuja., Caust., Sabina.

Feet : bathed in foul-smelling sweat.– Petrol., Graph., Sanic., Sil., Psor., Zinc.

Parchment-like dryness of skin. – Sabad.

Herpes of genital organs extending to perineum and thighs; itching, redness, skin cracked, rough, bleeding; dry or moist.– Petrol.

Skin of hands cracked; tips of fingers cracked, fissured.– Petrol.

Hastens suppuration.– Heper. S., Lech., Merc. Sol., Phyto., Sil.

Dry, scaly eruptions disappear in summer, return in winter. – Psor.

Acne : all forms.– Psor.

Eruptions, easily suppurate.– Psor.

Sty.– Puls., Lyco., Staph., Con., Thuja Occ.

Septic ulcers.– Pyrozen.

Corns.– Ran. Bulb., Acid Salicylic.

Herpes Zoster : vessicle have bluish appearance.– Ran. Bulb.

Vesicular erysipelus.– Rhus. Tox.

Skin : itching of various parts < by cold > wormth when undressing.– Heper. S., Nat. Sulph., Rumex. C.

Eruptions of face of young women, esp. during scanty menses.– Calc. C., Psor., Sang. Can.

Herpetic eruptions on all parts of the body.– Sarsa.

Dry, itching eruptions, prone to appear in spring; become crusty. – Sarsa.

Itching eruptions of forehead during menses. – Psor., Sang. Can., Sarsa.

Small boils : mature very slowly, and heal in the same manner.– Sec. Cor.

Rhagades : skin cracked on hands and feet; pain and burning; particularly on sides of fingers and toes; skin hard, in durated.– Sarsa.
Large ecchymoses; blood blisters; often commencement of gangrene.– Sec. Cor.
Herpes circinatus in isolated spots on upper part of body.– Sepia.
Itching of skin : of various parts; of external genetalia.– Sepia.
Unhealthy skin; every little injury supprates.– Graph., Hep. S., Petrol., Merc. Sol., Sil.
Ingrowing toe-nails.– Sil., TMV.
Crippled nails on fingers and toes.– Ant. Crude, Sil.
Sweat of hands, toes, feet and axillae, offensive.– Sil.
Herpes of anus.– Tab.
Ringworm. – Tuberculinum.
Leucoderma. – Ars. Sulph. Flavum.
Scirrhus of sigmoid or rectum, painful.– Spig., Alum.
Skin : itching; soreness of folds.– Lyco., Sulph.

NERVOUS SYSTEM

Nerve Tonic - Kali Phos.
Convulsion of teething children; child gnaws its fist, frets and screams.– Acon., Bell., Mag. Phos., Zinc Met.
Spasms : hysterical and epileptical.– Ast. Rub., Cim., Kali Brom.
Epileptic spasm with clenched thumbs, pupils fixed and dilated, foam at the mouth, jaws locked. – Aethusa Cyn., Bufo., Lach.
Involuntary movements while awake, cease during sleep; trembling of whole body. – Agar Mur.
Neuralgic pains.– Allium. Cepa.
Constant and violent motion of one arm and one leg. (Left arm and leg.– Bryo.)– Apoc., Helleb.
Convulsion.– Arg. Nit., Chamo., Nux. V., Cuprum Met., Hypericum., Lyssin., Heleborus Nig.
Paralysis, left-sided.– Arn. Mont., Rhus Tox.
Dilirium and hallucination.– Bell., Can. Ind., Cim., Hyos. Nig., Bryo., Ac. Phos.
Chorea, hysterical or epilepsy at puberty.– Actea Rece., Caubo., Crocus., Zinc Met.
Disturbed functional activity of brain and spinal cord, from exhausting disease or severe mental shock resulting in paralysis.– Caust.
Paralysis, right-sided.– Caust.
Convulsions : violent, with frightful distortions of limbs and whole body; with loss of consciousness of opisthotonos; renewed from slightest touch, noise or jar.– Cic. Vir.
Puerperal convulsions, continue after delivery.– Cic. Vir., Hyos. Nig.
Epilepsy : lockjaw, distortion of limbs; recurring, first at short, then at long intervals.– Cupr. Met., Cic. Vir.
Injurious chronic effects from concussions of the brain and spine.– Cic. Vir.
Trismus and tetanus from getting splinters into flesh.– Cic. Vir.
Unrefreshing sleep or constant sopor.– China.
Sciatica : from hip to feet.– Colo., Ganph.

Weakness and trembling; of tongue, hands, leg; of the entire body.– Gels.
Convulsions of childrens from cerebral congestion; meningitis.– Glonoin., Hyos. Nig.
Hydrocephalus.– Apis., Heleborus, Sulph., Tub.
Dilirium.– Bell., Hyos., Ran. Bulb., Stramo.
Spasms : without consciousness.– Hyos. Nig. (with consciousness.– Nux. Vom.)
Bad effects of unfortunate love; often followed by epilepsy.– Hyos. Nig.
Lascivious mania.– Hyos., Phos., Stramo., Ver. Alb.
Prevents lockjaw.– Hypericum.
Hands and fingers in constant motion; fidgety hands.– Kali Brom. (fidgety feet.– Zinc. Met.)
First stage of hydrocephaloid.– Kali. Brom.
Trembling the whole body.– Lach., Medo.
Epilepsy : comes on during sleep.– Bufo., Lach.
Hysteria : continual rising of white froth into the mouth.– Mag. Mur.
Spasm during dentition, no fever.– Mag. Phos. (with fever.– Bell.)
Diseases of spinal cord, ending in paralysis.– Medo.
Intense burning pain in brain, < in cerebellum; extends down spine.– Medo.
Intense restlessness and fidgety legs and feet.– Medo., Zinc. Met.
Convulsions : of children during dentition (Bell.); infantile spasm, eclampsia, epilepsy.– Melilotus Alb.
Trembling extremities; paralysis agitans.– Merc. Sol.
Mental traumatism; mental effects from injuries to head; chronic brain effects of blows and falls.– Nat. Sulph.
Opisthotonos.– Nat. Sulph., Ver. Vir.
Spinal meningitis : violent crushing pains at base of brain; spasms with mental irritability and delirium; violent congestion of blood to head.– Nat. Sulph.
Convulsions, with consciousness.– Nux. Vom., Stramo.
Tendency to faint; from odor, in morning, after eating.– Nux. Vom., Nux. Mos., Sulph.
Sleepy, but cannot sleep.– Bell., Chamo., Opium, Stramo.
Delirium tremens; screaming before or during a spasm.– Opium.
Brain-fag : of literary or business people.– Ac. Picric.
Diseases from spinal origin (Phos., Pic. Ac., Zinc.); general or partial paralysis. Muscular atrophy from sclerosis of spinal system.– Plumb. Met.
Spasms : clonic, tonic, from cerebal sclerosis or tumor; epilepsy or pileptiform convulsion.– Plumb. Met.
Erethism : with anxiety and faintness.– Sepia.
Sleepy all day, awake all night.– Staphis.
Delirium : loquacious, talks all the time, sings, makes verses, raves.– Bell., Hyos. Nig., Stramo.
Convulsion : without consciousness. – Bell., Cic. Vir., Hyos., Opium.
Twitching of single muscles or group of muscles, esp. upper part of body; chorea.– Stramo, Zinc. Met.
Trembling of limbs.– Tab.
Cerebral or basilar meningitis.– Tub., Ver. Vir.
Automatic motion of hands and head.– Apoc. Can., Bryo., Helleborus., Zinc. Met.
Weakness and trembling of extremities; of hands while writting.– Zinc. Met.
Cerebro-spinal diseases; spasm, dilated pupils, tetanic convulsions, opisthotonos.– Ver. Vir.

GENERALITIES

Marasmus of children. – Abrot., Iod., Sanic., Tub., Opium. Ars., Kreos., Sil., Calc. Phos., Arg. Nit., Ac. Acetic.

Haemorrhage : from every mucus outlet, nose, throat, lungs, stomach, bowels, uterus.– Acetic Acid., Ipec., China, Fer. Met., Phos., Mill., Canth, Carbo. Veg., Crot., Hor., Hamamelis.

Dropsy.– Acetic Acid., Ars., Dulc., Fer. Met., Lac. Def., Colchicum, Terebin.

Mascular soreness, from dancing, skating or other violent mascular exercise.– Act. Race.

Paliative in incurative diseases.– Amyl. Nit.

Jaundice.– Ant. Tart., Berb. Vulg., Chelid., Crot. Hor., Taraxa.

Dropsy, without thirst. – Apis Mel., Uran. Nit.

Dropsy, with thirst. – Acid. Acetic., Apoc. Can.

Pain : migrating from one part to another.– Apis., Puls., Kali Bich., Lac. Can.

Cancer of breast.– Aesteria Rub., Carbo An., Con., Sil.

Dwarfish children who do not grow.– Baryta Carb.

Destroys craving for tobacco.– Calad.

Measles.– Camphor., Dros., Eupat. Perf., Kali Carb.

Glands : indurated, painful, in neck, axillae, grain, mammae, etc.– Carbo. An., Con.

Variola, chiken-pox.– Am. Carb., Carbolic Acid.

Rawness or soreness : of scalp, throat, respiratory truct, rectum, anus, urethra, vagina, uterus.– Arn. Mont., Caust.

Unsteady walking and easy falling of little children.– Caust.

Cancerous and scrofulous persons with enlarged glands.– Con.

Glandular induration of stony hardness; of mammae and esticles in persons of cancerous tendency.– Aster. Rubens, Con. Mac.

Spasmodic contractions and twitching of single sets of muscles.– Agar., Crocus., Ign., Zinc.

Dissecting wounds insect stings.– Crot. Hor.

Bruised feeling as if broken, all over the body.– Arn., Bellis., Eupat. Perf., Pyrozen.

Bad effects from falls, contussions or mechanical injuries of external part.– Arn., Euphrasia.

Irritability : slight noises like crackling of paper drive him to despair.– Ferr. Met.

Sumstroke and sun headache. – Glonoin.

Chronic effects of mechanical injuries.– Con., Hamamelis.

Dropsy : of brain, chest, abdomen; after scarlatina, intermittents; with fever; suppressed urine; from suppressed exanthemata.– Apis., Heleborus., Zinc. Met.

Sweats : perspiration sour, offensive.– Heper. Sulph.

Cancer.– Hydras. Can., Lapis. Alba., Ast. Ruben.

Mechanical injuries of spinal cord; pains, after a fall on coccyx.– Hypericum.

Hypertrophy and induration of glandular tissue– thyroid, mammae, ovaries, testis, uterus, prostate or other glands, – breast may dwindle and become flabby.– Iod.

Affections of the mucous membrane–eyes, nose, mouth, throat, bronchi, gastro-intestinal tract and genito-urinary tract– discharge of tough stringy mucous.– Kali Bich., Lyssin.

Shifting pain.– Kali Bich., Puls., Kali Sulph., Lac. Can.

Obesity : fatty degeneration.– Lac. Def.

Scirrhus, carcinoma or cancer.– Medo.
Enlargement of lymphatic glands all over the body. – Medo.
Glandular swellings with or without suppuration.– Hep. Sulph., Merc. S., Sil.
Great debility : caused by heat of summer, chronic effects of sum-stroke.– Glon., Nat. Carb.
Children slow in learning to walk. – Nat. Mur.
Great emaciation : losing flesh while living well. – Abrot., Iod., Nat. Mur.
Very sensitive to rattle of wagons over paved streets. – Acid Nit.
Ailments : from riding in a carriage, railroad car, or in a ship.– Cocc., Petrol., Sanic.
The whole body painful, easily sprained and injured.– Psor.
All excretions – diarrhoea, leucorrhoea, menses, perspiration – have a carrion-like odor.– Psor.
Mumps : metastasis to mammae or testicle.– Puls.
Most effective remedies for the bad effects of alcoholic beverages.– Ran. Bulb.
Mascular pains about margins of shoulder blades in women of sedentary employment; from needlework, type-writting, piano-playing (Actea R.).– Ran. Bulb.
Bruised lame sensation all over, as after a fall or blow, < in limbs and joints.– Arn., Ruta. G.
Oedematous swelling in various parts of the body, esp. in legs, instep and feet.– Sambucus.
The slightest wound causes bleeding for weaks.– Lach., Phos., Sec. Cor.
Suffer from deficient nutrition, not because food is lacking but from imperfect assimilation.– Baryta Car., Calc. C., Sil.
Scrofulous, rachitic children with large head; open fontanelles and sutures; distended abdomen; weak ankles; slow in learning to walk.– Sil.
Craving alcohol, in any form. Hereditary tendency to alcoholism.– Tub, Asar., Syphil., Psor., Sulph., Ac. Sulph.
Hiccough, from tobacco chewing.– Ign.
Tumour, inlarged glands.– Thiosin.
Glandular swelling, malignant tumor.– Kali Mur., Kali Phos.
Hiccough.– Chin. Sulph.
Inflammation, swelling and suppuration of glands, cervical,axillary, parotid, mammary, inguinal, sebaceous, malignant, gangrenous.– Sil.
Has a wonderful control over the suppurative process– soft tissue, periosteum, or bone– maturing abscess when desired or reducing excessive suppuration.– Sil. (affecting chiefly the soft tissues.– Calad., Hep. Sulph.)
Promotes expulsion of foreign bodies from the tissues, fish bones, needles, bones splinters. – Sil.
Swelling and induration of glands; goitre.– Brom., Spongia.
Mechanical injuries from sharp-cutting instruments.– Staphis.
Chronic alcoholism; dropsy and other ailments of drunkards.– Psor., Sulph., Tub.
Hydrophobia.– Stramo.
To facilitates absorption of serous or inflammatory exudates in brain, plura, lungs, joints.– Bryo., Kali Mur., Sulph.
Constant heat on vertex; burning soles at night.– Sulph.
Tendency to gangrene following mechanical injuries.– Acid Sulph.

HEAD

Headache alternating with lumbago. – Aloe. Soc.
Acute hydrocephalus.– Apoc. Can., Arn. Mont.
Headache; ending in vomiting. – Arg. Nit.
Falling of hair.– Aurum Met., Nat. Mur., Sepia. Sil.
Headache– Bryo., Sep., Aloe Soc., Fer. Met., Nat. Mur., Sulph.
Headache : throbing of head and carotids.– Bell., China.
Vertigo : of old people.– Con., Kalmia L., Spig., Tab., Thuja Occ.
Headache : from bites of dog.– Lyssin.
Headache : from eye-strain.– Acid Phos., Calc. Phos., Nat. Mur.
Hair becomes frowsy, and tangled; splits, sticks together at the tips, cannot be combed again.– Acid Flour., Borax., Lyco., Psor., Tub.
Dandruff; falls out in clouds (Lyco.); hair falls out in bunches, baldness of single spots.– Phos.
Headache : preceded by flickering before eyes, by dimness of vision or blindness (Lac. Def., Kali Bich.), by black spots or rings.– Psor.
Hair dry, lustreless, tangles easily, glues together (Lyco.); Plica Polonica (Berb. V., Sarsa, Tub.); Scalp : dry, scaly or moist, foetid, suppurating eruptions; oozing a sticky, offensive fluid (Graph., Mez.).– Psor.
Vertigo < lying down.– Rhus. Tox. (> lying down.–Apis.)
Periodical sick-headache : begins in occiput, spreads upwords and settles over right eye. (over left eye.– Spig.).– Sang. Can., Sil.
Scaly dandruff on scalp, eyebrows, in the beard.– Sanicula.
Hair falls off; on head, eyebrows, genitals.– Selen.Headache : at menstrual nisus.– Sepia.
Plica polonica.– Borax., Psor., Tub.
Headache : from sunrise to sundown.– Nat. Mur., Spig., Tab.
Chronic sick headache : ascending from nape of neck to the vertex, as if coming from the spine and locating in one eye, esp. right.– Sil. (left eye.– Spig.)

MOUTH

Corner of mouth sore. – Arum Tri.
Aphthae of mouth. – Borax., Acid Sulph.
Malignant affections of mouth; studded with ulcers, deep, perforating; having a black or dark base : offensive, foul breath; intense prostration; diphtheria, scarlatina, cancer. – Acid Mur.
Ulcers : easily bleeding; in corners of mouth.– Acid Nit., Nat. Mur., Rhus. Tox.
Bright redness of lips.– Sulph., Tub.

TONGUE

Stammering children. – Bovista, Cuprum Met., Kali Brom Spig., Stramo., Ign.
Paralysis of tongue : imperfect stammering speech.– Cuprum Met.
Saliva. – Cyclamen Euro., Lac. Can., Merc. Sol.
Paralysis of tongue.– Acid Mur.

Ringworm on tongue.– Nat Mur., Sanicula.

TEETH AND GUM

Looseness of teeth, easily bleeding gums.– Acid Sulph., Carbo. Veg.
Toothache.– Chamo., Bismuth., Bryo., Coffea, Puls., Mag. P., Rhodo., Sepia, Nat. S., Mag. Mur., Merc. Sol.
Rapid caries of teeth; dental fistula.– Acid Flour.
Haemorrhage : after the extraction of teeth.– Hamamelis, Kreos., Trill. P.
Teeth begin to decay as soon as they appear. Gums spongy bleeding, ulcerated.– Kreos.
Toothache > by heat.– Mag. Phos. (> by cold.– Bryo., Coffea, Fer. P.)
Crowns of teth decay, roots remain. – Merc. Sol. (crowns intact, roots decay.– Mez)
Toothache, in caries teeth.– Kreos., Mez.
Distinct blue line along margin of gums; gums swollen, show a lead-coloured line.– Plumb. Met.
Toothache > by cold water.– Bryo., Coff., Puls.
Toothache : during early months of pregnancy.– Ratan.
Difficult dentition.– Rheum.
Toothache from tobacco smoking. – Spig.
Teeth become yellow.– Thuja.
Teeth : decay on edges.– Staphis., Syphil. decay at the root.– Mez., Thuja.

EYE

Eye : ciliary neuralgia.– Actea Rece.
Eyes : excessive lachrymations, burning. – Allium Cepa., Euphrasia.
Conjuntivitis, eye-strain, ophthalmia neonatorum.– Arg. Nit., Apis., Merc. Sol., Arn., Borax., Rhus., Tox.
Periodic orbital neuralgia, with excessive lachrymation; tears fairly gush out.– Chelid., Rhus. Tox.
Aversion to light without inflammation of eyes; < from using eyes in artificial light; often the students remedy for night work; intense photophobia.– Con., Psor.
Yellow colour of conjuctiva; clears up vision after keratitis or kerato-iritis.– Crocus Sat.
Painful soreness of eye-ball. – Eupat. Perf.
The eyes water all the time and are agglutinated in the morning. – Euphrasia.
Lachrymal fistula.– Acid Flour.
Dim vision, diplopia.– Gels., Syphil., Tab.
Traumatic conjuctivities.– Hamamelis.
Eye-ball sore to touch.– Heper. S.
Oedema : bag-like puffy swelling under the eyes.– Apis. Mel. (over the eyes.– Kali Carb.)
Severe stitching pain in right eye and orbit.– Kalmia L. (left eye.– spig.)
Contusions of eye and lids, conjuctivities.– Ledum. Pal.

Lachrymations : tears slream down the face whenever he coughs.– Euphrasia, Nat. Mur.

Granular lids : like small blisters; green pus and terrible photophobia.– Nat. Sulph., Staphis., Thuja.

Dryness of eyes; too dry to close the lids. – Nux. Mos.

Eyes : surrounded by blue rings; lid, puffy, swollen, oedematous.– Pos. (upper lid–Kali Carb.) (lower lid.– Apis. Mel.)

Dim vision, pain after using eyes, floating black spots.– Physostigma.

Photophobia; with inflamed lids; can't open the eyes.–Psor.

Day blindness; mist before eyes; pressure and smarting in eyeballs.– Phos., Ran. Bulb.

Aching in and over eyes, with blurred vision. Using eyes at fine works, watchmaking; dim vision; Amblyopia or asthenopia or anomalies of refraction eye-strain.– Ruta. G.

Fistula lachrymalis.– Sil.

Intolerable pressive pain in eyeballs; could not turn the eyes without turning the whole body.– Spig.

Pain in eye after a blow of an obtuse body.– Symphytum.

Ophthalmia neonatorum.– Syphil., Thuja Occ.

Amaurosis, from atrophy of retina or optic nerve.– Tabacum.

EAR

Deafness, with roaring and humming in ears. – Kreos.

Otorrhoea.– Aurum Met., Kali Mur., Merc. Dulcis., Merc. Solubilis., Psorinum.

Eustachian tube closed; catarrhal deafness, deafness of old age.– Kali Mur., Merc. Dulcis.

Chronic otitis, condylomata, polipi.– Thuja Occ.

NOSE

Violent sneezing on rising from bed.– Allium Cepa.

Nasal polyp.– Allium Cepa, Formica R., Sang. Can., Psor., TMV.

Coryza and sneezing.– Arum Tri., Tab.

Nasal polypi, rhinitis.– Lemna Minor.

Nosebleed. – Crocus., Sat., Kali Carb., Arn. M., Am. Carb., Melilotus Alb., Merc. Solubilis.

Nosebleed during menses. – Nat. Sulph. (instead of menses.– Coffea, Puls.)

Ozena : green casts from the nose every morning.– Acid Nit.

Sneezing in spasmodic paroxysms; followed by lachrymation; copious watery coryza.– Sabad., Tab.

Laryngeal or nasal polypi.– Sang. Can., Sang. Nit., Psor., TMV.

THROAT

Follicular pharyngitis.– Acs. Hip., Wyethia.

Putrid sore-throat; tendency to gangrenous ulceration of tonsils; glands engorged.– Am. Carb., Lac.Can., Lyssin., Medo., Spon.

Sensation of a splinter in throat when swallowing. – Arg. Nit., Dolich., Hep., S., Ac. Nit., Sil.
Painless sore-throat.– Bapt. Tinc., Phyto., Kali Bich.
Tonsillitis.– Baryta C., Capsicum, Lach., Lac. Can., Psor., Merc. Sol.
Oedema or gangrene of fauces or tonsils.– Crot. Hor.
Sensation of a splinter, fish bone or plug in the throat. (Arg. Nit., Ac. Nit.); quinsy, when suppuration threatens; chronic hypertrophy.– Baryta C., Plumb. M., Psor.
Hard goitre, in dark-haired persons.– Iod.
Hard goitre, in light-haired persons.– Brom.
Deep-eating ulcers in fauces.– Kali Bich.
Oedematous, bladder-like appearance of uvula.– Kali Bich., Rhus. Tox.
Diphtheria.– Lac. Can., Kali Bich., Lach., Phyto., Lyco. Merc.
Thyroid gland swollen, goitre.– Brom., Spong., Thyroidin., Iris. Vers.
Food easily gets into the windpipe.– Kali Carb.
Mumps.– Merc. Sol.
Tubercular pharyngitis.– Merc. Bon. Iod.
Throat affections where the cervical and parotid gland swollen.–Merc. Bin. Iod. (Left side) Merc. Proto Iod. (Right side.)
Hoarseness of voice.– Nux. Mox.
Aphonia : after long use of voice; husky when beginning to sing; oblized to clear the throat frequency of a transparent starchy mucus. Tubercular laryngitis.– Arg. Met., Stann Met., Selen.
Diphtheria, tonsillitis, dryness of fauces and throat; sensation of a skin hanging loosely in throat, must swallow it over.– Sabad.
Sensation of lump in throat. – Rumex C.

CLINICAL ORGANOTHERAPY

Chapter - 7
BEDSIDE MEDICINE

Gastro-Enterology

Hepatitis – Ferr. Phos. 3x (3g ′ 4); Veratrum Vir. q (5d ′4); Nat. Sulph 6x (3g ′ 4); Bryo q (3d ′ 5); Heper Sulph 1x, 3x (3g ′5)

Cirrhosis of Liver – Eunanyminum 3x (1g ′4); Chionanthus Virg. q (10d′3); Nux. Vom. q (5d ′3); Bryo. q (5d ′3).

Enlargement of the Liver – Carduus Marianus q (5d ′3); Chelidonq (10d ′3); Ptelea Trifoliate q (5d ′3); Chelone Glabra q (5d ′4).

Splenitis – Ceanothus Americana q (5d ′4).

Enlargement of the Spleen – Carduus Marianus q (5d ′6); Polymnia Uvedalia q (10d ′3).

Gallstone Colic – Hydrastis q (10d ′ 8); [Removes gall-stone = Podophyllin 3x (3g ′at night) + Olive Oil (3oz ′ in the morning); Euonyminum 3x (5g ′6); Chelidon q (20d ′ 8); Juglans Cinerea q (30d ′ 3).]

Jaundice – Chelidon (10d ′3); Chionanthus Virg. q (10d ′3); China q (5d ′ 3); Myrica Cerifera q (10d ′ 3).

Malaria – [Hydrastis q (30z) + Ars.q (10ml) = 1/2 t.s.f. after meal.]; [Xanthoxylum q (20drs.) + Aristolochia Serpentaria q (20 drops) + Capsicum q (5drs) = (5d ′5)]; Gels q (5d ′5); Boletus Laricis q (5d ′ 4); Chininum Ars. 3x (2g ′ 3); Chin. Sulp. 3x (2g ′4); Grindelia Squarrosa q, 30 (10d ′5).

Stomatitis (mouth) – [Ferr. Phos 3x + Kali Mur 3x (10g each) = (5g ′3)]

Aptheae – Bismuth Subnitrate 2x (3g′5); Kali Mur 3x (2g′6); (Local = Rhus Glabra q, Eupat. Aromaticum q, Hydrastin Mur 1x)

Ulcers in the Mouth – (Local = Zinc Sulph 1x, gargle with worm water.)

Glossitis (tongue) – Acon. q (3d ′4).

Dyspepsia – Alnus Rubra q (5d ′3); Alunin 1x (3g′3); Robinia Pseuda. q (5d′3); Nux Vom. q (5d ′3); Chelone Glabra q (5d ′ 4); Lyco. q (5d ′3); [Pepsinum q (5ml) + Bismuth Subnit. 2x (5g) + N.V. q (15ml) + Gentiana L.q (20z) = 1 t.s.f. after meals].

Acute Gastritis – Acon. q (3d ′ 4); Bismuth Submit 2x (3g ′5).

Chronic Gastritis – Arg. Nit q (5d ′4); Ars. q (2d′3); [N.V.Q (5ml) + Hydrastis q (15ml) + Glycerine (10z) = (1/2 t.s.f. ′ 3)]

Gastralgia – Melilolus Alba q (5d ′4); Gaultheria Oil 1x (5d ′3); Dioscorea V. q (20d′4).

Gastric Ulcer – Uranium Nit. 3x (3g ′4); Potash Bi-chromete 3x (3g′ 3); (Kali Bich) Arg. Nit 3x (3g ′4); Nat Phos 3x (3g′4).

Haemorrhage of the Stomach – Geranium Mac. q (5ml ′ 4).

Gastric Catarrh (nausea) – Nux. Vom. q (5d ′ 4).

Gastric Catarrh (gas) – Graph. 3x (3g ′ 4).

Appendicitis – Dioscorea q (20d ′ 6); [Ferr. Phos 3x (10g) + Kali Mur 3x (15g) = (5g ′5)]; Ipecac q (10d ′ 4); Ricinus Communis q (5d ′4).

Cholera Morbus – [Mag. Carb. 3x (1dr.) + Ammonium Causticumq (5ml). + Mentha Piperita q (15ml.) = (1/2 t.s.f. ′6)]; [Acon q (10d) + Nux V. (20d) = (5d ′6)].
Proctitis – [Gels q (20d) + Collinsonia q (20d) = (10d ′4)].
Proctalgia (with fissure at anal orifice) – Acid Nit q, 3x (5d′4).
Dysentery – [Acon. q (20drops) + Magnesia Sulph 1x (20 grains) + Ipecac q (20d) = (5d ′4)]
Dysentery (Old people) – Baptisia q (5d′4).
Diarrhoea – Podo. q (5d′5).
Chronic Diarrhoea – Epilobium August. q (15d ′4).
Prolapsus Ani – Aes. Hip q (3d ′4); (Local = Hamamelis q (5ml) + Veslinc (10z) = apply to anus thrice).
Anal Fissure – Krameria (Ratanhia) q (5d ′4); Paeonia officinalis q (10d′3); [Local = Ratanhia q (5ml) + Salicylic Acid (20g) + Veslinc OZ].
Haemorrhoids – Aes. Hip. q (5d ′4); Colinsonia q (4d′4); Hamamelis q (5d ′4); [Local = Conium q (5ml) + Tannic Acid 2x (10g) Morphin 3x (5g) + Vesline (oz).]; [Local = Acs. Hip. q + Plantago q].
Cholear Asiatica – Camphor q (5d′4); Acid Phos q (5d ′5); Bell. (5d ′5); Ver. Alb. q (5d′5); Cuprum Met. 3x (5g′6);
Cholera Infantum – Cuphea Visco q (5d ′2 hourly); Euphorbia Corollata q (5d ′5); Ferr. Phos 3x (3g′4);
Peritonitis – Acon. q, 3x (5d′4).
Peritonitis (Puerperal) – [Gels q + Cimicifuga R.q = (5d each ′4)].
General Peritonitis – [Ferr. Phos. 3x + Kali Mur 3x = (3g each ′4)].
Muco-Enteritis – Potash Bi-chromate 3x (3g′4).
Constipation – Nux. V. 3x (3d′4); Bryo q (3d ′4); Nat. Mur. 3x (5g′3); Hydrastis q (10d ′ before breakfast); Kali Mur 6x (10g ′ at bedtime).
Intestinal Haemorrhage – Carbo Veg. 1x (5g ′ 4); Ipecac q (10d ′5); Ferri Phos 3x (3g′4);
Lead Colic – [Mag. Sulph 1x + Acid Sulph.q + Potash Iodide 3x(Kali Iod 3x).];
Colic – Dioscorea V. q (20d ′4); Colocynth q (4d ′4); Mag. Phos 3x (5g′4).
Enteritis – [Ferr. Phos 3x +Kali Mur 3x = (5g ′4)].
Dropsy – Apocynum Can. q (10d′3); Digitalis q (5d′4); Convallaria Majalis q (10d ′4); Adonis q (5d ′3); [Elaterin 6x (2g) + Jalapa q (20d) + Squilla q (20d) = (10d ′4)]; Strychninum (for collapse) Sulph 6x (1g ′3).
Worms – [Santonin 3x (10g) + Podophyllin 3x (5g) = (5g ′3)]; Acid Sulph q (1 t.s.f. ′3).

Dermatology

Pimples – Nat. Sulph 3x (3g′4); Berberis Aquifolium q (10d′3); [Local = Nat Sulph 1x (10z) + Aqua (80z).]; [Local = Sulph q; Sulphurus Acid q; Ichthyolum 1x].
Erythema (abnormal flushing of the skin) – Bell. q (4d ′4); [Local = Hamamelis q].
Erythema Nodusum – (fever, joint pain, leg swelling)– Rhus Venenata q (5d ′4); Echinacea q (15d′4); [Local = Echinaca q (8ml)]
Urticaria – Urtica Urens q (10d′4); Apis q (10d′4); Antim. Crude 3x (3g′4); [Local = Sodium Bi-carbonate lotion.]

Acne – Berberis Aquifol. q (10d′4); Calcaria Sulph 2x (4g′4); Bell q (5d′4); [Local = Boracic Acid 2x (15g) + Kali Nitricum 3x (15g) + Aqua.]; [Local = Ichthol 1x + Vesline]. Juglans Regia q (5d′4);

Acne (Chronic) – [Juglandin 6x (1g) + Chin. Sulph 3x (1g) = (2g′4)]. [Local = Sulph q; Sulphurus Acid q]; Kali Ars. 3x (5d′4);

Eczema – [Podo q (15ml) + Kali Aceticum q (15ml) = (20d′4)]; [Local = Lobelia (for itching eczema) q]; [Rumex q (15ml) + Alnus Rubra (15ml) + Gentiana L. q (15ml) + Taraxacum q (15ml) = (2ml′5)]; **For babies** – [Local = Bismuth Sub-nitrate 1x oint] and Rhus Tox q (5d′ 4); Graph 3x (3g′3); Staphis q (5d′4); Bovista q (5d′4); Berberis Aquifal q (10d′4); [Local = Skookum Chuck q; Alnus q; Graph 1x; Vinca Minor q; Saxonite IX]

Salt Rheum (sore, bleeding, itching) – [Rumex q + Alnus q + Gentiana q + Taraxacum q (15ml each) = (2ml′5)].

Psoriasis – Thyroidinum 3x (2g′4); Lappa q (20d ′3); Berberis Aquifol q (20d′4); [Local = Nat. Sulph IX lotion + Alcohol 10z.]

Ichthyosis – Ars. Iod 3x (3g′3); Thyroidin 3x (5g′2); Thuja q (5d′4); Clematis Erecta q (5d ′4); [Local = Nat. Sulph IX, lotion.]

Herpes (facial) – Nat. Mur. 6x (3g′4).

Herpes Zoster - (nerve pain in face, chest, abdomen & followed by vesicles) – Ranunculus Bulbosus q (5d′4); Rhus

Tox q (5d′4); [Rumex q + Alnus q + Gentiana q + Taraxacum q (15ml each) = (2ml ′ 5)]; [Local = Nat. Sulph IX, lotion.]

Pityriasis Rubra (bran-like scales) – Erythrinus q (5d′4);

Pemphigus – (blisers form) – Caltha palustris q (5d′4); Rhus Tox. q (5d′4); Thuja q (5d′4); [Kali Ars. 3x (10g) + Berb. Aquifol q (20z) = 1/2 t.s.f. ′3].

Lichen (round hard lesions) – Juglans Cinerea q (5d′4); [Local = Grindelia Robusta q]; [Jugladin 6x (2g) + Chin. Sulph 3x (10g) = (3g′4)].

Barber's Itch – Sulph. Iodatum 3x (3g′4); [Local = Sulph Iod 1x + Vesline.]; [Local = Kreosote q + Alcohol.]; [Local = Acid Carbolic q + Glycerine.]

Crusta Lactea (hair mats, itching) – Viola Tricolor q (5d′4); Lappaq (8d′4);

Scald Head – Viola Tricolor q (5d′4); Sil 6x (3g′4); [Local = Salicylic Acid IX + Vesline.]; [Local = Phyto q + Lobelia q.]

Scabies – [Local = Ver. Vir. q + Sulph q + Ichtholum IX].

Ring Worm – Juglans Cinerea q (10d ′4); [Local = Acetic Acid q] [Local = Oleum Jecoris Aselli IX + Acetic Acid q].

Liver Spots (Chloasma) – Euoymus Atrop. q (1/2 t.s.f.′2). [Local = Lactic Acid q].

Rhagades (cracks) – Graph 3x (3g′3); [Local = Balsam Peru q].

Prurigo – Dolicos Pruriens q (5d′4); [Rumex q + Alnus q + Gentiana q + Taraxacum q (10ml each) = (1/2 t.s.f. ′3)]; [Local = Nat. Sulph IX + Lobelia q].

Warts (verruca) – Thuja q (5d′4); Mag. Sulph 3x (2g′4); [Local = Thuja q + Acid Nit q + Chronic Acid q + Sabina q].

Bromidrosis (offensive sweat) – Sil 6x (3g′3); Baryta Carb 3x (3g′3); Sepia q (5d′4); Acid Nit q, 3x (5d′4).

Vaccinosis (eruption after vaccination) – Thuja q (3d′4).

Prickly Heat – [Local = Carbolic Acid q + Borax 1x + Aqua.]

Anaemia – Ferrum Met. 1x (3g′3); Digitalin 3x (3g′3); China q (5d′4); Nat. Mur 6x (3g′3); Helonias Dioica q (5d′4); Calc. Phos. 3x (3g′3).

Cerebral Anaemia – Calc. Phos 3x (3g´3); Kali Phos 6x (3g´3).

Pernicious Anaemia – Picric. Acid 3x (3g´4); Ars. 3x (3g´3); Calc. Phos. 3x (3g´3); Carduus q (5d´3);

Scrofula – Alnus Rubra q (5d´3); Cistus Canadensis q (5d´3); Heper Sulph 3x (3g´3); Iodine 6x (10d´4); Sil 6x (3g´3);[Local = Phyto q + Myrica q + Lobelia q]; Ferr. Phos 3x (3g´3); Rumex q (5d´4). [Thuja q + Baptisia q = (15d´3)]; Rumin 1x (3g´4).

Abscess – Heper Sulph 1x (3g´3); Calc. Sulph 2x (3g´3); [Local = Lobelia q]; Echinacea q (10d´3); Alnus Rubra q (8d´3); [Local = Sil q].

Boils – Bell q (3d´5); Lappa q (10d´3); Echinacea q (5d´3); Calc. Sulph 3x (3g´3); [Local = for checking progress – Acon q + Hamamelis q + Arn.q]; [Local = Lobelia q + Sil q].

Carbuncles – Echinacea q (15d´3); [Local = Echinacea q + Acid Carbolic q].; Strychnia Sulph 6x (1d ´4); Heper Sulph 3x (3g´3); Kali Mur. 3x (2g´4); Tarantula C. q (5d´4);

Chlorosis (Severe anaemia) – Puls q (5d´4); Nat Mur. 6x (3g´3); Senecio Aurens q (10d´4); Alumina 1x (3g´3); Digitalin 6x (3g´3); Ferr. Met. 1x (3g´4);

Scurvy – [Rhus Glabra q (5ml) + Ferrum Carbonicum 6x (20g) = (1ml´5)] [Local = Rhus Glabra q + Glycerine.]

Purpura (Skin rash due to bleeding) – Hamamelis q (10d´4); Ergotin 6x (2g´4); Lach 6x (5d´4);

Leucocythemia – Picric Acid 3x (3g´3); Calc. Carb 1x (5g´3); Thuja q (4d´4); Aranea Diadema q, 3x (3d´4); Menispernum12 (1d´4).

Erysipelas – [Bell q +Rhus Tox q = (5d´4)]; [Local = Hamamelis q].

Glanders – (fever, inflamed lymph-node, nasal mucous membrane) – Kali Bich 3x (3g´3); Echinacea q (10d´4); Calc. Sulph 3x(3g´3);

Aneurism (artery swelling) – Kali Iodatum 3x (5g´4); Ver. Vir q (5d´4); Baryta Mur 3x (3g´4); Calc. Flour 3x (3g´4); [Local = Mag. Sulph IX + Aqua.].

Rheumatism – Colchicum q (5d´4); Rhus Tox q (5d´3); [Local = Iodineq]; Berberis V. q (5d´4); Rhododendron q (5d´4); [Cascara Sagrada q (10z) + Glycerine (10z) = (1 t.s.f. ´3)]. Acid Salicylicum 1x (3g´4); Bryo q (5d´4); [Cimicifuga q + Phytolacca q + Guiacum q (10z each) = (1 t.s.f. ´3)]. [Local = Capsicum q + Origanum q + Opium q + Camphor q].

Urology & Nephrology

Cystitis – (bladder) – (Desire to pass urine frequently and burning)– [Acon q (2ml) + Gels. q (2ml) = (1ml´4).]; Cantharis q, 3x (5d´4); Camphor q (3d´4); Nux. Vom. q (2d´4); Equisetum Hy. q (4d´4).

Suppression of the Urine – Apis Mel (5d´5);

Chronic Cystitis – Chimaphila Umbelata q (4d´5); [Gelsemin 6x (2g) + Hamamelin 3x (4g) + Pupulin 6x (2g) = (2g´4)]; Terebinthina q (5d´4); Cuprum Ars. 6x (2g´4).

Gravel – Thalaspi B.P. q (5d´4); Uric Acid, dysuria – Epigea Repens q (2od´4);

Calculus in the Bladder – Magnesia Boro Citrate 1x, 30(5g´4).

Acute Prostatitis – [Staphis q (30d) + Gels. q (30d) = (15d´4)].

Chronic Prostatitis – Sabal Serrulata q (10d ´4); Acs. Hip q (10d´4) Selenium 3x (3g´4);

Haematuria (bloody urine) – Terebinthina q, 3x(5d´4); Ferr. Phos. 3x (3g´4); Lycopus Virg. q (5d´4);

Diabetes – Lactic Acid q (1/2 t.s.f. ′3); Chionanthus q (20d′4); Acid Phos q (20d′4); Syzygium q (3d′4); Uranium Nit 3x (3g′4); Lycopus Virg. q (1/2 t.s.f.′4).

Spermatorrhoea – Eryngium Aquaticum q (10d′4); Lupulin 3x (2g′4); Disocorea q(8d′4); Ver. Alb. q (5d′4); Kali Phos. 3x (3g′4); [Strychine Sulph 6x (3g) + Gelsemin 6x (3g) = (2g′3)].

Kidney Complaint – Berberis Vulgaris q (5d′4); Acid Benzoic 3x (5g′4); Terebinthina q (8d′3).

Acute Bright's Disease (Nephritis) –Triticum Repens q (10d′3); Cantharis q (5d′4); Kali Mur. 3x(3g′4); Kali Phos. 3x (3g′4); Calc. Phos. 6x (3g′4); Calc. Sulph 3x (3g′4).

Chronic Bright's Disease – Helonias Dioca q (5d′4); [Helonin 3x + Chelonin 3x = (2g′4)].

Respiratory Medicine

Coryza – Acon q (2d′4); Euphrasia off. q (15d′4); Nat. Mur 3x (3g′4); Kali Mur 3x (3g′4);

Inlfuenza – Bell q (5d′4); Eupat. Perf. q (5d′4); Kali Mur 3x (3g′4); Strychnia Sulph 6x (1g′4);

Nasal Catarrh – [Calc. Phos. 3x + Nat. Mur 3x + Ferri Phos. 6x + Kali Mur 3x = (4g′4)].

Chronic Catarrh – [Iodine q + Carbolic Acid q + Ammonia Causticum q + Camphor q = (10d ′4)]; Sanguinaria Nitrica q, 3x (3d/g′4) Kali Bich q, 3x (5d/g′4); [gargle local = Natrum Sulphocarb. 1x.];

Nasal Polypus – Sanguinaria Can. q (10d′4).

Epistaxis – Ferr. Phos. 3x (3g′4); Melilotus Alba q (5d′4); Ferrum Aceticum 3x (3g′5); [Local = Geranium Mac. q, press it well up into nostril with cotton].

Pharyngitis – [Gels q + Phyto q =(10d′4)]; Guiacum q (8d′4); Arg. nit. 3x, q (3d/g′4); [Local gargle = Kali Chloricum (20g) + Zinc. Sulph 1x (10g)].

Tonsilitis – [Acon q + Phyto q = (8d ′4)]; Lac.Can. 30 (1d′4); Kali Mur. 3x (3g′4); Baryta Carb. 3x (3g′4);

Chronic Tonsilitis – Calc. Phos. 3x (3g′4); Baryta Iod 3x (3g′4);

Laryngitis – Acon 3x (5d′4); [Eucalyptus q + Jaborandi q = (5d′4)]. Sanguinaria Can. q (5d′4); Stillingia q (10d′4); Lobelia q (8d′4);

Chronic Laryngitis – Arum Triphyllum q (5d′4); Causticum q (5d′4); Lachesis q, 3x (5d′4);

Oedema Glottidis – Apis Mel. q (5d′4).

Acute Bronchitis – [Acon q + Asclepias Tuberosa q = (10d′4)]. Kali Mur 3x (3g′4); [Inula q + Asclepias Tub. q = (8d′4)]; Stillingia q (8d′4); Heper Sulph 3x (3g′4);

Chronic Bronchitis – Stannum Met 3x (3g′4); Strychnine Sulph 6x (1g′4);

Acute Pleurisy – Bryo q (5d′3); Asclepias Tub. q (10d′4); Kali Mur. 3x (3g′4);

Chronic Pleurisy – Kali Aceticum q (20d ′4); Ammon Carb. q (20d′4); Iodium q (3d′5); Chin. Sulph 3x (5g′4);

Asthma – Aspidosperma q (1/2t.s.f.′ 4); Lobelia Inflata q (10d′4) Grindelia Robusta q (25d′4); Senega q (5d′4); [Sumbul q + Gels q = (5d′5)].

Aphonia – Kali Bich q (5d′4); Erigeron q (5d′4); Strychina Sulph 6x (1g′4); Rhus Glabra q (15d′4).

Pneumonia – [Ver. Vir q + Asclepias Tub q = (1/2 t.s.f.′4)]; Kali. Mur. 3x (3g′4); Strychnine Sulph 6x (1g′4); Baptisia q (5d′4); Antim Tart 1x (3g′4); Chin. Sulph 3x(3g′4); Ipecac q (5d′4);

Typhoid Pneumonia – Chin. Sulph. 3x (3g´4); Baptisia q (10d´4);

Hay Fever – Sabadilla q (5d´4); Allium Cepa q (10d´4).

Whooping Cough – Drosera q (8d´4); Ipecac q (5d´4); Naphthaline 3x (2g´6); Corallium Rubrum q (5d´4);

Bronchocele – Iris Vers. q (5d´4); [Iodine q + Phyto q = (8d´3)]; Calcarea Iodata 3x (2g´5);

Diphtheria – Diphtheria Antitoxin 32 (1/4d ´3); [Phyto q + Gels q = (6d´4)] [Local gargle = Kali Chloricum 3x + Zinc Sulph 1x]; Acid Sulphurous q (8d´5) Apis Mel. q (5d´4); [Baptisia q + Eucalyptus q = (10d´4)]; Lach. q (5d´4); Arum Triphylum q (8d´4); Chin. Sulph 3x (3g´4);

Pulmonary Tuberculosis – Baptisin 3x (1g´4); [Drosera q + Ver. Vir q + Glycerine = (10d´5)]; Silicea 3x (3g´4); Ferr. Phos. 3x (3g´4); Millefolium q (8d´4); Myosotis Symphytifolia q (10d´4); Picrotoxin 6x (5g´3); Kali Mur. 3x (3g´4);

Gynaecology

Menses (delayed) – Caulophyllum q (8d´4); Ferr. Phos. 3x (3g´4); Puls q (4d´5); Acon. q (5d´4); Polygonum Punctatum q (10d´5);

Menses (Irregular) – Senecio Aurens q (20d´4); Trillium P. q (20d´4);

Menses (profuse) – Sabina q (10d´4);

Menses (Dark-coloured) – Ustilago Maydis q (10d´4); Crocus Sat. q (5d´5);

Menses (painful) – [Viburnum Opulus q + Gels q = (10d´4)]; Viburnum Prunifolium q (15d´4); Mag. Phos. 3x (4g´4); Dioscorea q (10d´4); Ver. Viride q (8d´4); Borax 1x (3g´4);

Os Uteri (congestion) – Bell q (8d´3); Sepia q (5d´4);

Os Uteri (Ulceration) – Bell q (8d´4); Kali Arsi. 3x (3g´4);

Leucorrhoea – Hamamelis q (10d´4); Kali Mur 3x (3g´4); Sec. Cor. q (5d´4); Fagopyrum Esculentum q (10d´4);

Pruritus Vaginae – [Borax 1x + Hydrastis q + Aqua = Local]

Os Uteri (prolapse) – Helonias Dioica q (10d´4); Sepia q (5d´4);

Os Uteri (Displacement) – Lilium Tigrinum q (8d´4);

Os Uteri (Enlargement) – Fraxinus Americans q (10d´4);

Metritis (womb) – [Gels q + Macrotin 3x = (5d´4)]; Aurum muriaticum 6x (3g´4).

Acute Salpingitis – [Ferr. Phos. 3x + Kali Mur. 3x = (4g´4)]; Macrotin 3x (2g´6);

Vaginismus – [Local = Cocaine Hydrochlorate + Vesline.] Platina Met. 6x (3g´3);

Ovary (congestion) – Lach 6x(5d´3); Apis Mel q (4d´4); Podophyllin 3x (3g´4).

Nymphomania – Murex Perpurea 6x (3g´4); Platina 6x (3g´3);

Sterility – Aurum Mur. Nat. 6x (4g´4); [Local = Ichlhyol 1x + Acid Boracicum 2x + Glycerine, to be applied by means of a tampon pressed up against the os. uteri.]; Borax 1x (3g´4); [Local = Nat. Bicarbonicum 1x + Glycerine.]

Female Frigidity – Sabal Serrulata q (10d´4);

Climecteric Flushing – Sepia q (5d´4); [Viburnum Opulus q + Vib. Pruntfoluim q = (10d´4)]; Ignatia q (5d´5);

Oedema of the feet and legs – Apocynin 6x (1g´4);

Pricking of the hands and feet – Kali Phos. 3x (3g´3); Zinc Met 3x (2g´5);

Headache – Veratrum Vir. q (5d´4); Bell q (4d´4); China q (4d´4); Glonoin q (5d´4); Kali Carb. 3x (3g´4);

With Stomach Complaints – Cimicifuga q (8d'4);
Enlargement of the Uterus – Fraxinus Americanus q (10d'4); Kali Carb. 3x (3g'3).
Dipsomania (alchol craving) – Apocynum Canabinum q (20d'4); Strychine Hypophos. 3x (1g'2); Strychine Nitricum 6x (1d'3);
Postpartum Haemorrahge and Convulsions – [Mitchella Repens q + Cimicifuga q + Sarsaparilla q = (1 t.s.f. '3) should be given the woman, about two months before the expected time.]
Weak Heart – Digitalis q (3d'5);
Constipation – Cascara Sagrada q (2 t.s.f.'2);
Haemorrhoids – Acs. Hip. q (5d'4);
Vomiting – Cerium Oxalicum 1x (5g'3); Ingluvin 6x (10g'3);
Horrible Dreams – Natrum Bromatum 3x (5g'3);
Cerebral Congestion – Ver. Vir. q (5d'4);
Hysterical Spasms – Camphor Bromide 1x (5g '15 minute intervals until relieved).
Micturation – Staphis q (5d'4);
Cramps in the calves of the leg – Vib. Opulus q (10d'4);
Cross, nothing please her – Chamo. q (5d'4);
Pain under the left breast – Macrotin 3x (2g'4);
Anaemia – Ferr. Phos. 3x (3g'4);
Dyspepsia, urine excessive or deficient – Helonias q (5d'4);
Salivation – Jaborandi q (8d'3);
Dropsy – Elaterium q (5d'4);
Heartburn – Lactopeptin 3x (3g'4);
Labor Pains – Cimicifuga q (10d'4);
After-pains – Gels q (5d'4); Cinnamon q (5d'4);
Diarrhoea – [Podophyllin 3x + Sac. Lac = (2g'4)]; [Rheum q + Zingiber q + Camphor q + Capsicum q + Opium q (8ml each) = (1t.s.f. '5)]; Acid Phos q (10d'4); Antin Crude 3x (3g'4); Colocynth q (4d'4); Cuprum Ars. 6x (4g'4); Mag. Carb. 3x (2g'6); Aloe q (6d'4); Henchera Americana q (10d'5);
Vomiting – Ipecae q (5d'5); Bismath Met 3x (3g'4); Ver. Alb. q (4d'4); Amygdalis Persica q (10d'4); Sepia q (4d'4); Colchicum q (10d'4).

Sexual Medicine

Impotency – Avena Sativa q (20d'4); Kali Phos 3x (3g'4); Strychninum Ars. 3x (1g'4); Acid Phos q (8d'4); Acid Picric q, 3x (5d/g'4); Lyco q (5d'4); Agnus Castus q (8d'4); Selenium 3x (3g'4); Sabal Serrulata q (20d'4);
Gonorrhoea – [Gelsemium q + Canabis Sativa q =(1/2 t.s.f. '4)]; Cubeba q (5d'4); Nat. Sulph 3x (3g'4); Sepia q (3g'4);
Orchitis – [Puls q + Phyto q = (10d'4)]; Clematis Erecta q (10d'5); [Ammon Mur q + Phyto q + Alcohol = Local];
Induration of the Testicle – Rhododendron q (10d'4); [Nat. Mur 6x + Aurum Mur 6x = (5g'4)]; [Local = Lobelia q + Mullein Oil.]

Buboss (swollen lymph-node in the armpit or grain, due to venereal disease) – Phyto q (5d´4); Kali Mur 6x (3g´4); Calc. Sulph 3x (2g´5); [Local = Iodine q + Phyto q + Lobelia q].

Chancre (painless ulcer on lip, penis, urethra, eyelid for syphilis) –[Ferrm Clorid q + Zinc Met 1x = Local].

Balanitis (glans penis) – [Zinc Sulph 1x = Local].

Stricture of the Urethra – Chimaphila Umbellata q (15d´4);

Hydrocele – Apis Mel q (5d ´4);

Syphilis – [Corydalin 3x + Chin. Sulph 3x = (5g´4)]; [Stillingia q + Podo. q + Phyto q + Iris Vers. q = (20d´4)]; Acid Nit q (4d´4); Kali Bich q (5d´4); Phyto q (10d´3); Corydalis Formosa q (15d´4); Berb. Aquifol. q (10d´d); [Local = Acon q + Conium q + Glycerine.]

Varicocele (dilation of spermatic veins) – [Local = Hamamelis q.]; Puls q (5d´4); Hamamelis q (10d´4);

Alopecia – [Local = Cantharis q +Ricinus Communis q + Oil Lemon + Oil Burgamont + Oil Lavender + Alcohol.]

Eye & Ear

Conjunctivitis (acute) – Ferr. Phos.3x (3g´4); Sulph 1x (3g´4); Heper Sulph 3x (3g´4); [Local = "eye wash", Zinc Sulph 1x (1g) + Morphinum Sulph 6x (1g) + Aqua.];

Purulent Conjunctivitis – Heper Sulph 1x (2g´4); Rhus T. q (5d´3);

Gonorrheal Conjunctivitis – Acon q (4d´3); Thuja q (5d´4);

Scrofulous Conjunctivitis – [Stillingia q + Kali Iodatum 3x = (5d´4)];

Catarrhal Conjunctivitis – Bell q (4d´4); Euphrasia q (5d´4); [Local = Hydrastin Mur 6x (1g) + Aqua.]

Granular Conjunctivitis – [Local = Eucalyptus q (5ml)].

Rheumatic Opthalmia – [Acon q + Spigelia q = (8d´4)].

Iritis – Jaborandi q (10d´4);

Choroiditis (blurred vision) – [Bell q (5d ´4), dry eye]; Kali Mur 6x (3g´4); Prunus Spinosa q (6d´4);

Suppurative Choroiditis – Rhus Tox q (6d´4); Viola Odorata q (5d´4);

Ulceration of the Cornea – Calc. Sulph 2x (3g´4); Bell q (5d´3); Corydalis q (10d´4); Kali Bich q (3d´5);

Retinitis – Ferrum Phos 3x (3g´4); Bell q (6d´4); Kali Mur 3x (3g´4); Picric Acid 2x, q (5d/g´4); Natrum Salicylicum 2x (4g´4);

Keratitis – (Cornea) – Apis Mel. q (5d´4); Kali Mur. 3x (5g´4); Aurum Met. 3x (3g´4); Heper Sulph 3x (2g´5);

Corneal Opacities – Cannabis Sativa q (10d ´3); Kali Bich 3x (4g´3); Calc. Flour 3x (3g´4).

Sty – Puls q (10d´3); Calc. Sulph 3x (3g´4);

Asthenopia (Eyestrain) – Ruto G q (5d´4); Asarum Europaeum q (6d´4); Sepia q (3g´4); Strychnine Sulph 6x (1g´4); Kali Carb. 3x (3g´4);

Oculo Motor Paresis – Rhus Tox. q (5d´4); Causticum q (3d´6);

Myopia (near-sightedness, night blindness) – Physostigma q (6d ´4);

Amblypia – (poor sight) – Aconite q (5d´4); Kali Phos 3x (3g´4); [Nux Vom. q + Acid Phos q = (10d´4)].

Cataract – Calcarea Flour 6x (4g´3); Phosphorus q, 6x (5d/1g´4); Sulphur Iodatum 3x (3g´4); Sil 3x (3g´4); Caust q, 3x (5d´4);

Otalgia (Pain in ear) – Plantago Major q (8d ´4); Ferr. Phos 3x (3g´4); Chamomilla q (5d´4);

Otitis – Acon q (5d´5); Calc. Sulph 3x (3g´4); Kali Mur 6x (3g´4); [Local = Puls q, cotton moistened with q, placed in the affected ear.]

Otorrhoea – [Local = Eucalyptus q]; [Local = Boracic Acid 2x + Glycerine = insert with cotton.]; Kali Phos 6x (3g´4); Kali Sulph 3x (3g´4); Sil. 1x (3g´4);

Polypus Aurium – Calc. Carb 3x (4g´3); [Local = Salicylic Acid IX + Vesline.].

Eczema Aurium – Rhus Tox q (5d´4); Calc. Sulph 3x (3g´4); [Local = Eucalyptus q + Vesline.].

Deafness – (Local = Ether q, to soften the wax.]; Kali Mur 6x (3g´4); Strychninum Sulph 6x (1g´4); Phos q, 6x (5d/g´3); Sil. 3x (3g´4); Kali Phos 6x (3g´4); Ferrum Picricum 3x (3g´4);

Head

Congestive Headache – Ver. Vir q (5d´4); Bell. q (5d´4); Melilotus Alba q (8d´3), relieved by nosebleed.; Glonoin q (4d´4); Gels. q (5d´4), > by urination; Acon q (5d´4); Sec. Cor q (10d ´5); Caffeinum 1x (3g´5); Nat. Carb. 3x (3g´4); Usnea Barbata q (5d´5).

Nervous Headache – Epiphegus Virginiana q (10d´5);

Brain Fag (headache of students & business) – Picric Acid q, 2x (5d´4); Ignatia q (4d´4); Kali Phos 6x (3g´3); Acid Phos q (10d´4); Codeinum 3x (3g´3); Spigelia q (6d´4); Coccinella Sept. q (5d´4);

Headache from Eye Strain – Ruta q (4d´4); Cimicifuga q (4d´4); Onosmodium q (5d´4)

Sick Headache – Chionanthus q (5d ´4); Cascara Sagrada q (5d´3); Niccolum Met 3x (3g´4); Epiphegus Virginiana q (10d´5);

Periodical Headache – Chin. Sulph 3x (2g´5); Bryo q (5d´4); Nat. Mur. 6x (3g´4);

Extrimity

Cold hands, frightened, starts at every sound – Calendula q (5d´3);
Gouty diposits in wrists, fingers & toes – Uric acid diathesis – Benzoic Acid 2x (3g´4);
Fidgety hands, can't keep them still – Kali Bromatum 3x (3g´3);
Sweating hands – Pilocarpinum Mur. 3x (3g´3);
Pricking & numbness of fingers – Kali Phos 3x (3g´4);
Oedeme of the left hand and foot – Cactus Grandi q (10d´3);
Writer's Cramp – Mag. Phos. 6x (3g´4); Strychnine Sulph 6x (1g´3);
Crackling of Joints – Nat. Phos. 3x(4g´3);
In caries of Bones – Calc. Flour 3x (3g´4);
Wrist joint swollen from rheumatism, motion impossible – Actea Spicata q (5d´5);
Weakness of hands, awkwardness, everything falling from the hands – Bovista q, 3x(5d´4);
Walking seems likely to fall to one side – Cocculus Indicus q (6d ´4);

Cold hands, feet with profuse menstruation – Calc. Carb 3x (3g′4);
Trembling of the hands in paralysis, sometimes hereditary – Lolium Temulentum q (4d′4);
Sprains & straining of the muscles of hands and arms from overlifting – Rhus Tox q, 3x (5d′4);
Periosteal inflammation of long bones, < at night, in damp weather – Mezerium q (5d ′4);
Periosteal inflammation of long bones, complicated with syphilis – Stillingea Sylvatica q (10d ′4);
Mascular rheumatism, < on motion, followed by numbness – [Kalmia Latifolia q + Gels. q = (20d ′3)].
Rheumatism, with painful sore muscles – [Jaborandi q + Cimicifuga q + Gels q = (10d ′4)].
Chronic rheumatism – Franciscea Uniflora q (30d′4);
Articular rheumatism – Gaultheria Oil q (10d ′4); [Local = Camphor q + Absinthium q + Alcohol];
Gout – Urtica Urens q (15d′4);
Cramps in the legs of pregnant women – Vib. Pruni q (5d′4);
Knee jerk walking difficult and unsteady – Lathyrus Sativus q (5d′4);
Hip Disease – Cistus Canadensis q (8d′3);
Phlebitis (Vein) – [Puls q + Hamamelis q = (10d ′4)];
Arthritis Deformans, with stiffness of the knee – Caust q (3d ′5).
Sciatica – [Colocynth q + Phyto. q + Gnaphalium q = (20d′4)].
Varicose veins upon the legs, due to enlargement of Spleen – Carduus M. q (8d ′3);
Varicose ulcers – [Local = Lobelia q + Baptisia q + Zinc Sulph 1x.]
Recent fractures of Bones – Symphitum q (10d ′3);
Old fractures – Sil. 3x (3g ′4);
Paralysis Agitans or tremors of multiple sclerosis – Hyoscyamine Hydrobromate 6x (3g ′3);
Hemiplegia (one-sided paralysis) – [Strychninum Sulph 6x (3g) + Xanthoxylin 3x (6g) = (3g ′3)].

Orthopaedic Medicine

Burning soles of the feet – [Local = Ammonium Mur q].
Burning soles of the feet under cover – Sulph 3x (3g ′3);
Rheumatism begins in the feet and travel upwards – [Ledum Pul. q + Gaultheria Oil q = (10d ′4)].
Corns and Callosities – Antim Crude 3x (3g′4); Rheumatism of feet.
Tingling of toes and burning feet – Bell q (5d′4);
Weak ankles – Calc. Phos. 3x(3g′3);
Bunions (swelling of the joint between the great toe and the first metatarsal bone) – [Ver. Vir. q = Local.]
Old people with oedema of the feet – Apocynin 6x (2g′ 3);
Numbness of the feet – Alumina 3x (3g′3);
For chilblians of the feet – Agaricus Mus. q (5d′4); [Local = Oleum Cajuputum q].
Fidgety feet – Zinc Met 3x (3g′3);

Offensive sweat of the feet – [Local = Kali Chloricum 3x]; Silica 3x (3g´3);
Feet Cold – Calc. Carb. 3x (3g´3);
Cramps in feet – Sulph 3x (3g´4);
Ingrowing toe-nails - (Local = Ferrum Cloride 1x.]. Acid Picricum 3x (3g ´3);
Feet cold and hands hot or vice versa – Sepia q (5d´4);
Every muscle in the body twitches from the eyes to the toes – Hyos. q (10d´4);
Spasms begins in the fingers and toes – Cuprum Met 3x (2g´4);
Toe nails grow out of shape and become thick – Graph 3x (3g´4);
Ankle joints are swollen and the soles of the feet are so painful that the patient can hardly step on the ground – Ledum Pal. q (5d ´5);

Cardiology

Pericarditis (pain in heart) – [Acon q + Asclepias Tub. q = (10d´5)]; Bryo. q (4d´4); Kali Mur 6x (4g´4); Spigelia q (5d´4); [Cimicifuga q (5d´5), when complicated with rheumatism.]; Jaborandi q (8d ´4); [Phyto q + Kali Iodatum 3x = (10d ´4)].

Hydropericardium – Digitalis q (5d´4); Apocynum Can. q (5d´4); Convallaria Maj q (5d´4); Apis Mel q (8d´3); Helonias Dioica q (5d´4); [Podophyllin 3x (1g) + Leptandrin 3x (2g) + Capsicum q (2ml) = (10d´4)];

Endocarditis – Cimicifuga q (8d´3); Ver. Vir. q (8d ´3); Acon. Redix q (5d´4); Kali Mur 6x (4g ´3); Spigelia q (8d ´3); Cereus Bonplandi q (10d´3); Calc. Flour 3x (3g´3);

Myocarditis – Iberis Amara q (8d ´4); Kali Mur 6x (4g´4); Calc. Flour 3x (3g´3); Crataegus Oxyacantha q (10d´4);

Hypertrophy of the Heart (enlargement) – Ver. Vir q (8d´4); Arnica q (5d ´3); [Cactus Grand q (15d ´4), for abuse of tobacco]; Lycopus Virg q (20d ´3); Collinsonia q (10d ´4); Colchicum q (5d´4);

Dilatalion of the Heart – Crataegus Oxy. q (10d ´4); Phaseolus q (10d´4); Digitalis q (10d ´3); Ignatia q (10d ´3); Collinsonia q (5d´4);

Fatty Heart – Vanadium 3x (3g ´4); Phyto q (10d ´4); [Ricinus Com. q + Opium q =(20d´3)]; [Cimicifuga q + Gels q + Puls q = (20d´3), pain, palpitation, shortness of breath of women.]

Angina Pectoris – Lobelia q (25d ´4); Spigelia q (10d ´4); Crataegus q (15d ´4); Glonoin q (2d ´5);

Exophthalmic Goitre – Lycopus Virg. q (20d ´4); Fucus Vesiculosus q (50d ´4); [Local = Iodine q + Phyto q.]

Weak Heart – Digitalin 6x (3g´4); Ferr. Phos 3x (3g ´4); Phaseolus Nana q (10d ´4); Glonoin q (2d ´5);

Valvular Disease of the Heart – Calc. Flour 3x (3g ´4); Spongia q (5d´4);

Dyspnoea – Aspidos q (30d ´4); Naja Tripudians q (20d ´3); Adonis Vernalis q (8d ´3); Crataegus q (10d ´2);

Arterio Sclarosis – Calc. Flour 3x (3g ´3); Ver. Vir. q (5d ´4); Strychnine Sulph 6x (1g ´4); Ars. Iod. 3x (3g ´4); Acid Phos. q (5d´ 4).

Palpitation of the Heart – Moschus q (5d ´4); China q (8d´ 3); Acid Phos q (8d ´4); Kali Phos. 6x (3g ´4).

Hiccough – Mag. Phos. 3x (3g ′4); [Sugar + Vinigar]; Caulophyllum q (10d ′1 hourly); Morphin Sulph 6x (1g ′5);

Neurology

Neuritis – Acon. Rad. q (4d ′3); [Cannabis Ind. q (5d ′4), for hyperesthesia (excessive sensibility, esp. of the skin)]; Hypericum q (5d ′4);

Neuralgia – [Gels q + Kalmia Lat. q = (15d ′4)]; Spigelia q (5d ′4); Bryonia q (4d ′3); Mag. Phos. 6x (4g ′4); Zinc Valerianicum 3x (3g′4); Aconitine 3x (1g ′3); [Scutullarin 3x + Cypripedium Pubescens q + Chin. Sulph 3x = (5d ′4)].

Hysteria – Capsicum q (8d ′4); Ammonia Valerian. 6x (3g ′5); [Asafoetida q + Valeriana Officinalis q + Cypripediumq + Lobelia q = (10d ′4); Pothos Foetida q (10d ′4); [Ignatia q (4d ′3), laughs and cries alternately, has globus hystericus.]; Moschus q (8d ′4);

Neurasthenia – Avena Sativa q (10d ′3); Acid Phos q (10d ′4); Acid Picricum q, 3x (5d/g ′4); Kali Phos 6x (3g ′4); Sil 3x (3g ′3).

Epilepsy – Oenanthe Crocata q (5d′4); [ammon. Brom. 3x + Bell q + OEnanthe Crocata q + Puls q = (15d ′3)]; Ver. Vir. q (5d ′3); Indigo 6x (4g ′4); Artemisia Vulgaris q (8d ′3); Kali Mur 6x (4g ′4); Lobelia q(10d ′4); Solanum Carolinense q (15d ′3); Calc. Phos 3x (3g ′4), [Kali Phos 3x + Mag. Phos. 6x = (4g ′4)]; Nat. Sulph 3x (3g ′3).

Chorea (jerky involuntary movement, affecting shoulders, hip & face) – [Mag. Phos. 6x + Calc. Phos 3x = (4g ′3)]; [Cimicifuga q + Gels q + Kali Ars. 3x = (10d ′4)]; [Scutallaria q + Cypripedium q + Ferr. Carbonicum 6x = (10d ′4)]; Agaricus M.q (15d ′4).

Catalepsy (abnormal maintenance of postures) – Cannabis Indica q (5d′4); Puls q (10d ′4); Stramonium q (8d ′3);

Facial Paralysis – Acon q, 3x (8d ′3); Caust. q (5d ′4);

Paraplegia (paralysis of both legs) – Arg. Nit. q 3x (5d/g ′4); Lathyrus Sativus q (8d ′3); Oleander q (8d ′4); Kali Phos 6x (3g′4); Conium Mac. q (5d ′3); Gels q (5d ′4);

Hemiplegia (one-sided paralysis) – Avena Sativa q (10d ′3); Lachesis q (5d′ 4); Causticum q (5d ′3); [Strychime Sulph 6x (1g) + Xanthoxylin 3x (5g) = (2g ′3)]. Zinc. Phos 3x (1g ′2); [Local = Origanum q + Capsicum + Stillingia q].

Writer's Cramp – Nat. Phos. 3x (3g ′4); Mag. Phos. 6x (4g′ 3); Conium Mac. q (5d ′4).

Puerperal Convulsions –Viburnum Prunifolium q (20d ′5); Glonoin q (10d ′4); Ver. Vir. q (20d ′5); Eupat. Perf. q (15d ′4).

Brain and Spine

Spinal Irritation – Bell q (3d ′5); Chin Sulph. 3x (3g ′2); [Local = Iodine q].

Spinal Meningitis – Bell q (4d ′4); Ver. Vir. q (8d ′3); Bryonia q (5d ′4);

Myelitis (spinal cord inflammation) – Acid Oxalicum 6x (3g ′4); Abrotanum q (10d ′3); Lathyrus Sativus q (5d ′4); Hyoscyamine Hydrobrom. 6x (2g ′6);

Cerebro Spinal Meningitis – Ferr. Phos. 6x (3g′ 4); Nat. Sulph

3x (3g ′3); Kali Phos. 6x (4g ′3); Bell q (4d ′4); [Gels q + Cimicifuga q = (10d ′4)]; Ver. Vir q (4d ′4); Echinacea q (10d ′5); Passiflora Incarnata q (10d ′5); [Sulph 3x + Sil 3x = (3g ′4)];

Locomotor Ataxia – Alumina 3x (3g ′3); Bell q (10d ′3); Arg. Nit q, 3x (3d/g ′4); Zinc Phos. 3x (1g ′3); Canabis Indica q (5d ′4);

Equisetum q (8d ′3); Secale Cor. q (5d ′4); Stramonium q (8d ′3); Sil. 3x (3g′3);

Tetanus – Angustura q (5d′ 1/2 hourly); Hypericum q (15d ′4); [Capsicum q + Lobelia q = (10d′ 4), for lock-jaw]; [Passiflora q + Gels q = (10d ′4)];

Hydrophobia – (Local = Kali Causticum q]; Echinacea q (10d ′4); [Scutellaria q + Cypripedin 3x + Lobelia q + Chin Sulph 3x = (10d ′4)];

Multiple Sclerosis (unsteady gait, shaky movements of the limbs, rapid involuntary movements of the eyes & defects in speech pronunciation) – Lathyrus Sativa q (5d ′4); Hypericum q (8d ′3);

Concussion of the Brain – Bell q (8d ′4);

Cerebral Congestion – Acon q (4d′4); Ver. Vir q (5d ′4); Bell q (5d ′4);

Meningitis – Ferr. Phos. 6x (3g ′4); Kali Mur 6x (4g ′3); Helleborus Nigre q (5d ′3); Kali. Phos. 3x (3g′ 4);

Apoplexy (stroke) – Acon q (5d ′3); Ferr. Phos. 3x (3g ′4); Kali Mur. 6x (4g ′3); Kali Phos. 3x (3g ′4);

Vertigo – Acon q (4d′4); [Ammonium Iodatum 3x (2g ′4), for tinitus aurium, Meniere's disease (deafness).]; Sec. Cor. q (10d ′3); Kali Phos. 3x (3g ′4); Digitalis q (5d ′4); Iodine q, 3x (5d ′4);

Delirium Tremens – Hyoscyamus q (8d ′4); Cannabis Indica q (30d ′ with sugar 1 hourly); Kali Phos 6x (3g ′4);

Mania – Kali Bromatum 3x (3g′4); Ipecac q (8d ′3); Cascara Sagrada q (1 t.s.f.′4); Hyoscyamus q (20d ′4); Bell q (8d′3); Sepia q, 3x (5d ′ 4); Cimicifuga q (10d′4); Stramonium q (8d′4); Ver. Alb. q (10d′4); Kali Phos 6x (3g′4).

Suicidal Mania – Ignatia q (4d′ 4); Cimicifuga q (8d ′3); Lillium Tig q (Iod ′4); Aurum Met. 3x (3g′ 4); Ars. Alb, 3x (3g ′4);

Fever

Exanthemata (typhoid fever) (skin rash with eruptive disease or fever) – Ferr. Phos. 6x (4g ′4); Kali Mur. 3x (3g ′4); Baptisia q (5d′4); Echinacea q (10d ′4); Acid Hydrochloric q (5d ′4); Carbo Veg. 3x (5g ′3); Hyoscyamus q (5d ′4); Kali Phos. 6x (3g′ 4); Kali Mur 6x (4g ′3).

Typhus Fever – Baptisiaq (8d ′4); Hyoscyamus q (8d ′4); Echinaceaq (10d ′6); Bell q (5d ′4).

Remittent Fever – Gels. q (4d′4); Rhus. Tox. q (4d′4); Chin. Ars. 3x (3g ′4);

Bilious Fever – [Acon q + Nux Vom. q = (10d ′ 4)].

Scarlet Fever = [Acon. Radix q (15d) + Bell q (15d) = (8d ′4)]; [Local gargle = Kali Chloricum 6x + Zinc. Sulph 3x.]; Ferr. Phos. 6x (4g ′3); Kali Mur 6x (4g ′4); Arum Triphyllum q (3d ′4); [Phyto q + Echinacea q =(10d ′4)]; Ammon Carb. q (5d ′4); Ailanthus Glandulosus q (8d ′3);

Yellow Fever – [Acon q + Bell q = (10d ′4)]; Ipecac q (10d ′3); Camphor q (10d′6); Cadmium Sulph 3x (3g ′4); Crotalus Horridus q (5d ′4)

Chapter - 8
DEFINITE MEDICINES

Acromegaly
Thyroidin - One tablet of the crude preparation thrice daily.
Conchiolinum - 5 grains of the 3-rd trituration every 8 hourly.

Actinomycosis
Hippozaeninum - 5 drops of 6-th attenuation every 8 hourly.

Amblyopia
Phosphoricum Acidum - As a result of sexual excess, use 1X potency 4 times a day.
Ruta G - From over use of the eyes, use 3-rd potency 3 times a day.

Anidrosis
Plumbum - Dry skin, with absolute lack of perspiration, administer 30-th potency every 4 hourly.

Aphasia
Stramonium - has to exert himself a long time before he can utter a word, use 30-th potency thrice daily.
Gelsemium - Loss of memory with incoherent talk, use 30-th every 4 hourly.

Ascites
Apocynum Cannabinum - If the symptoms indicate no other remedy, whenever the ascites is the principal trouble, prescribe mother tincture 2 drops every 4 hourly.

Balanitis
Jacaranda Caroba - Try with 6-th potency thrice daily.

Blepharospasm
Codeinum - Involuntary twitching of eyelids, administer 3rd potency twice dailly.
Physostigma - With ciliary spasm, patient unable to read without pain and frontal headache, aggravated by light,
use 3X potency every 6 hourly.

Borborygmi
Jatropha Curcas - Preceding a loose stool, prescribe 3-rd potency every 4 hourly.
Lycopodium - With constipation and abdominal distention, use 6-th potency thrice a day.

Brain-fag
Zincum aceticum - From loss of sleep, use 10 drops of 1X potency every 4 hourly.
Anacardium - Loss of memory 'funk' before an examination, use 3-rd potency every 3 hourly.

Catalepsy
Ignatia - with opisthotonus; with emotional disturbance, use 6-th potency every hourly.

Cellulitis
Silicea - Inflammation of connective tissue characterized by first step of abscess, administer 6-th potency every 4 hourly.

Cheloid
Fluoricum Acidum - 6-th potency twice daily.
Graphites - 5 drops of 3-rd potency every 8 hourly.

Chilblains
Sulphur - Patients with irritable skins, use 3-rd attenuation three times a day.

Chorea

Agaricus Muscarius - The most commonly indicated remedy, use 3-rd potency every 4 hourly.

Veratrum Viride - When Agaricus fails to cause improvement within a considerable period, prescribe 3-rd attenuation every 3 hourly. Also externally apply to the spine, with the hand, night and morning, of a lotion consisting of equal parts of Veratrum Veride mother tincture, spirit of wine, and water.

Coccygodynia
Causticum - Bruised pain, use 6-th potency twice daily.

Corns
Ferrum Picricum - 3-rd attenuation every 6 hourly.

Radium Bromidum - Recent or painful, use 30th potency once a fortnight.

Delirium Tremens
Scutellaria Lateriflora - 10 drops of mother tincture in hot water every half-an-hourly.

Dupuytren's Contraction
Gelsemium - Recent cases, use 1st potency every 8 hourly.

Thiosinaminum - 3X trit., 2 grains night and morning.

Elephantiasis Arabum
Hydrocotyle Asiatica - Tincture, every 6 hourly.

Emphysema
Lobelia - 3-rd potency thrice daily.

Erotomania
Origanum - Great sexual excitement driving to onanism, use 3-rd potency every hourly.

Erythema Nodosum
Apis Mel. - 3X potency every 2 hourly.

Exostosis
Calcarea Fluor. - 6-th potency twice daily.

Fibroma
Silicea - Three grains of 3-rd trituration thrice daily.

Hydrastininum Muriaticum - Bleeding from, use 2 grains of 2X trituration every 4 hourly.

Fracture
Symphytum - To promote the union of, prescribe 1X every 4 hourly.

Ganglion
BenzoicumAcidum - 3X potency every 4 hourly. Also apply lotion prepared from pure Benzoic Acid (15 grains) with 3 drachms of rectified spirit and eight ounces of distilled water, in night and morning.

Sulphur - The highest CM potency once a week.

Gastrodynia
Oxalicum Acidum - Cutting pain, use 3-rd potency every 2 hourly.

Bismuth - Cramplike and pressive pains in stomach after eating, use 6-th potency every 2 hourly.

Gleet
Thuja Occ. - 12-th attenuation thrice a day.

Gum-boil
Merc. Sol. - 6-th potency every 2 hourly.

Gumma
Kali Iodatum - 5 grains of 3X trit. Every 8 hourly.

Haematemesis
Hamamelis - Dark blood, administer 1-st potency every 15 minutes.
Ipecac - Bright blood, use 1-st potency every 15 minutes.
Arnica Mont. - From mechanical injury, use 1-st potency every 15 minutes.
Haematuria
Terebinthina - 3-rd Attenuation every 2 hours.
Haemoglobinuria
Picric Acid - 3X trituration, 2 grains every 4 hourly.
Hay Fever
Sabadilla - Violent sneezing with lachrymation, redness and swelling of eyelids, contracting stupefying headache, use 30-th attenuation 4 times a day.
Gelsemium - Excessive sneezing, 3-rd potency every 4 hourly.
Head Lice
Natrum Mur. - 6-th attenuation thrice daily. Also the hair to be bathed with a lotion of Sabadilla Tincture, an ounce to the pint.
Heartburn
Capsicum - During an attack, prescribe 3-rd potency every 15 minutes.
Harpes Circinatus
Tellurium - 6-th attenuation every 4 hourly.
Herpes Zoster
Variolinum - 6-th potency 4 times a day.
Prunus Spinosa - If the pain is intractable, use 30-th attenuation every 3 hourly.
Hodgkin's Disease
Pertinum - 30-th potency twice daily.
Housemaid's Knee
Sticta Pulmonaria - Acute, use 1-st potency every two hours.
Hydrothorax
Apis Mel. - If the inflammation has been recent, use 3X every 3 hourly.
Hystero-epilepsy
Moschus – During the attacks, administer 3-rd potency every 10 minutes.
Zincum Valerianicum – During the intervals, use 3-rd trituration 4 times a day.
Arsenicum Iodatum – Where selected remedy fails, use 4 grain of 3X trit. Immediately after meals.
Impetigo
Viola Tricolor - Of the face, recent, administer 3-rd attenuation thrice a day.
Calcarea Muriatica - Of the head, use 1X trituration every 4 hourly.
Antimonium Tart. - General impetigo, 6-th potency 4 times a day.
Impotence
Phosphoric Acid - When due to sexual excess, 4 drops of 1st potency every 6 hourly.
Lycopodium - Impotence of long standing, use 30-th potency every 8 hourly.
Influenza
Influenzinum - 30-th attenuation every 4 hourly.
Leucocythaemia
Assenicum Iodatum - Where selected remedy fails, use 4 grains of 3X trit. Immediately after meals.
Lichen

Apis Mel - Lichen urticatus, prescribe 3X every two hourly.
Lienteria
Ferrum Met. - 6-th potency every 2 hourly.
Oleander - 3-rd potency every 2 hourly.
Liver-spots
Sepia - 6-th potency every 4 hourly.
Lycopodium - 6-th potency thrice a day.
Lupus
Tuberculinum Kochii - 4 globules of 200-th potency once a week.
Meniere's Disease
Natrum Salicylicum - Giddiness and noises in the ears, with deafness, use 3-rd trituration every 4 hourly.
Chininum Sulph. - 2 grains of 3X trit. Four times a day.
Miliaria
Aconite - 3-rd potency every 1 hourly.
Cactus Grandiflora - When oppression at the heart is very distressing, administer 3-rd potency every 1 hourly.
Mollities Ossium
Calcarea Iodata - 3X trituration every 4 hourly.
Myelitis
Plumbum - Chronic spiral paralysis, use 6-th attenuation every 4 hourly.
Myopia
Physostigma - 3X potency every 4 hourly.
Myxoedema
Thyroidin - 5 grains of 3X trituration twice a day.
Arsenicum Album - Great chilliness, scaly skin, restlessness, anxiety, use 200-th potency thrice daily.
Naevus
Radium Bromidum - 6 globules of 30-th attenuation once a week.
Vaccininum - 200-th potency twice a week.
Nettle-Rash
Chloral Hydrate - 3X potency three times a day. Use it for recent cases.
Astacus Fluviatilis 6-th attenuation every 4 hourly.
Nightmare
Paeonia Officinalis - 1-st potency every 4 hourly.
Noma Pudendi
Arsenic - 3-rd attenuation every 4 hourly.
Nyctalopia
Belladonna - 3-rd potency thrice a day.
Helleborus Niger - 3-rd attenuation every 4 hourly.
Osteo-myelitis
Gunpowder - 4 grains of 3X trituration every 4 hourly.
Ozaena
Leuticum - 200-th potency at bed-time.
Locally, spray of a solution of Muriate of Hydrastia, 1 grain to the ounce.
Cadmium Sulphuratum - 2 grains of 3X trit. Thrice a day.

Hippozaeninum - 6-th potency every 4 hourly.
Pancreatitis
Atropinum Sulphuratum - 2 grains of 3X trit. Every 4 hourly.
Pellagra
Ars. Sulph. Rub. - 4 grains of 3X trituration 4 times a day.
Perimetritis
Merc. Cor. - 3-rd potency every 1 hourly.
Plague
Pestinum - 30-th attenuation every 4 hourly.
Plica Polonica
Vinca Minor - 3-rd potency every 4 hourly.
Viola Tricolor - 3-rd attenuation every 4 hourly.
Prurigo
Radium Bromidum - 30-th potency once a week.
Psilosis
Fragaria Vesca - 5 drops of tincture, every 4 hourly.
Calcarea Lactica - 8 grains of 3X trituration thrice a day.
Psoriasis
Arsenic - General, acute, or chronic, prescribe 30-th potency every 4 hourly.
Pyelitis
Uva Ursi - mother tincture every hourly.
Pyorrhoea
Merc. Sol. - Spongy gums, bad odor from mouth, use 4 grains of 3X trit. Every 4 hourly.
Gunpowder - Free suppuration, use 4 grains of 3X trit. Every 4 hourly. A mouthwash of Peroxide of Hydrogen, one teaspoonful with water
Quinsy
Guaiacum - Acute tonsillitis, use 3X potency every 2 hourly.
Gunpowder - Septic tonsillitis, use 4 grains of 3X trit. Every 4 hourly.
Raynaud's Disease
Bacillinum - 30-th attenuation once a week and prescribe also Ferrum Phos., 8 grains of 6X trit. Twice a day.
Roseola
Belladonna - 3-rd potency every 2 hourly.
Rupia
Kali Iodatum - 5 grains of 3X trit. Every 6 hourly.
Lueticum - 5 globules of 200-th attenuation twice a week.
Aethiops Antimonialis - 2 grains of 1X trit. Thrice a day.
Scurvy
Merc. Sol. - 5 grains of 3X trituration every 4 hourly. As a wash for the mouth, a solution of Kali Chloricum, 10 grains to the half-pint.
Shock
Veratrum Album - Cold sweat on forehead and body, use 3-rd potency every half-an-hourly.
Coffea Cruda - Especially from sudden joy, administer 3-rd potency every half-an-hourly.
Stammering
Stramonium - 3-rd potency every 6 hourly.
Stomatitis

Capsicum - Simple exudative inflammation of the mouth, use 3-rd potency every 2 hourly.
Strangury
Camphora - Acute cases, administer 1 drop of 1X potency every 5 minutes.

Copaiba - In women especially, use 3-rd potency every half-an-hourly.
Tenesmus
Merc. Cor. - Incessant tenesmus most distressing, nothing but mucus and blood pass, prescribe 3-rd attenuation every half-an-hourly.
Throat-Deafness
Hydrastis - 3-rd potency every 2 hourly.

Merc. Sol. - 6-th attenuation four times a day.
Tennitus Aurium
Kali Iodatum - Chronic cases, use 30-th attenuation a single dose to the allowed to act.

Natrum Salicyl. - Roaring, with giddiness and difficult hearing, prescribe 3X trit. Every 4 hourly.
Torticollis
Lachnanthes Tinctoria - spraining on moving it, head twisted to one side, use 30-th attenuation every 4 hourly.
Uraemia
Cuprum Aceticum - When there are convulsions, use 3X trituration every 15 minutes.
Vaginismus
Plumbum - 6-th potency thrice a day.
Wens
Baryta Carb. - On scalp, sensitive and scurfy, use 6-th potency every 6 hourly.

Conium - Recurrent, administer 30-th attenuation every 6 hourly.
Woolsorter's Disease
Anthracinum - 30-th potency every 2 hourly.

HOMOEOPATHIC REPERTORY

Chapter - 9
CLINICAL REPERTORY

PSYCHIATRY

Ailments after anger, vexation, anxious delirium – Apis., Cocc., Coff., Nat. M. Staph., Sulph., Tarent. , Zinc.

Anxiety, in the morning – Ars., Graph, Lach, Nux.V., Phos., Ver. Alb., Zinc.

Anxiety, during evening – Bar.Mur., Carbo. Veg., Caust., Mur. Ac., Stam., Tab.

Anxiety alternating with indifference – Nat. Mur.

Anxiety, hypochondriacal – Canth., Kali Phos., Mosch, Nat. M., Nit. Ac., Valer.

Anxiety, when about to journey by – Ars. Alb., Psor., Sepia.

Aphasia, an impairment of expression or comprehension of language caused by injury or disease in the language centres of the brain – Glon., Kali. Br.

Aversion, to the opposite sex – Lyc., Puls., Sulph.

Cheerful, convulsions after – Sulph.

Concentration, dificult – Alum., Carb. S., Cimic., Lac. Can., Led., Nat. Carb., Rhus. V., Sep., Spong., Tab.

Confusion, loses his way in well-known streets – Glon., Merc., Nux. Mos., Petr., Ran. Bulb., Thuja.

Dancing, alternating with sighing – Bell.

Delirium, alternating with colic – Plumb.

Delirium, epilepsy, during –Opium.

Delirium, hysterical, intermittent –Con.

Delirium, during sleep – Apis., Chamo., Gels, Lach, Mur. Ac., Opium., Stramo.

Delusions, fancy, illusions of – Acon., Ambr., Ars. Iod., Can. Ind., Chin. S., Hyos., Ign., Kali C., Mag. M., Plat., Phos. Ac., Visc.

Catalepsy, a state of myotonia in which a person's muscles are partly rigid, sometimes manifested in hypnosis, in people with catatonia and in people with certain forms of brain damage, notably cerebellar lesions – Can. Ind., Cic., Hyos., Mosch., Opium, Sabad., Stramo.

Delirium, lascivious furor – Canth., Hyos., Stram.

Dementia, impairment or loss of memory, esp. evident in the learning of new information, and of thinking, language, judgement and other cognitive faculties, without clouding of consciousness – Agar., Can. Ind., Acid Phos., Picr. Ac., Plumb. Met., Staph., Ver. Vir., Zinc. Met.

Delusions, strangers seemed to be in the room. –Tarent., Thuja.

Emotions, shame, mortification, reserved displeasure, vexation. – Gels., Ign., Nat.M., Staph.

Fears, death, fatal diseases, impending evil – Apis., Cim., Nux. Vom., Plat., Psor., Sabad.

Fears, lactophobia – Can. Sat.

Fear of people, anthropophobia – Acon., Bar. C., Gels., Iod., Nat. C., Sep., Stann., Staph.

Fear of self-control, losing – Arg. Nit., Gels., Staph.

Hypochondriasis, a somatoform disorder characterized by pathological hypochondria, intense preoccupation and delusional disorder. – Aur.M., Helon., Zinc. Oxy.

Hysteria – Ambra., Camph. Monobr., Ign., Lil. Tig., Mosch., Nux. Mos., Orig., Phos., Puls., Strych. P., Ther.

Idiocy, before epilepsy – Caust.

Imagination, being pregnant, or something alive in the abdomen – Croc., Cycl., Sabad., Sulph., Ver. Alb.

Hallucination, auditory, bells, music, voices. – Ars., Can. Ind., Elaps, Naja., Stramo., Thea.

Hallucination, visual, animals faces. – Absinth., Atrop., Kali Br., Morph., Val., Ver. Alb.

Kleptomania, an impulse-control disorder by repeated stealing of objects, as ego-dystonic behaviour. – Absin., Art. Vulg., Nux. Vom., Oxytr., Plat., Sep., Staph., Stramo., Sulph., Tarent.

Loquacity, changing quickly from one subject to another. - Agar., Cim., Lach., Lyc.

Mania, erotomania, nymphomania, satyriasis. – Bar. Mur., Canth., Hyos., Murex, Plat., Salix Nig.

Melancholia, pubertic – Ant. C., Helleb., Nat. Mur.

Memory, forgetful, weak or lost. – Anac., Arg. Nit., Calc.Carb. Can. Ind., Kali Br., Lac.C., Medo., Nux. Mos., Selen., Sil., Sepia., Zinc. Phos.

Memory, difficulty or inability of fixing attention. – Agn., Apis., Caust., Gels., Helleb., Indol., Ac. Phos., Picr. Ac., Sep., Zinc. Met.

Mind, absence of moral and will power – Can. Sat., Irid., Lac. Can, Lecity., Mancin. Selen., Zinc. P.

Mood, disposition, aversion to mental and physical work. – Aloc., Aur. Mur., Caps., Nat. C., Oxytr., Selen., Sep.

Obstinate, against whatever was proposed, he had the queerest objection. – Arg. Nit.

Taciturn, morose, sulky, sullen, unsociable. – Ant. C., Cupr., Cycl., Lil.T., Mag. Mur., Sep., Sil, Stam.

Speech, lost or paralysis, aphasia, an impairment of expression or comprehension of language caused by injury or disease in the language centres of the brain. – Bar. C., Caust., Colch., Lach. Mey., Plumb. Met., Stramo.

Taedium Vitae, disgust of life. – Cinch., Lac. Can., Nit. Ac., Sulph., Tab., Thuja., Ver. A.

Somnambulism, sleep walking. – Art.V., Kali Br., Zinc. Met.

Weeping, nervous, feels so, she would scream unless she held on to something. – Sep.

NEUROLOGY

Adynamia, worse in women worn out from hard mental and physical work, or from indolence and luxury. – Helon.

Epilepsy, followed by rage, automatic impulse. – Opium.

Epiteptic vertigo. – Bell., Cupr., Sil., Stramo.

Paralysis, ascending, spinal. – Alum., Con., Ox. Acid., Phos., Acid. Picr.

Hemiplegia, paralysis of one side of the body caused by disease of the body caused by disease of the opposite, contralateral hemisphere of the brain. – Arn., Aur. M., Carbon. S., Cocc., Nux. V., Rhus. Tox., Sec. C., Stann., Vipera.

Infantile hemiplegia, poliomyelitis anterior. – Acon. Bell., Chrom. S., Lathyrus., Plumb. M., Sec.

Incubus, nightmare. – Aur. Br., Cina., Ptel., Sulph.

Insomina, sleeplessness, difficulty in falling asleep, waking up in the middle of the night and having difficulty going back to sleep. – Ant. C., Avena., Can. Ind., Coff., Ign., Lupul., Passifl., Selen, Sulph., Zinc. V.

Hereditary tendency, alcoholism. – Asar., Cic., Cupr., Ferr. Cy., Latrod., Psor., Sumb., Ver. V.

Chorea, St. Vitus's dance, a jerky involuntary movement particularly affecting the shoulders, hips and face, due to disease of the basal ganglia. – Agar., Calc. P., Cic., Ferr. Cy., Ign., Nat. M., Spig., Zinc. Br.

Convulsion, clonic. – Antipyr., Cupr. M., Nicot.

Convulsion, tonic, opisthotonos, the position of the body in which the head, neck, and spine are arched backward. – Cupr. Ac., Mag. P., Plat., Plumb.Met., Stramo., Ver.V.

Morvan's disease – Aur. Mur., Lach., Sec. Cor.

Nervous affections, from tobacco, in sedentary persons; dyspepsia, right prosopalgia. – Sepia.

Nervousness, tremulousness, faintness. – Aquil., Caul., Murex., Puls., Raph., Ac. Sulph., Val.

Neurasthenia, nervous prostration, set of symptoms including fatigue, irritability, headache, dizziness, anxiety and intolerance of noise caused by organic damage like head injury or due to neurosis. – Asar., Can.Ind., Ac. Flour., Helon., Kali Hypoph., Lecith., Picr. Ac., Scutel., Zinc. Picr.

Neurasthenia, nervous prostration, set of symptoms including fatigue, irritability, headache, dizziness, anxiety and intolerance of noise caused by organic damage like head injury or due to neurosis. – Asar., Can.Ind., Ac. Flour., Helon., Kali Hypoph., Lecith., Picr. Ac., Scutel., Zinc. Picr.

Nervous prostration, cerebral symptoms, unable to apply mind. – Anac., Calc.C., Ac.Phos.

Neurasthenia, hypochondriacal tendency. – Coca., Kali Br., Nat. Mur.

Nervous prostration from sexual origin. – Agn., Graph., Onosm., Plat., Sabal., Staph.

Neuroses, of children. – Passif.

Tremors, twitching, trembling, a rhythmical alternating movement that may affect any part of the body, which is a prominent symptom of parkinsonism with disease of the cerebellum. – Absinth., Arg. Nit., Caust., Hyosc., Hydrobr., Latrod., Morph., Oxytr., Plumb. M., Stramo., Vir. Vir., Zinc. P.

Senile tremors. – Avena., Can. Ind. Phos.

Tremors, disseminated sclerosis. – Acet. Ac., Ars., Hyosc. Hydrobr.

Neuritis, lumbo-sacral plexus. – Berb. Vulg.

Neuritis, inflammation, retro-bulbar, with sudden loss of sight. – Chin. Sulph.

Neuralgia, severe burning or stabbing pain often, trigeminal. – Gnaph., Morph., Ox. Acid., Prun. Sp., Rhod., Zinc. V.

Neuralgia, cervico-occipital. – Bell., Chin. S., Zinc. P.

Sciatica, by degeneration of an intervertebral disk, pain felt down the back and outer side of the thigh, back is stiff and painful, compress a lower lumber or an upper sacral spinal nerve root. – Am. Mur., Bell., Carbon. S., Gels., Ign., Kali. Iod., Plumb.M., Ran. B., Ruta., Sulph., Ver. Alb., Xanth.

Sciatica, vertebral origin. – Lac.C., Phos., Sil., Tellur.

Sciatica, tearing, shooting, darting like chain lighting, ending in sharp, vice-like grip. – Cact.

Spasmodic sciatica, muscular contraction. – Am. M., Bell., Nux. Vom., Plat., Plumb.M., Zinc.M.

Spinal cord, concussion. – Arn., Bellis., Cic., Con., Hyper., Kali P., Physost.

Sclerosis, softening, degeneration, due to fibrosis after inflammation, affecting the lateral columns of the spinal cord and the medulla of the brain, causing progressive muscular paralysis. – Bar. Mur., Carbon. S., Naja., Ox. Acid., Phos., Plumb. Iod., Zinc. M.

Hyperesthesia, from using arms in sewing typewriting, piano-playing. – Agar., Cim., Ran. Bulb.

Meningitis, inflammation of the meninges due to viral infection, headache, intolerance to light and sound, convulsions, vomiting and delirium. – Bry., Kali Iod., Merc., Ox.Acid., Rhus.T., Sec.

Myelitis, chronic, inflammation. – Crot., Lathyr., Plumb. M.

Locomotor ataxia, tabes dorsalis, form of neuro - syphilis destroying the sensory nerves, an unsteady gait, stabbing pains in the legs and trunk and loss of bladder control. – Alum., Ars. Br., Chrom. S., Ferr. Picr., Ac. Flour., Ign., Kali Iod., Onosm., Phos. hydr., Ruta., Thall.

Tetanus. – Angust., Cupr., Gels., Morph., Stramo., Tab.

Weekness of the spine. – Arg. N., Con., Selen., Sil.

ONCOLOGY

Cancer, of glandular structures. – Hoang. Nun.

Cancer, of breast. – Ars. Iod., Brom., Carbo. An., Con., Graph., Phyto., Plumb. Iod., Nat. Cacodyl.

Cancer, of uterus. – Aur. M.N., Carbo. An., Fuligo., Iod., Lapis Alba., Ac. Nit.

Tumours, cystic. – Apis., Bary C., Brom., Calc. C., Graph., Sil.

Tumours, atheroma, degenaration of the walls of the arteries due to formation of fatty plaques and scar tissue. – Bary. Carb.

Cancer, of bones. – Aur. Iod., Phos., Symphyt.

Cancer, of stomach. – Acet. Ac., Condur., Hydor., Kreos., Ornithog., Phos.

Tumours, erectile. – Lyc., Nit., Ac., Phos., Staph.

Epithelioma, a tumor of epithelium, the covering of internal and external surface of the body, benign tumors. – Ars. Iod., Calc. P., Con., Kali S., Lyc., Ran. B., Sep., Sil., Thuja Occ.

Cancer, to relieve pain. – Apis., Ars., Calc. Ox., Ced., Euphorb., Hydr., Morph., Ova. T., Ac. Phos., Sil.

Scirrhous, carcinoma that is stony hard to touch.– Arg. M., Carbo., An., Con., Carb. S., Graph., Lapis A., Phos., Sep., Sil. Sulph.

Tumours, fibroid. – Calc. C., Calc. Flour., Con., Phos., Sil.

Tumours, sarcoma, cancer of connective tissue. – Baryt.C., Calc. Flour.

Encephaloma, having the appearance of brain tissue, encephaloid carcinoma. – Ars. Iod., Carbo. An., Caust., Kali Iod., Lach., Thuja.

Cancer, of antrum. – Aur., Symphyt.

Cancer, of bowel. – Ruta. G.

Tumours, neuroma. – Calc. C., Staph.

Tumours, steatoma, suppurating. – Calc. C., Carbo. Veg.

Cancer, of caecum. – Ornithog.

DERMATOLOGY

Acne Rosacea, skin disorder in which the sebaceous glands become inflamed, the face in which the blood vessels enlarge having a flushed appearance. – Ars. Brom., Carb. An., Kali Iod., Petrol, Psor. Rhus. R., Sul. Iod.

Acne Simplex, in anaemic girls at puberty, with vertex headache, flatulent dyspepsia, better by eating. – Calc. Phos.

Acne Simplex, with menstrual irregularities. – Aur. M. N., Berb. Aq., Graph., Kali Carb., Puls., Sang. Sarsa.

Actinomycosis, affects the jaw, causing the slow formation of abscesses and ulcers. – Hekla., Kali Iod., Acid Nit.

Alopecia, hair falls out in patches. – Ars., Ac. Flour., Nat. Mur., Phos., Acid Phos., Pix L., Sep., Vinca.

Anthrax, carbuncle, malignant pustule. – Anthrac., Apis., Bufo., Cinch., Echin., Lach., Ac. Mur., Rhus. T.

Blood boils. – Arn., Crot. Tig., Lach., Phos. Ac.

Bromidrosis, offensive sweat. – Bapt. T., Con., Hep., Ac. Nit., Petrol., Sepia., Sil., Tellur.

Callosities, corns. – Ant. C., Graph., Ran. Bulb., Thuja.

Chilblains, red sound itchy swelling. – Agar., Canth., Crot. Tig., Ledum., Petrol., Rhus. Tox., Sulph., Terab.

Chloasma, liver spots, moth patches. – Arg. Nit., Caulo., Laur., Lyc., Nat. Hyposul., Plumb. M., Sep.

Coldness, one side of the body during convulsions. – Sil.

Decubitus ulcer, bed sores. – Bapt. T., Carbo. Veg., Hippoz., Lach., Ac. Mur., Pyr., Ac. Sulph.

Eruptions, alternating with dysentery. – Rhus. Tox.

Eruptions, alternating with asthma. – Calad.

Erysipelas, an infection of the skin and underlying tissues with the bacterium strptococcus pyogens. – Ant. C., Bell., Carb. S., Clem., Euph., Graph., Kali Chl., Lach., Merc. S., Nat. C., Ran. Bulb.

Eczema, of scalp. – Calc. C., Clem., Oleand., Selen.

Eczema, of rheumatico-gouty persons. – Alum., Ac. Lactic., Uric. Ac.

Eczema, with pigmentation in circumscribed areas following. – Berb. Vulg.

Eczema, worse at sea-shore, ocean voyage, excess of salt. – Nat. Mur.

Foreign bodies, to promote expulsion of fish bones, splinters, needles. – Heper., Sil.

Furuncle, recurrent tendency. – Arn., Calc. Mur., Calc. Pier., Tub.

Gangrene, decay of part of the body due to cessation of blood supply. – Ant. C., Ars., Canth., Echin., Ferr. P., Kali Chlor., Ac. Sulph., Sec. Cor.

Herpes, with pimples or pustules surrounding spread by coalescing. – Heper.

Herpes zoster, zones, shingles, with pain along the nerve followed by vesicles. – Aster., Carbon. Ox., Dolich., Prun. Sp.

Hyperidrosis, excessive sweating. – Acet. Ac., Bapt. T. Lact. Ac., Nat. C., Nux. V., Piloc., Selen.

Ichthyosis, fish skin disease. – Ars. Iod., Kali Iod., Phos., Thuja.

Itching, walking in open air. – Cinnb., Sulph.

Keloid, often increase in size, hard prominent irregular scar tissue. – Ac. Flour., Graph., Sab., Sil.

Leprosy, Hansen's disease, affecting the skin and nerves. – Calopt., Cupr. Ac., Hura., Hydrocot., Oenanthe., Pip.M.

Leucoderma. – Ars. S.Fl., Nat. M., Sumb., Zinc. P.

Lichen Planus. – Apis., Jugl. C., Led., Sarsa.

Lupus Vulgaris. – Cistus., Guarana., Formica., Jequir., Kali Bich., Phyt., Steph.

Nails, inflamation, around root, paronychia. – Alum., Calc. S., Hep., Nat. Sulph.
Onchogryposis, nails deformed, brittle, thickened. – Ant. C., Ac. Flour., Graph., Sil.
Pityriasis, dermatitis exfoliative. – Berb. Aq., Kali Ars., Mang. Ac., Mez., Nat. Ars., Pip. M., Tellur.
Pruritus, worse from underssing. – Alum., Dulc., Kreos., Menisp., Merc. I. Fl., Psor., Rumex., Tub.
Psoriasis, itchy scaly red patches, form on the forearms, elbows, knees, legs and scalp. – Ars., Bor., Coral., Graph., Hep., Iris., Kali Br., Mur. Ac., Nat. Ars., Phos., Sep., Strych. P., Tereb.
Purpura Haemorrhagica. – Crot. T., Millef., Rhus. Ven., TBP.
Scabies. – Aloe. Soc., Crot. T., Hep., Rhus. V.
Sebaceous Cysts. – Benz. Ac., Calc. Sil., Con., Hep. Nit. Acid., Phyto., Thuja.
Tinea Versicolor, chromophytosis. – Chrysar., Mez., Nat. Ars., Tellur.
Trichophytosis, in intersecting rings over great portion of body. – Tellur.
Ulcers, syphilitic. – Asaf., Cistus., Flour Ac., Kali Bich., Merc. C., Nit Ac., Sarsa., Still.
Ulcers with vesicles, surrounding it, red shining areolae. – Flour. Ac., Hep., Mez.
Urticaria, hives, nettle rash. – Apium Gr., Berb. V., Bombyx., Cina., Dulc., Ichth., Kali. C., Rhus., Ven., Sanic., Stam., Tereb., Ustil.
Verucca, warts. – Ant. C., Calc. Carb., Caust., Dulc., Ferr. Picr., Mag. S., Ac. Nit., Thuja.
Whitlow, felon, panaritium. – Anthrac., Dios. V., Hep., Led., Merc., S., Myrist., Nat. S., Sil.

GYNAECOLOGY
Abortion, third month. – Cim., Sabin., Sec. Cor., Ust.
Atrophy, overies, due to degeneration of cells. – Bar. M., Con., Helon., Iod.
Ball, overy feels like a heavy, right. – Carb. An.
Coition, fainting. – Murex., Orig., Plat.
Coition, oversion to. – Graph., Kali Sulph., Med., Nat. M., Psor., Sep., Tarent.
Coition, orgasm delayed. – Berb. V., Brom.
Coition, painful, sexual contact, copulation between a man and a woman during which the erect penis enters the vagina and is moved within it by pelvic thrusts until ejaculation. – Apis., Plat., Staph.
Conception, difficult, sterility. – Agn., Bar. M., Con., Gossyp., Graph., Medo., Nat. P., Sabal.
Desire, increased sexual, nymphomania. – Calc. P., Hyos., Lach., Murex., Orig., Plat., Stramo., Xerophyl.
Excoriation, menses, during. – Am. Carb., Caust., Sarsa., Sil.
Itching, menses, during. – Kreo., Lyc., Petrol., Zinc. M.
Leucorrhoea, acrid, corroding burning. – Alum., Ars., Calc. C., Graph., Iod., Kreos., Merc., Ac. Nit., Puls., Sep., Sil., Ac. Sulph.
Leucorrhoea, flesh coloured, like washing of meat, non-offensive. – Ac. Nit.
Leucorrhoea, occurrence, after menstruation and between periods. – Aesc. Hip., Cocc., Eupion., Kreos., Sab., Sep., Thlaspi.
Mastitis, inflammation. – Crot. T., Hep., Phyto., Sil.
Mastodynia, pain in breasts. – Aster., Lac. Acid., Plumb. Iod.
Menstruation, amenorrhoea, abscence or stoping of the menstrual period. – Apis., Calc. C., Cycl., Ferr. Red., Kali Perm., Ova. T., Polgy., Sence.
Menstruation, amenorrhoea, suppressed from transient, uterine congestion, followed by chronic anaemic state. – Sabal. Ser.

Dysmenorrhoea, from overian irritation, non-obstructive. – Apis., Ham. Xanth.
Menorrhagia, profuse, premature flow, after miscarriage, parturition. – Cim., Helon., Kali C., Ustil.
Masturbation, in children, due to pruritus vulvae. – Calad., Orig., Zinc. M.
Menopause, Climacteric period, change of reproductive life. – Amyl., Cact. G., Ign., Oophor. Sang., Sul. Ac., Ther., Vipera.
Ovaritis, acute inflammation, with peritoneal involvement. – Acon., Canth., Chin. S., Merc. C.
Parturition, labor, convulsions, eclampsia, shifting across abdomn, doubling her up, pricking in mammae, shivers during first stage. – Cim.
Lochia, bloody in gushes, worse from motion. – Erig.
Septicaemia, puerperal fever, septic. – Bapt., Pyroz., Rhus. T., Ver. Vir.
Prolapsus uterus, displacements. – Alet., Aur. M.N., Ferr. Iod., Graph., Lil. Tig., Murex., Onosm., Plat., Podo., Puls., Senec., Stann.
Pruritus, itching of vagina, soreness, tenderness. – Canth., Collins., Graph., Orig., Radium., Rhus. Ven., Urt. U.
Sterility, excessive sexual desire from. – Kali Br., Orig., Phos., Plat. M.
Metrorrhagia, haemorrhage, with blood clotted or fluid, paroxysmal flow, nausea, palpitation, pulse quick, vital depression; fainting on raising head from pillow. – Apoc. Can.
Vagina, aphthous, patches, ulcers, erosions. – Arg. Nit., Hydr., Acid Nit., Sep.
Vaginismus, sensitiveness, pain, stinging, stitching, shooting, tearing. – Cimex, Ferr. M., Ign., Lyssin, Murex, Nux. Vom., Plumb., Thuja.

PHYSICAL MEDICINE
Back, bent, arch-like, opisthotonos. – Cic., Nicot., Phyt., Strych.
Backache, aching, dull, constant. – Agar., Berb. V., Calc. Fl., Cim, Nat. M., Still., Tereb., Zinc. M.
Back pain, between scapulae. – Apomorph., Con., Medo., Sep.
Pain, falling apart sensation, involoving small of back, sacro-iliac synchondroses. – Trill.
Coccyx, neuralgia, worse rising from sitting posture. – Lach.
Upper extremities, jerking, or involuntary motion, of one arm, and leg. – Apoc., Bryo., Helleb., Myg.
Cramps (writer's) : piano or violin players, typists. – Arg. Met., Gels., Mag. Phos., Stann.
Lumbago, low backache, due to prolapsed intervertebral disk or strained muscle. – Aesc. Hip., Arn., Eupat. P., Hydr., Macrot., Pampin., Radium, Ruta G.
Tendo-Achilles pain. – Ac. Benz., Medo., Upas.
Joints, contraction, painful, of tendons, hamstrings. – Caust., Cimex., Guaiac. Kali Iod., Nat. M., Tellur.
Arthritis, inflammation, acute. – Acid Benz., Colch., Gnaph., Iod. Led., Lith C., Puls., Rhus T.
Arthritis deformans, chronic.– Am. Benz., Chin. S., Formica, Mang. Ac., Ox. Acid., Sab., Sulph. Taxus., Uric. Acid., Urtica. U.
Govt. inflammation, of hands, feet, little swelling, subacute. – Led. P.
Elbows, numbness, pains. – Arg. Met., Ferr. Mur., Menisp.
Knee-joint, synovitis, bursitis, housemaid's knee. – Bry., Heper., Phos., Ruta. G.
Shoulder-scapulae, deltoid, pain, rheumatism. – Medo. Nux. Mos., Ac. Oxal.

Rheumatism, fibrous tissue, sheaths, tendons. – Arn., Ac. Formic., Rhodo., Rhus. T.
Neck, cracking of cervical vertebrae, on motion. – Cocc., Nat. Carb., Niccol., Thuja.

GASTRO-ENTEROLOGY

Hyperchlorhydria, acidity, flautulent food. – Arg. N., Carbo. V., Iris. V., Nux. V., Orexine. Tan., Robin., Ac. Sul.
Dyspepsia, gastric juice scanty. – Alum., Lyco., Phos., Sulph.
Eructations, sour., burning, acid, bitter. – Carbo. V., Ac. Lactic., Robin.
Stomach, flatulent distention. – Abies. C., Calc. C., Cinch., Graph., Kali Bich., Nux. Mos.
Gastritis, inflammation, acute from alcoholic abuse. – Ars., Cupr., Gaulth., Nux. Vom.
Nausea, from nervousness, emotional exitement. – Menthol.
Gastrodynia, pain cutting, lancinating, stitching, spasmodic, proxysmal, darting, tearing shooting. – Act. Sp., Bryo., Chin. Ars., Colo., Cupr. Ac., Mag. P., Sep., Thall.
Stomach, ulcer of. – Arg. Nit., Geran., Kali Bich., Kreo., Pho., Symphyt., Uran., Nit.
Vomiting, with chronic tendency. – Lob. Inf.
Appendicitis, typhilitis, nausea, pain. – Bell., Dios. V., Iris Ten., Lach. Merc., C., Nux. V., Plumb., Sil.
Flatulence, rumbling, borborygmus. – Cinch., Graph., Ac. Phos., Ricin C.
Rectum, burning before and during stool. – Aloe. S.
Prolapsus ani, with piles, in alcoholies, leading sedentary life. – Aesc. Gl.
Cholera infantum, summer complaint.– Bism., Cupr. Ars., Ipec., Ver. Alb.
Constipation, from torpor, inertia, dryness of intestines. – Alum., Bryo., Opium., Mez. , Syphil.
Deodenitis, catarrhal inflammation. – Ars., Chel., Kali Bich.,Podo.
Cholelithiasis, gall-bladder stone, biliary colic.– Berb. V., Card. M., Chionanth., Dios. Vill., Fel. Touri., Tarax.
Haemorroids, piles, protruding, grape-like, swollen. – Aloe. Soc., Collins., Ac. Mur., Ratanhia, Sep., Thuja Occ.
Hernia, strangulated. – Acon., Bell., Lyc., Nux. V., Plumb.
Jaundice, icterus, malignant. – Ars., Crot. Tig., Lach., Phos.
Liver, cirrhosis. – Aur. Mur., Kali Iod., Nasturt Aq.
Hepatitis, pain, inflammation. – Bryo., Chelid., Merc. D., Nat. S., Phos., Psor., Sil., Sulph., Thuja.
Liver, fatty degeneration. – Aur. M., Kali Bich., Phlorid.
Spleen, enlargement. – Calc. Ars., Ferr. Iod., Mag. Mur., Ac. Phos., Querc., Urt. U.
Umbilicus, naval, bleeding from, in newborn. – Abrot., Calc. Phos.
Wroms, taenia, ascaris lumbricoides, oxyuris vermicularis.– Chelone., Ferr. Mur., Filix Mas., Kuosso., Nat. P., Sabad., Santonin., Spig., Sumb., Teucr., Viola Od.

CARDIOLOGY

Arterio-sclerosis, atheroma of arteries. – Am. Iod., Crat., Glon., Vanad.
Apoplexy, rupture of artery. – Cact., Junip. V., Laur., Ver. Vir.
Heart, affections, rheumatic. – Benz. Ac., Colch., Lith. Carb.
Cardiac dyspnoea.– Acon. fer., Adon. V., Calc. Ars., Dig., Iberis., Naja. T., Spig.
Hypertrophy of heart.– Brom., Crat., Lil. Tig., Spong.

Myocarditis, acute or chronic inflammation of heart muscles.– Adon. V., Iod., Lach., Vipera.
Pericardities, acute.– Apis., Asclap. Tub., Can. Sat., Kali Iod., Naja. T., Ver. Vir.
Angina pectoris, from organic heart disease.– Ars. Iod., Calc. Fl., Stront.
Palpitation, cardiac, from emotional causes.– Acon., Anac., Coff., Ign., Sep.
Pulse, rapid, tachycardia.– Adon. V., Conv., Latrod., Kal. L., Phaseol., Rhodo., Stroph., Thyr.
Pulse, slow, bradycardia.– Apoc., Can. Ind., Lupul., Morph., Naja., Opium., Spig., Ver. Alb.
Syncope, from odors, in morning, after eating.– Nux. Vom.
Heart, volvular diseases.– Aur. Iod., Dig., Glon., Laur., Lycop., Sang., Spong., Stroph.
Veins, inflamed, phlebitis.– Agar., Ham., Lach., Vipera.

NEPHROLOGY & UROLOGY

Eneuresis, nocturnal, incontinence.– Arg. N., Benz. Ac., Kali Br., Kreos., Medo., Rhus. Ars., Sabal., Thyr.
Cystitis, with fever, strangury.– Acon., Bell., Canth., Merc. C., Sabal.
Urinary bladder, irritable, radiating to spermatic cord.– Clem., Lith.C., Puls., Spong.
Nephrolithiasis, kidney stone. – Berb. V., Epig., Eupat. Perf., Ipomoea, Ac. Nit., Ocimum, Piperiz., Sarsa., Stigm., Uva.
Nephritis, parenchmatous, acute and subacute.– Apis., Chimaph., Hydrocot., Kali Chlor., Ol. Sant., Tereb.
Uraemia, with convulsions. – Cic., Cupr. Ars., Piloc., Ver.Vir.
Nephralgia, pain in renal region, tearing, radiating, lancinating.– Berb. V., Canth., Coccinal., Lyc., Sarsa., Tab., Tereb., Thlaspi.
Dysuria, difficult, slow, painful.– Ant. T., Ac. Benz., Caust., Epig., Fabiana., Kreos., Ocimum, Plumb., Selen., Uva.
Urination, involuntary, when coughing, sneezing, walking, laughing.– Caps. Caust., Ferr. Mur., Selen.
Ischuria, urinary retention, from spasmodic constriction of neck of bladder. – Bell., Cact., Hyos., Opium., TBP.
Strangury, in females.– Eupat. Perf., Sab., Vib. Op.
Haematuria, bloody, burning, scalding, hot.– Acon., Canth., Merc. C., Ac. Nit.
Diabetes, gastro-hepatic origin, assimilative disorder, pancreatic origin.– Adren., Borac. Ac., Coca, Crot., Helon., Kreos., Lact. Ac., Mosch., Ac. Phos., Rhus. Ar., Uran. Nit.

SEXOLOGY

Bubo, indurated.– Alum., Carbo. An., Merc. S.
Coitus, painful, followed by vertigo.– Bov., Sep.
Desire increased, erethism, satyriasis.– Canth., Hyos., Mosch., Nux. Vom., Orig., Ac. Picr., Plat., Salix N.
Desire increased in old men but impotent.– Lyc., Selen.
Gonorrhoea, muco-purulent, yellowish-green, acute inflammatory stage.– Arg. N., Clem., Doryph., Hep., Merc. C., Nit. Ac., Petros. Sul.
Gleet, orchitis, epididymitis.– Aur. M., Ham., Rhodo., Spong.
Impotence, spermatorrhoea. – Agn. C., Calad., Cinch., Con., Damiana., Lyco., Nux. Vom., Onosm., Ac. Picr., Selen. Yohimb.
Penis, glans, epithelioma.– Ars., Con., Thuja.

Prepuce, constriction, paraphimosis, phimosis.– Arn., Con. Sat., Caps., Ac. Nit., Rhus. T., Sarsa., Sulph.
Prostate gland, hypertrophy.– Bar. C., Calc. Fl., Hydrang., Merc. D., Medo., Sabal., Thiosin.
Prostatorrhoea, weaknss, discharge during stool, urination, straining.– Agn., Can. S., Eryng., Junip., Pertrol., Selen., Tereb., Thymol.
Hydrocele, oedema, haematocele, acute.– Arn., Con., Erig., Nux. V., Puls.
Spermatorrhoea, deficient physical power, nocturnal pollutions.– Arg. N., Calad., Chlorum., Gels., Lyco., Medo., Onons., Salix N., Sil., Strych., Thymol., Yohimb.
Sexual debility, with emission and orgasm absent.– Calad., Calc. C., Selen.
Syphilis, chancre and primary lesions.– Ars., Cinnob., Kali Iod., Lyco., Merc. S., Ac. Phos., Plat. Mur.
Testicles, induration, hard.– Bar. C., Brom., Iod., Ac. Oxal., Phyt., Rhodo., Sil., Spong.
Undescended testicles in boys.– Thyr.

RESPIRATORY MEDICINE
Asthma, with bronchial catarrh.– Ant. T., Bryo., Eriod., Grind., Lob., Inf., Nat. Sulph., Sabal.
Bronchitis, capillary.– Am. Carb., Ant. T., Cupr. Ac., Kali Iod., Senega, Tereb., Ver. A.
Cough, catarrh, post-nasal, in children and adults.– Hydr., Pop. C., Spig.
Croup, spasmodic, paroxysmal, nervous, violent, suffocative.– Ambra., Aral.R., Caust., Coral., Cupr. M., Justicia., Nat. Mur., Phos., Rumex., Scilla., Viola. Od.
Pertussis, whooping cough, cyanosis.– Ant. T., Cupr. M., Ipec., Ver. A.
Laryngitis, inflammatory membranous exudate.– Acet. Ac., Calc. Iod., Dros., Kali Bich., Phos., Sang., Spong.
Laryngismus stridulus, spasm.– Ars. Iod., Chlorum., Gels., Ign., Mosch., Samb., Strych., Zinc. M.
Voice, hoarse, aphonia.– Am. C., Caust., Eupat. Perf., Kali C., Ac. Nit., Rumex., Stann.
Hoarseness, from overusing voice, especially public speakers, professional singers.– Arg. M., Arum., Caust., Merc. Cy., Phos., Rhus T., Selen., Still.
Emphysema, lungs, dilation of cells.– Am. C., Chin. Ars., Dros., Grind., Lob. Inf., Myrtus., Phos., Sulph.
Haemoptysis, haemorrhage, bright red blood.– Aran., Cact., Geran., Millef.
Tuberculosis, phthisis pulmonalis.– Ars. Iod., Chin. Ars., Form., Ac., Iodof., Kali C., Millef., Phell., Phos., Spong., Stann. Iod., Tub.
Dyspnoea, aggravated during damp, cloudy weather. – Nat. Sulph.
Pleurisy, pleural effusion, diaphragmatic.– Acon., Bryo., Cact., Ran. Bulb.
Trachea, burning, constricted feeling, rawness, irritation, tickling.– Ars., Lach., Merc., Rumex., Still.

DENTISTRY - E.N.T. - OPTHALMOLOGY
Dentition, teething difficult, dalayed.– Calc. P., Hekla., Kreos., Sil.
Fistula dentalis.– Calc. Fl., Ac. Flour., Sil., Staph.
Toothache, odontalgia, from cold exposure.– Acon., Bryo., Chamo., Puls., Sil.
Odontalgia, from tobacco-smoking.– Clem., Ign., Plant., Spig.
Teeth, decayed.– Ant. C., Chamo., Kreos., Mez., Nux. V., Staphis., Spig., Thuja.
Bleeding protractedly, after tooth extraction.– Ars., Ham., Kreos., Phos., Trill.

Pyorrhoea alveolaris, ulceration.– Bapt. T., Cistus., Merc. C., Phos., Plant., Sep., Staph., Ac. Sulph.
Deafness hardness of hearing, caused by adenoids and hypertrophied tonsils.– Agraph., Bar. C., Ac. Nit., Staph.
Eustachian tube inflamed, sub-acute, great pain.– Bell., Caps.
Labyrinth inflamed, otitis interna.– Kali Iod.
Membrana typmpani, calcareous deposits.– Calc. Flour.
Otitis media, suppurative, acute.– Bell., Kali Mur., Merc., Puls.
Otorrhoea, muco-purulent, fetid, acrid or bland.– Borax., Calc. S., Hep., Puls., Sil.
Tinnitus aurium, noises in ears. – Adren., Bar. Mur., Carbon. S., Chenop., Graph., Jabor., Kali M., Lecith., Merc. D., Sang. Nit., Sil., Sulph., Ac. Sulph., Viola. Od.
Epistaxis, bleeding nose.–Arn., Bryo., Elaps., Ferr. Picr., Ham., Millef., Phos., Thalaspi.
Nasal polyp, ulcerations, excoriations.– Calc. Iod., Kali Bich., Lemna. M., Merc. I.R., Sang., Teucr., Wyeth.
Rhinitis, inflamed, acute, catarrhal.– Ambros., Cepa., Euphres, Lach., Nat. Iod., Psor., Sabad., Sticta.
Pain, pressing at root of nose.– Cinnab., Kali Bich., Net. Ars.
Posterior nares, naso-pharynx, chronic with droping of mucous.– Alum., Calc. Sil., Lemna M., Phyto., Spig., Teucr., Wyeth.
Sinusitis, catarrh of frontal sinus, antrum, frontal, sphenoidal.– Asaf., Aur. M., Iod., Merc., Mez., Phos., Spig., Sticta., Teucr.
Sneezing, sternuation.– Aral., Cycl., Ipec., Kali Iod., Rosa D., Sang. Nit., Senega.
Diphtheria, with spasm of glottis.– Mosch., Samb.
Oesophagitis, pain, burning.– Bell., Naja., Phos., Ac. Sulph.
Dysphagia, deglutition painful, difficult. – Agar., Cajup., Ac. Flour., Kali C., Kali Perm., Merc. Cy., Phyt., Stramo.
Pharyngitis, inflammation, follicular, acute.– Apis., Kali Mur., Phyto., Wyeth.
Throat, hawking, with gelatinous, vicid, gluey mucus,difficult raising.– Arg. N., Coccus., Iberis., Lach., Nat. S., Petrol., Rumex.
Tonsillitis, acute catarrhal and follicular.– Acon., Bapt. T., Caps., Guaiac., Kali Bich., Merc.S., Sabad.
Peritonsillar abscess, gangrenous.– Calc. S., Merc. Cy.
Uvula, constricted feeling, pain, sore spot behind.– Kali Bich., Merc. C., Wyeth.
Cataract.– Calc. Fl., Chimaph., Kali M., Mag. C., Phos., Senega, Sil, Thiosin., Zinc.
Ciliary neuralgia, accommodation disturbed, spasm.– Agar., Lit. Tig., Physost.
Conjunctivitis, acute and subacute catarrhal.– Acon., Chloral., Euphras., Upas.
Cornea, staphyloma, after suppurative inflammation.– Apis., Euphras., Ilex., Physost.
Fistula lachrymalis.– Calc. C., Ac. Flour., Petrol., Phos.
Optic disks, pallor, visual field contracted, retinal vessels shrunken.– Acetan.
Eye-balls, burning, smarting.– Asaf., Clem., Indol., Ran. B.
Photophobia.– Arg. N., Benzol., Graph., Nux. M., Ac. Phos., Puls., Scrophul., Ther.
Myosis, pupils contracted.– Morph., Physost., Solan. N.
Retinitis, apoplectic.– Glon., Lach.
Amaurosis, blindness.– Chin. S., Momord., Plumb. Ac.
Vision, retro-bulber neuritis.– Iodof.
Amblyopia, objects appear as looking through mist or veil.– Croc., Lil. T., Puls., Ruta G.

Eye-strain, asthenopia, with spasm of accommodation.– Am. Carb., Caust., Cim., Lac. F., Macrot., Onosm., Rhod., Ruta.

Optical illusions, chromopsia, photopsia, black before eyes.– Atrop., Carbon. S., Mag. Carb., Nat. M., Physost., Stront., Tab.

Vitrous opacities, turbid.– Kali Iod., Senega, Solan. N.

Diplopia, double vision.– Cic., Cycl., Gels., Ac. Nit., Sec. Cor., Stramo., Ver. Vir.

FUSION HOMOEOPATHY

Chapter - 10
COMBINED REMEDIES

1. For anaemia and general debility. –
   Calc. Phos. 3x
   Nat. Mur. 6x
   Calc. Iod. 3x
   Kali. Phos. 6x
   China 3x
   Lyco. 12x

2. For throat disorders and tonsillitis. –
   Sil. 6x
   Ferr. Phos. 6x
   Baryta Carb. 6x
   Guiacum 3x
   Bell 3x
   Lachesis 12x

3. For rheumatism and arthritis. –
   Sil. 6x
   Lapis Alb. 6x
   Ferr. Phos. 6x
   Formica 6x
   Drosera 6x

4. For Blood disorders, toxaemia, skin diseases and septic conditions. –
   Calc. Sulph. 6x
   Nat. Phos. 6x
   Nat. Sulph. 6x
   Sulph 6x
   Rumex 3x
   Echinacea 6x

5. For acute liver affections. –
   Nat. Sulph. 6x
   Merc. V. 6x
   Nux Vom 3x
   Podo 3x
   Opium 6x

6. For disorders of the skin –
   Graphitis 6x
   Sulph. 6x
   Silicea 6x
   Echinacea 3x

Euphorbium 3x

7. For chronic catarrh, colitis., leucorrhoea. –

Kali. Mur. 6x
Calc.Carb. 6x
Kali Bich 6x
Juniperus C 3x
Hydrastis 3x

8. For flatulence and nervous dyspepsia. –

Mag. Phos. 3x
NuxMos. 3x
Ignetia 3x
Asafaet. 6x

9. For infant's disorders. –

Calc. Phos. 3x
KaliPhos. 6x
Mag.Phos 6x
Nat Phos 3x
Chamo. 2x

10. For all female diseases. –

Kali Phos. 6x
Mag.Phos. 6x
Sepia 12x Puls. 3x
Cauloph. 3x
Lil Tig 3x

11. For dyspepsisa, indigestion and acidity of the stomach. –

Arg. Nit 6x
Nux Vom. 6x
Robin 6x
Carbo. Veg. 6x
Bismuth 3x
Hydrastis 3x
Abies Nig. 1x

12. For impotency. –

Calc. Phos. 6x
Kali Sulph. 6x
Nat.Phos. 6x
Sil 6x
Selen. 6x
Agnus C. 3x

13. For prolapse of uterus and nymphomania –

Calc. Fluor. 6X
Aletris F. 1x
Murex 6x
Ferr. Phos. 6x
Fraxinus A 3x

14. For high blood pressure. –

 Aur. Mur 6x
 Glonoin 6x
 Sumbul 6x
 Viscum Alb. 6x
 Hydrastis 6x

15. For asthma, bronchitis, coughs and breathlessness. –
 Kali Mur 6x
 Lobelia 3x
 Ipecac 3x
 Drosera 3x
 Spongia 3x
 Grindelia 3x

16. For feverish cold and influenza. –
 Ferr. Phos. 6x
 Cad. Sulph. 6x
 Cinnam. 6x
 Gels. 3x
 Baptisia 3x
 Bell 3x
 Eupat Perf. 6x

17. For insomnia and nervous excitement. –
 Kali Phos. 6x
 Daphne 6x
 Coffea 6x
 Passiflora 1x

18. For warts and skin growths. –
 Antim. Crude. 6x
 Kali Sulph. 6x
 Silicea 6x
 Thuja Occ. 3x
 Euphorbium 3x

19. For haemorrhoids and rectal symptoms. –
 Calc. Flour. 6x
 Ruta G. 3x
 Hydrastis 3x
 Galium 3x
 Hamam. 3x

20. For pin and thread worms. –
 Nat. Phos. 2x
 Antim Crude. 3x
 Cuprum 6x
 Santonin 3x

21. For alopecia. –
 Calc. Phos. 3x
 Silicea 6x
 Lyco. 6x

22. For traumatic accidents. –

    Pilocarpus 3x
    Kali Phos. 6x
    Mag.Phos. 6x
    Calendula 3x
    Hypericum 3x
    Arnica Mont. 3x

23. For kidney affections. –

    Nat. Sulph. 6x
    Berb. Vulg. 3x
    Juniperus C. 3x
    Opium 6x
    Triticum 3x

24. For catarrhal deafness and otitis media. –

    Nat. Mur. 6x
    Kali Mur. 6x
    Merc. Sol. 3x
    Bell. 3x
    Chenopod. 3x

25. For any type of pain, neuralgia and sciatica. –

    Bell. 3x
    Mag. Phos. 6x
    Acon. Nap. 3x
    Spigelia 3x
    Apis Mel. 3x
    Lyco. Clav. 12x

These above 25 compound formulas is being prescribed successfully for scores of cases with the help of these 'secondary remedies'. One could only expect deep-seated chronic conditions to respond with a course of the similimum remedy in a higher potency.

DOSAGE : Medicines (available either triturations, attenuations or tablets) have to be in the trituration form for easy dispensing. For chronic conditions, use three grains twice daily. Acute conditions needed two grains every three hourly.

Chapter - 11
MASTER GUIDE

ABORTION
Cinnamon
Induces complete abortion in cases of unwanted pregnancy when prescribed within first two months in physiological doses.
Dose : 30 drops of mother tincture every twelve hours. Four doses are needed.

ABSCESS
Natrum Salicylicum
Used for axillary abscess.
Tarentula Cubensis
Marked action in any abscess where there is very severe pain.

ACNE
Kali Bromatum
Acne, of face.
Berberis Aquifolium
Acne. Tincture in rather material doses.

ALOPECIA
Vinca Minor
Spots on scalp, oozing moisture, corrosive itching of scalp.
Bald spots. Use lower potencies.

APPENDICITIS
Dioscorea Villosa
Relieves pain in inflamed appendix.
Dose : Use 20 drops of mother tincture.
Iris Tenax
Specifically prescribe for all appendicitis.

ARTHRITIS
Actea Spicata
Rheumatism of small joints. Use 3X potency.
Berberis Vulgaris
For polyarthritis. Use high potency.

ASTHMA
Adrenalin
For any types of asthma. Use 3X potency.

BALDNESS
Jaborandi
For baldness. Even white and blonde hair have been observed to turn black by this medicine.

BEDWETTING
Sycotic Co. (Paterson)
Efficacious when other indicated remedies fail.

BOILS
Echinacea
For the condition of the system which sets up the boil habit.
Dose : 10 drops to be taken thrice a day.
Miristica Sebifera
For carbuncles.
Ichthyolum
Especially for crops of boils.

BURNS
Causticum
Relieves pain in cases of burns and scalds immediately.

CANCER
Euphorbia Lathyris
Can help the burning pain in cancer.
Carcinosin
For cancer. Use high potency once a week.
Asteria Rubens
Useful in treating cancer of breast.

CERVICAL SPONDYLOSIS
Latrodectus Mactans
Pain with numbness and tingling.
Lachnanthis
Helps to cure cervical spondylitis.

CHRONIC CATARRH
Bacillinum
Tendency to take cold and easy expectoration.

CIRCUMCISION
Staphysagria
Given before the incision allays the pain following incision and prevents inflammation.

CONSTIPATION
Silica Marina
Prescribe to patients in crude form of all ages for obstinate constipation.

CONVULSIONS
Cicuta Virosa

Used for convulsions which are violent whether epileptic, cataleptic, clonic or tonic, eclampsia.

COUGH
Mentha Piperita
For dry cough. Use tincture, 10 drops thrice daily.

DIABETES
Uranium Nitricum
Cured many cases of diabetes.
Dose : Usually given in lower triturations.

DYSENTRY
Chaparro Amargoso
Bloody dysentery with marked pain.
Dose : Use 3-rd attenuation.

EPISTAXIS
Millefolium
Use tincture
Ferrum Picricum
Use third trituration.

FELON
Iris Versicolor
Useful to abort the felon. Administer 30-th potency. Also apply on the part externally.

FEVER
Eucalyptus Globulus
Efficacious for all kinds of fever.
Dose : Ten drops of tincture to be taken thrice daily.

FISSURE ANUS
Ratanhia
Use sixth potency. Locally, the cerate has proved invaluable in rectal complaints.

GOITRE
Fucus Vesiculosus
A specific remedy for exopthalmic goitre.
Dose : Use tincture, 20 drops thrice daily before meals.

HEART
Acetic Acid
For terminal stages of heart disease.

HICCOUGH

Scutellaria
Administer in case of severe and rapid hiccough.
Take 60 drops of the mother tincture every two hours.

HOARSENESS
Populus Candicans
Instantaneous voice producer. Use tincture.

HYDROCELE
Ampelopsis
For moderate size hydrocele.

IMPOTENCY
Agnus Castus
Cures impotency in the male and sterility and uterine atony in the female.

JAUNDICE
Myrica
Use tincture.

KELOIDS
Thoisinaminum
Helps in healing, shrinking and softening of keloids. Use internally and externally.

LEPROSY
Calotropis
Use 6X potency. Also apply tincture, 5 drops three times a day.

LEUCORRHOEA
Cubeba
Leucorrhoea in litte girls.

LICE
Staphysagria
Apply externally, tincture mixing with hair-oil.

LUMBAGO
Ginseng
Almost a specific in lumbago, sciatica and chronic rheumatism.

MASTURBATION
Gratiola
Marked action in masturbation and nymphomania in females.

MEASLES

Pulsatilla
Great reputation as a prophylactic against measles.

MOUTH
Kali Chloricum
For foul odour from mouth. Use lower potencies.

MUMPS
Parotidinum
Often used as a preventive for mumps.
Administer 30-th potency.

NAILS
Magnetis Polus Australis
For ingrowing toe-nails.
Use 200-th and higher.

PARALYSIS
Morph Acet.
Paralysis caused by electricity is relieved by this drug.

PENIS
Coca
Sensation as if the penis is absent.

PHOTOPHOBIA
Conium
Is of great value in intense photophobia and excessive lachrymation.

PHIMOSIS
Cannabis Sativa
Cures many cases of phimosis. Use tincture and lower.

PILES
Plantago
Most useful local remedy for inflamed piles.
Mullein Oil
Apply at bedtime for itching piles as ointment made of mother tincture.
Hypericum
A specific in painful bleeding piles.
Both externally and internally.

PREGNANCY
Amygdalus Persica
Allay the vomiting of pregnancy than any other remedy.

Dose : Tincture, 5 drops thrice a day.

PROPHYLACTICS
Lathyrus Sat
For poliomyelitis.

Pertussin
For whooping cough.

Diphtherinum
For diphtheria.

Belladonna
Surest preventive of hydrophobia.

Chionanthus
Prevents formation of gall-stones and promotes the discharge of already formed. Use tincture.

PROSTATE
Populus Tremuloides
Use tincture for enlarged prostate with severe pain, tenesmus and scalding urine containing muco-purulent discharge.

PUBERTY
Pituitrin
For delayed puberty with non-development of breast.

RHEUMATISM
Gaultheria
Quick result in treatment of inflammatory rheumatism and neuralgia.
Dose : Tincture, 10 drops to be taken four times a day.

SCABIES
Styrak Balsam
Use tincture externally in scabies, dry or moist, once a day.

SEMINAL DISCHARGE
Thuja
Te drops of mother tincture at bedtime controls nocturnal emissions better than any other remedy.

SEX
Titanium
Two early ejaculation of semen in coitus.

SINUSITIS

Nat. Mur.
For frequent attack with loss of smell. Use high potency only.

SPERMATORRHOEA
Eryngium Aquaticum
A very useful remedy for emission of sperms without erection.
Dose : Preferably tincture. Also use lower potencies.

SPINAL CURVATURE
Baryta Muriatica
Use 3-rd trituration. Bears repetition of dosage well.

SPRAINS
Bellis Perennis
For musculo-tendinous sprains and bruises.

TEETH
Hirudo Medicinalis
Indicated for bleeding of gums.

URINE
Turnera Aphrodisiaca
Helps brilliantly in cases of dribbling of urine day and night.

Mullein Oil
Use Mullein Oil 3X for nocturnal enuresis and painful micturation.

Formica Rufa
For bedwetting.

VOMITING
Iris Versicolor
In cases of vomiting of all kinds.

WARTS
Calcarea Calcinata
Before searching a similimum, use confidently this remedy for all kinds of warts.
Dose : Use 3X trit.
Anagellis
Low potencies have the power of softening flesh and destroying warts.

WHOOPING COUGH
Naphthaline
Third trituration found more useful than any other remedy.

WORMS

Chelone
It is an enemy to every kind of worm infesting the human body. Specific for round and thread worms.
Dose : Five drops of tincture thrice daily.
Calotropis
Highly efficacious for tape worms. Use tincture.
Tuberculinum
For ascarides.

Chapter - 12
SPECIFIC MEDICINE

ABSCESS
Hepar Sulph. - When there is throbbing pains, during the forming stage of an abscess.
Dose : 3 tablets of the 1-st decimal every 3 hours.
Calcarea Sulph.- Has discharged long enough and the suppuration shows no signs of checking.
Dose : 3 tabs, once in 4 hours.
Echinacea - 10 drops tincture once in 3 hours.
Alnus Rubra - In elderly people.
Dose : 1-st decimal 4 tabs. Once in 4 hours.

APHONIA
Bi-chromate of Potash - In hoarseness as a result of cold.
Dose : 4 tabs. Of the 3-rd decimal once in 3 hours.
Strychnine Sulph - For partial paralysis of the vocal cords.
Dose : 1/30th grains before each meal and at bedtime.
Rhus Glabra - With soreness in the throat.
Dose : Tincture in 10 drop doses every 2 hours.

APPENDICITIS
Dioscorea - When the bowels seem full of gas and a twisting pain.
Dose : 60 drops in a glass of water every hour until relieved.

ASTHMA
Aspidosperma - Associated with emphysema.
Dose : 10 drops of tincture every 6 hourly.
Lobelia Inflata - When there is difficulty of breathing.
Dose : 10 drops of third decimal dilution every two hours.
Grindelia Robusta - Cough attended with tenacious mucus.
Dose : 10 drops of tincture once in two hours.
Senega - In old people.
Dose : 5 drops of tincture every 4 hours.

BRONCHITIS
> Tr. Aconite, gtts. V
>> Fl. Ext. Asclepias Tub.
>>> Aqua
> Mix Sig. Teaspoonful once an hour.

COLIC
Dioscorea - for wind colic, pain< by bending forward, relieved by standing erect and giving pressure on the bowels.
  Dose : Give 60 drops of tincture in a glass of hot water every hour.
  Colocynth - Agonizing pain causing the patient to bend double.
  Dose : 2 drops of tincture every 15 minutes.

Phosphate of Magnesia - Cramping pain > by heat and belching of gas which does not lessen the pain.

Dose : add 5 grains of the 3-rd decimal trituration to a half cup of hot water and give the patient a teaspoonful every few minutes.

CONSTIPATION

Nux. Vom. - Frequent desire to have the movement of the bowels but pass only a small amount each time.

Dose : 3 tabs. Of the 3-rd decimal trituration after each meal and at bedtime.

Bryonia - No desire for stool, bowels are inactive, the stools large, hard and dry.

Dose : 3 drops of tincture 3 times a day.

Natrum Muriate - Stools are difficult of expulsion and straining causes flow of blood, leaves fissure and soreness of the anus.

Dose: 5 grains of the 2-nd decimal trituration 3 times a day.

Hydrastis - Patients who lead a sedentary life.

Dose : tincture, 5 drops before breakfast.

ECZEMA

Treat chronic cases by :
Mix. Sig. Teaspoonful three times daily.
Fl. Ext. Podophyllum ,
Acetate Potash
Aqua
Berberis Aquifolium - In scaly eczema in various parts of the body.
Dose : 10 drops of tincture once in 4 hours.

For severe itching of inflamed parts, use this prescription:
Carbolic Acid gtts.,
Sulph. Morphia grs. Iii,
Glycerine,
Aqua q.s.
Mix. Sig. Apply locally thrice daily.

FEVER (Typhoid)

Ferri Phos. - For the fever in the first stage.

Dose : Add 5 grains of the 3-rd decimal to a cup of warm water and give a reaspoonful every hour.

Baptisia - When there is stupor and delirium, tongue dry and breath is offensive.

Dose : Add 20 drops tincture to 4 ounces of water ; mix and give a teaspoonful every hour.

GASTRIC ULCER

Nitrate Uranium - There is burning pain and flatulence with vomiting, and the ulcer is near the pyloric extremity of the stomach.

Dose : 3-rd decimal trituration in 2-grain doses three times a day.

Bi-chromate of potash - When there is distress immediately after eating with vomiting of ropy mucus and blood.

Dose : 4 tabs. Of the 3-rd decimal trit. Once in 4 hours.

DIABETES
Lactic Acid - When there is great thirst and voracious hunger, pofuse urine loaded with sugar.
Dose : One teaspoonful in a glass of water three times a day.
Chionanthus - When the liver is involved, with pain the right hypocondrium.
Dose : 10 drops once in 4 hours.
Lycopus Virg. - In diabetes with great thirst, passing large quantities of urine.
Dose : tincture, 5 drops 4 times a day.
Nitrate Uranium - With symptoms of dyspepsia.
Dose : 3 tabs. Once in 4 hours. Use 3-rd decimal trit.

DIARRHOEA
Tr. Camphor,
Tr. Capsicum,
Tr. Ginger,
Tr. Opium, a.a.
Sig. Teaspoonful in a little hot water every hour until relieved.
Cuprum Arsenicum - Profuse diarrhoea with vomiting of watery material with colicky pains.
Dose : 4 tablets of the 6-th decimal every hour.
Henchera Americana - Watery stools containing traces of blood with tenesmus.
Dose : 5 drops of tincture once in two hours.

DYSPEPSIA
Pepsin (pure)
Subnitrate bismuth,
Tr. Nux. Vom. 3ss.
Comp. Tr. Gentiana
Mix. Sig. One teaspoonful after meals in a little bit of water.

GONORRHOEA
The following prescription covers the indications for the acute stage:
Tr. Gelsemium,
Tr. Canabis Sativa, a.a. 3ss.
Spts. Nitre Dulce,
Aqua q.s. ad,
Mix. Sig. Teaspoonful every hour.
Cubeba - For the chronic stage with a discharge of thick, yellow pus-like matter.
Dose : 3 tablets of the 2-nd decimal trituration once in 4 hours.

HAEMORRHOIDS
Aesculus Hip. - When there is knife-like pains shoot up the rectum, with severe dull backache in lumbo-sacral region.
Dose: 5-drop doses once in 4 hours.
Collinsonia - Bleeding from the rectum, with great flatulence having sensation of a foreign body and when there is constipation alternating wi th diarrhoea.

Dose : 10 drops of tincture in half a glass of water and give a teaspoonful every two hours. Where the parts are sore and sensitive, apply the following ointment:

    Ext. Conium, grs. x..
    Tannic Acid, grs. xii.
    Morphine , grs. iv. –
    Vesline,

Mix. Sig. Apply to the parts night and morning.

HICCOUGH

Magnesia Phos. - Cures most cases.

Dose : Place 10 grains in a cup of hot water and give a teaspoonful every few minutes until relieved.

A lump of sugar wet with vinegar, placed in the mouth and allowed to dissolve will often give relief.

HAEMATURIA

Terebinthina- When the urine is mixed with black blood, sediments like coffee grounds and burning drawing pains in the kidney and bladder.

Dose : Place 25 drops of the 3-rd decimal dilution in a cup of water and give a teaspoonful of hour.

Ferri Phos. – In haematuria with bright red blood.

Dose : Add 10 grains to a glass of hot water and give teaspoonful every 1:5 minutes.

Lycopus Virg.- . - Blood in urine with calculus in the bladder.

Dose : 10 drops in a glass of water once in two hours.

HYDROCELE

Liquid Ergot- Remove the fluid from scrotum, with trocar and canula, then inject two fluid drachms of Normal Liquid Ergot into the cavity. Many fine cures have been made in old men with very little discomfort from the use of the remedy.

Apis Mel.- Indicated where there is considerable edema of the parts.

Dose : 8 drops of the 3-rd decimal dilution once in two hours.

IRITIS

Jaborandi- The best internal remedy which allays inflammation, controls spasms of the muscle of accommodation.

Dose : tincture Jaborandi, gtts. Xx, aqua. Mix. Sig. Teaspoonful once in two hours.

Sulph. Atropia - For local application from the very start it may be made in the strength of 4 grains to an ounce of 1 water which should be used 3 times a day.

JAUNDICE

Chelidonium - With severe right-sided pain, yellow skin stools clay coloured, urine loaded with bile.

Dose : 10 drops of tincture three times a day.

Chionanthus Virg. -Cramp-like pains in the abdomen constipation, urine dark is the guiding indications.

Dose : 20 drops of tincture, three times a day.

Myrica - For catarrhal jaundice.
Dose : 2 grains on the tongue twice daily.

LEUCORRHOEA
Kali Mur. - Where the discharge is milky white and non irritating.
Dose : 2 tabs. of the 3-rd decimal trit. Once in two hours.
Secale Cornutum - For the leucorrhoea that comes on every few days in torrents of thick, yellowish discharge.
Dose: 4 tablets of the 3-rd decimal trit. r 3 times a day.
Fagopyrum Esculentum - When there is yellow leucorrhoea, itching of the parts covered with hair, and o bruised painful feeling in the overies.
Dose: 3 tablets of the 3-rd decimal trit. Once in 2 hours.

MEASLES
       Tr. Aconite, gtts. V,
       Tr. Ipecac. Gtts. X,
       Aqua
Mix Sig. Teaspoonful every hour.

MENSES (delayed)
Polygonum Punctatum : In amenorrhoea of young girls with aching pains in the hips arid loins.
Dose : Add tincture Polygonum 3ii to aqua and give teaspoonful once in 4 hours.

MENSES (irregular)
Senecio Aureus - For irregular menstruation with uterine leucorrhoea.
Dose : Add 3i of the tincture with aqua and give in once in 4 hours.

MENSES (painful)
       Tr. Gelsemium gtts. xx.
       Tr. Viburnum Qp. 3ii
       Simple syrup, q.s.
Mix Sig. Teaspoonful once in two hours until relieved.

NEURALGIA
       Use following prescription:
       Tr. Gelsemium
       Tr. Kalmia, a.a. 3ss.
       Aqua q.s. ad.
Mix. Sig. Teaspoonful once in 15 minutes until the pain is relieved.

NYMPHOMANIA
Murex- Where the least touch of the sexual Organs causes violent sexual excitement and menses are irregular with large clots.

OTORRHOEA
If there is a chronic bad smelling discharge from the ear, use the following prescription :

        Fl. Ext. Eucalyptus,
        Aqua,
Mix. Sig. Inject one drachm into the ear 3 times a day with an ear syringe.
Kali Sulph. - In catarrh of the ear with earache and thin yellow, watery discharge.
Dose : 4 tabs. Of the 3-rd decimal every three hours.

PEMPHIGUS
The following prescription is the best for the chronic variety of this affection:
        Fl. Ext. Berberis Aquifolium ,
        Fowler's Solution Arsenic, 3ii
        Simple Syrup, q.s.
Mix. Sig. Half teaspoonful after each meal.

PHARYNGITIS
        Tr. Gelsemium
        Tr. Phytolacca, a.a. gtts/Xx :
        Aqua
Mix. Sig. Teaspoonful once an hour.
Guaiacum - When there is dryness of the throat, swallowing is painful and burning in the throat.
Dose: 3 grains of the 2-nd decimal once in 4 hours.
Argentum Nit. - For chronic pharyngitis.
Dose : 6th decimal trit., 3 tabs. Every 4 hours.

PRICKLY HEAT
A good local application for this condition is the following mixure :
        Carbolic Acid sol.
        Pulv. Borax, a.a.3ii
        Aqua,,
Mix. Sig. Apply locally as often as is needed. .

RHEUMATISM
Colchicum- Limbs stiff and feverish, pains shift from place to place, worse at night.
Dose : 5 drops of, three times a day. For lumbago, I have found the following prescription valuable:
        Tr. Cimicifuga
        Tr. Gels.
        Tr. Bryonia, a.a
Acidum Salicylicum- - Use in articular rheumatism with serous effusion.
Dose : 5 grains every 4 hours.
As a liniment for rheumatism I like the following prescription:
        Tr. Capsicum,
        Oil Origanum 3i,
        Tr. Opium
        Spts. Ammonia, a.a.3ii
        Tr. Camphor. 3i

Mix. Sig. Rub well into the affected parts 3 times a day.

Obstinate cases of chronic rheumatism will often yield to comp. Tr. Cimicifuga made as follows:

>Tr. Cimicifuga, Oi
>Juice of Phytolacca berries,
>Tr. Guaiacum,
>Mix. Sig. Half teaspoonful four times daily.

RINGWORM

Acetic Acid - The best local application in this affection is glacial acetic acid. Apply to any portion of the body except the scalp.

Juglans Cinerea - Is the most useful internal remedy.

Dose : 5 drops of tincture, once in 3 hours.

SCABIES

>Oil Tar,
>Tr. Veratrum Vir ,
>Lanolin,
>Sublimed sulphur sufficient to make the mass of the consistency of an ointment. .

Mix. Sig. Apply 3 nights in succession, then take a bath and skip three nights, then apply it 3 nights more.

SCURVY

>Rhus Glabra 1x. grs. v
>Ferri Carbonas, grs. Ss.
>Mix. Make one powder. Sig. Give one of these powders every 4 hours.

SPERMATORRHOEA

Eryngium Aquaticum - Used in seminal emissions without erection.

Dose : 2 grains of the 3-rd decimal trit. 3 times a day.

Fine cures have been made by using this prescription:

>Sulph. Strychnine, gr. 1/30-th
>Gels. Gr. 1/16-th
>Mix. Sig. Give one pill at bedtime.

STY

Pulsatilla- For the acute stage.

Dose : 2 drops tincture, once in 4 hourly.

Calcarea Sulph. - Use after the acute stage has passed.

Dose : 4 tablets of the 2-nd decimal every 4 hourly.

SYPHILIS

>Fl. Ext. Aconite, 3ii
>Fl. Ext. Conium
>Glycerine q.s. ad,
>Mix. Sig. Apply 3 times a day.

TONSILITIS
In acute tonsilities, use the following prescription :
>Tr. Aconite, gtts. V.
>Tr. Phytolacca, gtts. Xx
>Aqua,

Mix. Sig. gig. Teaspoonful every hour.
Iodide Baryta - For indurated tonsils with chronicity of symptoms.
Dose : 3 tablets every 4 hourly.

URTICARIA
Urtica Urens -When the skin is elevated, a white central spot and a red areola with a burning stinging sensation.
Dose : Add 20 drops of tincture, to 4'ounces of water and give a teaspoonful once in 4 hours.

VAGINISMUS
Hydrochlorate Cocaine - For the newly married woman.
Dose : Use as an ointment of 5 grains to the ounce of Vaseline to be applied to the inside of the vagina before retiring.

VERTIGO
Ammonium Iodatum - Vertigo with unsteady gait.
Dose : Give two grains once in 3 hours.
In vertigo with noises in the ears, prescribe Fl. Ext Ergot gtts. X, three times a day.

VOMITING
Ipecac - With persistent nausea, not relieved by vomiting.
Dose : Put 5 drops of tincture, in a cup of water and give one teaspoonful every hour.
Bismuth - The water is thrown off the stomach as soon as it is swallowed, although solid food is retained for some time.
Dose : 3 tabs of the 2-nd decimal every hour.
Amygdalis Persica - For gastric irritability in small children. Also for morning sickness in pregnant women.
Dose : 5 drops of tincture, once in 2 hours.

WARTS
Thuja – If the warts come in crops.
Dose : 5 drops of tincture every 4 hours. Tincture Thuja and equal parts of of Chromic Acid with a little bit of water makes a good local application.
Nitric Acid- For syphilitic warts and condylomata, keep the parts constantly moist with dilute nitric acid.

WORMS
>Santonin, grs. x.
>Podophyllin, grs.ii.
>Sacch. Alba., grs. xxx

Mix. Devide into powder. Sig. One powder night and morning until the bowels move freely.
Aromatic Sulpulphuric Acid - Specific for tapeworms.
Dose : Put a teaspoonful in a glass of sweetened water and drink at once. Take 3 such doses in 24 hours that will bring worms.

DEFINITE ORGANOTHERAPY

Chapter - 13
INTERNAL DEFINITE PRESCRIPTION

A

Aphtheae — Bismuth Subnitrate 2X (3g × 4) Rhus Glabra ø (Local) ; Hydrastin Mur 1x (Local).Kali Chloric. 30 (4h).

Acute Gastritis — Acon. (3d × 4h); Arg. Nit. ø (5d × 3h)

Appendicitis — Dioscorea q (20d × 6h) ; Arg. Nit. (5d × 3h).

Appenditicitis — Dioscorea (20d × 6h) ; Ricinus Communis ø (5d × 4h)

Anal Fissure — Paeonia Officinalis ø (10d × 3h) ; Krameria ø(Local).

Acne — Berberis Aquifol. ø (10d × 4h) ; Juglandin 6x (2g × 4h); Kali Nitricum 3x (Local) ; Boracic Acid 2x (Local) ; Sulphurus Acid ø (Local) ; Ichthol 2x (Local).

Anaemia — Ferrum Met. 1x (3g × 4h) ; Digitalin 3x (3g × 3h) ; China ø (5d × 4h) ; Nat. Mur 6x (3g × 4h) ; Helonias Dioica ø(5d × 3h) ; Plumb. Acet. 30 (4h).

Abscess — Alnus Rubra ø (8d × 4h) ; Echinacea (10d × 4h) ; Lobelia ø (Local) ; Tarent. Cub. 30 (3h).

Aneurism — Baryta Mur. 3x (3g × 4h) ; Kali Iodatum 3x (5g × 3h); Ver. Vir. ø (5d × 3h). Carbo Animalis 30 (5h).

Acute Prostatitis — Staphis ø (10d × 4h) ; Gels ø (10d × 3h).

Acute Bright's Disease — Triticum Repens ø (10d × 4h). Cantharis ø (5d × 3h) ; Calc. Sulph 3x (3g × 4h). Apis Mel 30 (4h).

Acute Bronchitis — Asclepias Tuberosa ø (10d × 4h) ; Heper Sulph 3x (3g × 4h) ; Stillingia ø (8d × 3h).

Asthma — Aspidosperma ø (50d × 3h) ; Lobelia ø (10d × 3h) ; Grindelia Robusta ø (25d × 3h) ; Senega ø (5d × 4h).

Acute Pleurisy — Asclepias Tub. ø (10d × 3h). Heper S. 30 (3h).

Aphonia — Erigeron ø (5d × 3h) ; Kali Bich ø (5d × 3h) ; Rhus Glabra ø (15d × 4h) ; Strychnine Sulph 6x (1g × 6h).

Acute Salpingitis — Macrotin 3x (2g × 3h).

After-pains — Cinnamon ø (5d × 4h) ; Caulophyl. 30 (2h).

Alopicia — Ricinus Communis ø (Local) ; Burgamont Oil. (Local).

Asthenopia — Kali Carb. 3x (3g × 4h) ; Ruta G. ø (5d × 4h) ; Asarum Europaeum ø (6d × 3h) ; Lil. Tig. 30 (6h).

Amblyopia — Acon. ø (5d × 3h) ; Nux Vom. ø (10d × 4h); Acid Phos. ø (10d × 4h) ; Ruta. G. 30 (4h).

Angina Pectoris — Glonoin ø (2d × 3h) ; Crataegus ø (15d × 4h); Lobelia ø (25d × 3h) ; Spigelia ø (10d × 3h).

Arterio Sclerosis — Ars. Iod. 3x (3g × 3h) ; Strychnina Sulph 6x (1g × 4h) ; Ver. Vir. ø (5d × 3h).

Apoplexy — Acon. ø (5d × 4h) ; Kali Mur. 6x (4g × 4h); Opium 30 (6h).

B

Barber's Itch — Sulph. Iod. 3x (3g × 3h) ; Acid Carbolic q (Local); Kreosote ø (Local). ; Heper Sulph 30 (6h).

Bromidrosis — Baryta Carb. 3x (3g × 4h) ; Acid Nit ø (5d × 3h); Sepia ø (5d × 3h) ; Sil 6x (3g × 4h).

Boils — Lappa ø (10d × 4h) ; Echinacea ø (5d × 4h) ; Bell ø (3d × 3h); Sepia ø (5d × 3h) ; Sil 6x (3g × 4h).

Bronchocele — Calcarea Iodata 3x (2g × 4h); Iris Vers. ø (5d × 3h), Iodine ø (8d × 4h).

Buboes — Phytolacca ø (5d × 3h) ; Calc. Sulph 3x (2g × 3h) ' Lobelia ø(Local) ; Carbo Animalis 30 (5h).

Balanitis — Zinc. Sulph 1x (Local).; Jac. Car. 30 (8h).

Bunions — Ver. Vir. ø (Local) ; Rhododendron 30 (4h).

Bilious Fever — Acon. ø (10d × 2h) ; Nux. Vom. ø (10d × 3h).

C

Cirrhosis of Liver — Bryo. ø (5d × 4h) ; Chinanthus Virg q (10d × 4h) ; Euonyminum 3x (1g × 3h).

Chronic Gastritis — Arg. Nit ø (5d × 2h) ; Phos. 30 (4h).

Cholera Morbus — Ammonium Causticum ø (25d × 3h) ; Mentha Piperita ø (30d × 2h).

Chronic Diarrhoea — Epilobium August. ø (15d × 3h).

Cholera Asiatica — Camphor ø (5d × 3h); Acid Phos. q (5d × 2h); Ver. Alb. ø (6d × 3h); Cuprum Met. 3x (4g × 4h).

Cholera Infantum — Cuphea Visco ø (5d × 2h) ; Euphorbia Corollata ø (5d × 3h) ; Aethus Cyn. 30 (2h).

Constipation — Nux Vom. ø (3d × 4h); Bryo. ø (3d × 3h) ; Natrum Mur. 3x (4g × 4h) ; Hydrastis ø (10d × before breakfast) ; Kali Mur. 6x (10g × at bedtime).

Colic — Dioscorea Vil. ø (20d × 2h) ; Colocynth ø (5d × 3h); Mag. Phos. 3x (5g × 4h) ; Plumb. Acet. 30 (2h).

Crusta Lactea — Lappa ø (8d × 3h); Viola Tricolor ø(5d × 3h)

Cerebral Anemia — Calc. Phos. 3x (3g × 4h).

Carbuncles — Heper Sulph. 3x (3g × 4h); Tarantula C. ø (5d × 3h); Echinacea ø (Local) ; Acid Carbolic ø (Local).

Chlorosis — Alumina 1x (3g × 4h); Digitalin 6x (3g × 4h) ; Ferr. Met. 1x (3g × 3h) ; Senecio Aurens ø (10d × 3h).

Cystitis — Cantharis ø(5d × 3h); Equisetum Hy. ø (4d × 3h).

Chronic Cystitis — Chimaphila Umbelata q (4d × 4h) ; Pupulin 6x (2g × 4g) ; Terebinthina ø (5d × 3h) ; Cuprum Ars. 6x (2g × 4h) ; Copaib. 30 (3h).

Calculus in the Bladder — Magnesia Boro Citrate 1x (5g × 4h)

Chronic Prostatitis — Acs. Hip ø (10d × 4h) ; Selenium 3x (3g × . 3h) ; Sabal Serrulata ø (10d × 4h) ; Thuja 200 (8h).

Chronic Bright's Disease — Helonias Dioca (5d × 4h) ; Chelonin 3x (2g × 4h) ; Plumb. 30 (5h).

Coryza — Euphrasia ø (10d × 4h) ; Nat. Mur. 3x (3g × 3h).

Chronic Catarrh — Ammonium Causticum ø (10d × 4h) ; Kali Bich. ø (5d × 3h) ; Sanguinaria Nit. 3x (3g × 4h) Natrum Sulphocarb. 1x (Local Gargle).
Chronic Tonsilitis — Baryata Iod. 3x (3g × 4h).
Chronic Laryngitis — Arun Triphyllum ø (6d × 3h) ; Causticum q (8d × 4h) ; Lachesis 3x (5d × 4h).
Chronic Bronchitis — Stannum Met. 3x (3g × 3h) ; Strychnine Sulph. 6x (1g × 4h). ; Senega 30 (4h).
Chronic Pleurisy — Kali Aceticum ø(20d × 4h) ; Iodium ø (3d × 5h); Chin. Sulph. 3x (5g × 4h) ; Ammon. Carb ø (20d × 4h).
Climacteric Flushing — Ignatia ø (5d × 4h) ; Sepia ø (5d × 4h) ; Viburnum Opulus q (10d × 4h).
Chancre — Ferrum Clorid. ø (Local). ; Merc. Sol. 200 (6h).
Catarrhal Conjunctivitis — Euphrasia q (5d × 4h)
Choroiditis — Prunus Spinosa ø (6d × 3h) ;
Cataract — Phosphorus 6x (1g × 4h) ; Sulph. Iodatum 3x (3g × 4h) ; Causticum ø (5d × 3h);
Chorea — Calc. Phos. 3x (4g × 4h) ; Ignatia 30 (3h).
Catalepsy — Cannabis Indica ø (5d × 4h) ; Stramonium ø(8d × 3h).
Cerebro-Spinal Meningitis — Cimicifuga q (10d × 4h) ; Nat. Sulph 3x (3g × 4h) ; Passiflora Incarnata q (10d × 4h).
Concussion of the Brain — Bell ø (8d × 4h) ; Kali Phos. 30 (3h).
Cerebral Congestion — Acon ø (4d × 2h) ; Ver. Vir. ø (5d × 3h).
Chicken Pox — Hydrastis ø (5d × 4h) ; Chin Ars. 3x (3g × 4h).

D

Dyspepsia — Alnus Rubra ø (5d × 4h) ; Robnina Pseudo ø (5d × 3h). Chelone Glabra ø (5d × 3h) ; Gentiana L. ø (60d × 4h). Pepsinum v (20d × 3h). Potash Bi-Chromate 30 (4h).
Diarrhoea — Podo. ø (5d × 4h) ; Henchera Americana ø (10d × 4h).
Dysentery — Mag. Sulph 1x (g × 3h) ; Ipecac ø (8d × 4h) ;
Dropsy — Apocynum Can. ø (10d × 4h); Digitalis q (5d × 4h) ; Convallaria Majalis ø (10d × 4h) ; Adonis ø (5d × 4h) ; Elaterin 6x (2g × 3h) ; Squilla ø (8d × 3h) ; Strychinine Sulph. 6x (1g × 3h) ; Jalapa ø (10d × 4h) ; Tereb. 30 (4h).
Diabetes — Lactica Acid ø (50d × 3h); Chionanthus ø (20d × 4h); Acid Phos. ø (20d × 3h) ; Uranium Nit 3x (3g × 4h) ; Lycopus Virg. ø (60d × 3h) ; Silica 30 (8h).
Dipsomania — Apocynum Canabinum ø (20d × 3h) ; Strychinine Hypophos. 3x (1g × 6h) ; Strychnine Nitricum 6x (1g × 4h).
Deafness — Ferrum Picricum 3x (3g × 4h) ; Sil. 3x (3g × 4h). Ether ø (Local) ; Nat. Salicyl. 30 (3h).
Dialatation of the Heart — Crataegus Oxy. ø (10d × 4h) ; Collinsonia ø(5d × 4h) ; Digitalis ø (10d × 4h) ; Phaseolus Nana q (8d × 3h).
Dyspnoea — Adonis Vernalis ø (8d × 4h) ; Crataegus ø (10d × 6h); Naja Tripudians ø (20d × 4h) ; Basil ø 200 (8h).
Diaphragmitis — Cactus Grand. ø (25d × 4h).
Delirium Tremens — Hyoscyamus ø (8d × 4h) ; Kali Phos. 6x (3g × 4h).

E

Enlargement of the Liver — Carduus Marianus ø (5d × 4h) ; Chelone Glabra ø (5d × 3h) ø Chelidon. ø (10d × 4h); Ptelea Trifoliata ø (5d × 4h).

Erythema — Bell. ø (4d × 3h) ; Hamamelis ø (Local).

Erythema Nodusum — Rhus Venenata (5d × 4h) ; Echinacea ø (Local).

Eczema — Kali Aceticum ø (20d × 4h) ; Bovista ø (5d × 4h) ; Taraxacum ø (30d × 4h) ; Lobelia ø (Local) ; Vinca Minor ø (Local); Morhpin Sulph 6x (Local).

Erysipelas — Bell ø (5d × 3h); Heper Sulph 200 (6h).

Epistaxis — Melilotus Alba ø (5d × 3h) ; Ferrum Aceticum 3x (3g × 4h) ; Geranium Mac. ø (Local, press it well up into nostril with cotton.) ; Millefol. 30 (1h).

Enlarged Uterus — Fraxinus Americanus ø (10d × 4h).

Eczema Aurium — Rhus Tox. ø (5d × 4h); Calc. Sulph 3x (3g × 4h); Eucalyptus ø (Local).

Endocarditis — Cimicifuga ø (8d × 4h) ; Acon. Radix ø (5d × 4h); Calc. Flour. 3x (3g × 4h) ; Cereus Bonplandi ø (10d × 4h), Spigelia ø (8d × 4h); Naja Trip. 200 (8h).

Epilepsy — Oenanthe Crocata ø (5d × 4h); Ammon. Brom. 3x (10d × 4h) ; Indigo 6x (4g × 4h) ; Artemisia Vulgaris ø (8d × 3h); Solanum Carolinense ø (15d × 3h); Bufo Rana 200 (6h).

Exanthemata — Baptisia ø (5d × 4h); Ferr. Phos. 6x (4g × 4h); Acid Hydrochloric ø (5d × 3h); Carbo. Veg. 3x (5d × 3h); Hyoscyamus ø (5d × 4h).

F

Female Frigidity — Sabal Serrulata ø (10d × 4h).

Fidgety Limbs — Kali Bromatum 3x (3g × 3h).

Fatty Heart — Vanadium 3x (3g × 4h); Phytolacca ø (10d × 4h); Ricinus Com. (20d × 4h); Cimicifuga (15d × 3h).

Facial Paralysis — Acon. 3x (8d × 4h); Causticum ø (5d × 4h).

G

Glossitis — Acon. (3d × 4h); Merc. Viv 30 (6h); Oxal. Acid 200 (8h).

Gallstone Colic — Podophyllin 3x (3d × 6h) Chelidon. q (20d × 2h); Euonyminum 3x (5g × 3x); Juglans Cinerea q (30d × 3h) ;

Gastralgia — Melilotus Alba ø (5d × 3h); Dioscorea ø (2d × 4h); Gaultheria Oil 1x (5d × 3h).

Gastric Ulcer — Uranium Nit. 3x (3g × 4h); Arg. Nit 3x (3g × 3h); Potash Bi-chromate 3x (3g × 3h).

Gastric Catarrh (nausea) — Nux. Vom ø (5d × 4h).

Gastric Catarrh (gas) — Graph. 3x (3g × 3h)

General Peritonitis — Kali Mur. 3x (3g × 3h); Lyco. 200 (8h)

Glanders — Potash Bi-cromate 3x (3g × 4h); Echinacea ø(10d ×4h).

Gravel — Thalaspi B.P. ø (6d × 3h); Epigea Repens ø (20d × 4h).

Gonorrhoea — Gels. ø (60d × 4h); Canabis Sativa ø (30d × 3h); Cubeba ø (5d × 4h); Nat. Sulph 3x (3g × 3h); Sepia ø (3d × 4h); Petrosel 30 (4h).

Gonorrheal Conjunctivitis — Thuja Occ. ø (5d × 3h).

Granular Conjunctivitis — Kali Mur. 6x (4g × 4h).

Gouty Deposits — Acid Benzoic 2x (3g × 4h).

Gout — Urtica Urens ø (15d × 4h); Ledum Pal 30 (6h).

H

Hepatitis — Ferr. Phos. 3x (3g × 4h) ; Ver. Vir. (5d × 3h); Nat. Sulph. 6x (3g × 4h); Bryo. (3d × 3h); Heper Sulph 3x (3g × 4h); Merc. Sol. IM (12h).

Haemorrhage of the Stomach — Geranium Mac. ø (5d × 3h).

Haemorrhoids — Acs. Hip. ø (5d × 4h); Colinsonia ø (4d × 4h). Hamamelis ø (5d × 4h); Conium Mac. ø (Local); Plantago ø(Local); Nit Acid 200 (6h).

Herpes (facial) — Nat. Mur. 6x (3g × 4h); Sarsaparilla 200 (8h).

Herpes Zoster — Ranunculus Bulb. ø (5d × 4h); Alnus q (30d × 4h), Rhus Tox ø(5d × 4h); Taraxacum ø (50d × 6h); Nat. Sulph 1x (Local); Variolinum 30 (8h).

Haematuria — Ferr. Phos. 3x (3g × 4h); Lycopus Virg. ø (5d × 4h); Terebinthina q (5d × 3h); Allium Cepa q (8d × 2h).

Hay Fever — Sabadilla ø (5d × 3h); Allium Cepa ø (8d × 2h).

Hydrocele — Apis Mel ø (5d × 4h).

Headache (eye-strain) — Ruta G. ø (4d × 3h); Cimicifuga ø (4d × 3h), Onosmodium ø (5d × 3h).

Hemiplegia — Strychnine Sulph 6x (1g × 4h); Apocynum Can. ø (5d × 4h). Convallaria Maj. ø (5d × 4h); Apis Mel. ø (8d × 3h); Helonias Dioica ø (5d × 4h); Leptandrin 3x (6g × 3h).

Hypertrophy of the Heart — Ver. Vir (8d × 4h); Arnica (5d × 4h); Cactus Grand ø (15d × 4h); Colchicum ø (5d × 5h); Lycopus Virg. ø (20d × 4h).

Hoccough — Mag. Phos 3x (3g × 4h); Caulophyllum ø (10d × 1h); Morphin Sulph 6x (1g × 2h); Moschus 30 (1h).

Hysteria — Capsicum ø (8d × 4h); Ammonia Valerian. 6x (3g × 4h); Asafoctida ø (20d × 4h); Valariana Officinalis ø (15d × 3h); Cypripedium (20d × 4h); Pothos Foetida (10d × 4h); Moschus (8d × 4h); Senecio Aurens 30 (6h).

Hydrophobia — Scutellaria (10d × 4h); Cypripedin 3x (2g × 3h); Chin. Sulph. 3x (2g × 3h); Hydrophobinum 30 (8h).

I

Intestinal Haemorrhage — Carbo. Veg. 1x (5g × 4h); Ipecac q (10d × 4h); Ferr. Phos. 3x (3g × 4h).

Ichthyosis — Ars. Iod. 3x (3g × 4h); Thyrodin 3x (5g × 6h) Thuja ø (5d × 4h); Clematis Erecta ø (5d × 4h); Nat. Sulph. 1x (Local); Medorrh. 200 (6h).

Influenza — Bell (5d × 3h); Eupat. Pref. (5d × 3h); Kali Mur. 3x (3g × 4h); Influenzinum 30 (4h).

Impotency — Avena Sativa ø (20d × 4h); Strychninum Ars. 3x (1g × 4h); Acid Phos. ø (8d × 4h); Lyco. ø (5d × 4h); Acid Picric. 3x (4g × 4h); Agnus Castus ø (8d × 4h); Selenium 3x (3g × 4h); Sabal Serrulata ø (20d × 4h).

Ingrowing toe-nail — Picric Acid 3x (3g × 4h); Ferrum Cloride 1x (local).

J

Jaundice — Chelidon. ø (10d × 4h); Chionanthus Virg. ø (10d × 3h); China ø (5d × 4h); Myrica Cerifera ø (10d × 4h). Crot. Hor. 30 (6h).

K

Kidney Complaint — Berberis Vulgaris ø (5d × 4h); Acid Benzoic 3x (5g × 4h); Terebinthina q (8d × 4h).
Keratitis — Apis Mel. (5d × 4h); Kali Mur. 3x (5g × 4h); Aurum Met. 3x (3g × 4h); Heper Sulph 3x (2g × 4h).

L

Lichen — Juglans Cineria ø (5d × 4h); Chin. Sulph. 3x (3g × 4h); Grindelia Robusta ø (Local). Rumex. Crispus 30 (6h).
Laryngitis — Eucalyptus ø (5d × 4h); Lobelia ø (8d × 4h); Sanguinaria Can. (5d × 4h); Stillingia ø (10d × 4h).
Labor Pains — Cimicifuga ø (10d × 4h).
Locomotor Ataxia — Alumina 3x (3g × 4h); Bell. ø (10d × 4h); Arg. Nit. 3x (3g × 4h); Zinc Phos. 3x (1 × 4h); Cannabis Indica q (5d × 4h).
Leucorrhoea — Sec. Cor. ø (5d × 4h); Fagopyrum Esculentum q (10d × 4h).

M

Malaria — Aristolochia Serpentaria ø (10d × 4h); Boletus Laricis ø (5d × 4h); Chininum Ars. 3x (2g × 3h); Grindelia Squarrosa ø (10d × 4h); Chin. Sulph 3x (2g × 4h).
Menses (delayed) — Caulophyllum ø (8d × 4h); Puls. ø (4d × 4h); Polygonum Punctatum ø (10d × 4h).
Menses (irregular) — Senicio Aurens ø (20d × 4h); Trillium Pend. ø (20d × 4h); Sabina 30 (6h).
Menses (profuse) — Sabina ø (10d × 4h).
Menses (painful) — Viburnum Opulus (10d × 4h); Mag. Phos. 3x (4g × 4h); Dioscorea ø (10d ×4); Borax 1x (3g × 4h); Ver. Vir. ø (8d × 4h).
Metritis — Macrotin 3x (5d × 4h); Aurum Mur. 6x (3g × 4h).
Micturation — Staphis. ø (5d × 4h).
Myopia — Physostigma ø (6d × 4h).
Myocarditis — Iberis Amara ø (8d × 4h); Calc. Flour. 3x (3g × 4h); Crataegus Oxyacantha ø (10d × 4h).
Myelitis — Acid Oxalicum 6x (3g × 4h); Abrotanum ø (10d × 4h); Lathurus Sativus (5d × 3h); Hyoscyamine Hydrobrom. 6x (2g × 6h).
Multiple Sclarosis — Hypericum ø (8d × 4h);; Lathyrus Sat. q (5d × 4h).
Meningitis — Kali Mjr. 3x (3g × 4h); Helleborus Nig. ø (5d × 4h).
Mania — Hyoscyamus ø (20d × 3h); Kali Bromatum 3x (3g × 4h); Stramonium ø (8d × 4h); Kali Bromatum 3x (3g × 4h); Cimicifuga ø (10d × 4h); Cuprum Met. 30 (6h).
Measles — Camphor ø (5d × 4h); Asclepias Tuberosa ø (8d × 4h); Kali Mur. 3x (3g × 4h); Euphrasia (5d × 4h). Cuprum Acet. 30 (8h).

N

Nasal Catarrh — Nat. Mur. 3x (4g × 4h); Ferri Phos. 6x (3g × 4h).
Nasal Polypus — Sanguinaria Can. ø (10d × 4h).
Nymphomania — Murex Perp. 6x (3g × 5h); Platina 6x (3g × 4h).
Nervous Headache — Epiphegus Virgiana ø (10d × 4h).
Neuritis — Acon. Radix ø (4d × 4h); Cannabis Indica ø (5d × 4h); Hypericum ø (5d × 3h); Lachesis 200 (6h).
Neuralgia — Kalmia Latifolia (8d × 3h); Spigelia (5d × 4h); Aconitine 3x (1g × 4h); Zinc. Valerian. 3x (2g × 3h); Silicea 3x (3g × 4h); Radium Brom. 30 (6h).

O

Os Uteri (Congestion) — Bell q (8d × 4h); Sepia q (5d × 4h).
Os Uteri (Ulceration) — Kali Ars. 3x (3g × 4h).
Os Uteri (Prolapse) — Helonias Dioica q (10d × 4h). Sepia q (5d × 4h).
Os Uteri (Displacement) — Lilium Tig. (8d × 4h).
Os Uteri (enlargement) — Fraxinus Americans (10d × 4h).
Overy (Congestion) — Lachesis 6x (5d × 4h); Apis Mel. ø (4d × 4h); Podophyllin 3x (3g × 4h).
Oculo Motor Paresis — Rhus Tox. ø (5d × 4h); Causticum ø(3d × 5d).
Otalgia — Plantago Major ø (8d × 4h); Ferr. phos. 3x (3g × 4h); Chamomilla ø (5d × 4h).
Otitis — Acon. ø (5d × 4h); Calc. Sulph 3x (3g × 4h); Kali Mur. 6x (3g × 4h).
Otorrhoea — Kali Phos. 6x (3g × 4h); Kali Sulph 3x (2g × 3h); Sil 1x (3g × 4h); Eucalyptus ø (Local); Tellurium 30 (3h).
Old Fractures — Sil. 3x (3g × 4h).
Offesnsive Sweat — Sil. 3x (3g × 5h); Kali Chloricum 3x (Local).

P

Proctitis — Collinsonia ø (10d × 3h); Gels ø (15d × 5h).
Prolapsus Ani — Aes. Hip. ø (3d × 3h); Hamamelis ø(Local).
Peritonitis — Acon. 3x (5d × 4h).
Peritonitis (Peurperal) — Cimicifuga ø (5d × 4h).
Pimples — Nat. Sulph. 3x (3g × 4h); Berberis Aquifolium ø (10d × 4h); Sulphurus Acid q (Local); Ichthyolum 1x (Local).
Psoriasis — Thyroidinum 3x (3g × 4h); Lappa ø (20d × 4h); Berb. Aquifol ø (20d × 4h); Nat. Sulph 1x (Local).
Pityriasis Rubra — Erythrinus (5d × 4h); Kali Ars. 3x (3g × 4h); Thuja (5d × 4h); Merc. Cor. 30 (4h).
Prurigo — Dolicos Pruriens ø (5d × 4h); Taraxacum ø (20d × 4h); Nat. Sulph 1x (Local); Radium Brom. 30 (12h).
Prickly Heat — Carbolic Acid ø (Loca); Borax 1x (Local).

Pernicious Anaemia — Picric Acid 3x (3g × 4h); Ars. 3x (3g × 4h); Carduns ø (5d × 4h);Calc. Phos. 3x (3g × 4h). Carcinosin 30 (6h).
Purpura — Hamamelis ø (10d × 4h); Ergotin 6x (2g × 4h); Lach. 6x (5d × 4h); Kali Chloricum 3x (Local).
Pneumonia — Asclepias Tub. ø (30d × 4h); Baptisia ø (5d × 4h); Antim. Tart. 1x (3g × 4h); Chin. Sulph. 3x (3g × 4h); Ipecac ø (5d × 4h); Tuberculinum Kochii 30 (6h).
Pulmonary Tuberculosis — Baptisin 3x (1g × 4h); Millifoliumø (8d × 4h); Picrotoxin 6x (4g × 4h); Sil. 3x (3g × 4h); Myosotis Symphytifolia ø (10d × 4h).
Pruritus Valvae — Borax 1x (Local); Hydrastis ø (Local).
Postpartum Haemorrhage and Convulsions — Sarsaparilla q (40d × 4h); Mitchella Repens ø (30d × 4h);
Purulent Conjunctivitis — Heper Sulph 1x (2g × 4h); Rhus. Tox. q (5d × 3h).
Polypus Aurium — Calc. Carb. 3x (4g × 4h); Salicylic Acid 1x (Local).
Periodical Headache — Chin. Sulph 3x (2g × 3h); Bryo. ø (5d × 4h); Nat. Mur. 3x (3g × 4h); Leptandra 30 (3h).
Periosteal Inflammation — Mezerium ø (5d × 4h).
Phlebitis — Hamamelis ø (10d × 4h); Puls. ø (5d × 4h).
Paralysis Agitans — Hyoscyamine Hydrobromate 6x (3g × 4h).
Pericarditis — Kali Iodatum 3x (2g × 3h); Asclepias Tub. q (10d × 4h); Spigelia ø (5d × 4h); Cimicifuga ø (5d × 4h); Jaborandi ø (8d × 4h); Merc. Sol. 1M (12h).
Palpitation of Heart — Moschus ø (5d × 4h); China ø (8d × 3h); Phos. Acid (8d × 4h); Kali Phos. 6x (3g × 4h).
Paraplegia — Arg. Nit. 3x (4g × 4h); Lathyrus Sativa q (8d × 4h); Oleander ø (8d × 4h); Conium Mac. ø (5d × 5h); Kali Phos 3x (3g × 4h).

R

Rhagades — Graph 3x (3g × 4h); Balsam Peru ø (Local).
Rheumatism — Colchicum ø (5d × 4h); Rhus Tox. ø (5d × 4h); Iodine (Local); Rhododendron ø (6d × 4h); Cimicifuga ø (10d × 4h); Guiacum ø (30d × 3h); Phytolacca ø (8d × 4h); Capsicum ø (Local); Origanum ø (Local); Stellaria Media q (Local).
Rheumatic Ophthalmia — Acon. ø (5d × 4h); Spigelia ø (8d × 3h).
Retinitis — Picric Acid 2x (4g × 4h); Kali Mur. 3x (5g × 4h); Bell. ø(6d × 4h); Natrum Salicylicum 2x (4g × 3h).
Remittent Fever — Gels. ø (4d × 3h); Chin. Ars. 3x (3g × 4h); Rhus Tox. ø (5d × 4h); Ipecac 200 (6h).

S

Splentis — Ceanothus Americana (5d × 3h); Agaricus 30 (5h).
Stomatitis — Kali Mur. 3x (3g × 4h); Arum Triphy. 30 (6h).
Salt Rheum — Rumex Crispus ø (25d × 4h); Alnus q (30d × 4h); Taraxacum ø (30d × 3h).
Scald Head — Viola Tricolor (5d × 3h); Sil 6x (3g × 4h); Salicylic Acid 1x (Local); Lobelia (Local).

Scabies — Ver. Vir. ø (local); Sulph ø (local); Ichtholum 1x (Local).

Scrofula — Alnus Rubra ø (5d × 4h); Cistus Canad. ø (5d × 4h); Rumin 1x (2g × 4h); Heper Sulph 3x (3g × 3h); Sil 6x (3g × 4h); Phytococca ø (Local); Myrica ø (Local).

Scurvy — Rhus Glabra ø (35d × 3h); Ferr. Carbonicum 6x (3g × 4h); Rhus Glabra ø (Local); Bryonia 30 (4h).

Septicemia — Kali Mur 3x (3g × 4h); Echinacea (10d × 4h); Calc. Sulph 3x (3g × 4h) ; Pyrogen 200 (6h).

Suppression of Urine — Apis Mel (6d × 4h).

Spermatorrhoea — Gelsimin 6x (2g × 4h); Eryngium Aquaticum ø (10d × 4h). Lupulin 3x (2g × 4h); Dioscorea ø (8d × 4h); Ver. Alb. (5d × 4h); Kali Phos. 3x (3g × 4h).

Sterility — Aurum Mur. Nat. 6x (4g × 4h); Borax 1x (3g × 4h); Acid Boracic. 2x (Local); Nat. Bicarbonicum 1x (Local).

Suppurative Chroiditis — Rhus Tox. ø (6d × 4h); Viola Odorata ø (5d × 4h).

Scrofulous Conjunctivitis — Stillingia ø (5d × 4h); Kali Iodatum 3x (3g × 4h).

Syphilis — Corydalin 3x (4g × 4h); Iris Vers. ø (20d × 4h); Acid Nit ø (5d × 4h); Kali Bich ø(5d × 4h); Berb. Aquifol. ø (10d × 4h); Corydalis Formosa ø (15d × 4h); Acon. ø (Local); Conium ø (Local); Kali Iod. 200 (8h).

Sty — Puls (10d × 4h); Calc. Sulph 3x (3g × 4h).

Nervous Headache — Epiphegus Virginiana ø (10d × 4h).

Sick Headache — Chionanthus ø (5d × 3h); Niccolum Met. 3x (3g × 3h). Cascara Sagrada ø (5d × 3h).

Sweating Hands — Pilocarpinum Mur 3x (3g × 4h).

Scitica — Colocynth ø (15d × 5h); Gnaphalium ø (20d × 3h); Phyto. ø (20d × 3h); Ars. Sulph. Rub. 30 (6h).

Spasms — Cuprum Met. 3x (3g × 4h).

Spinal Irritation — Bell ø (3d × 4h); Chin Sulph 3x (3g × 4h); Iodine q (Local); Actea Racemosa 200 (6h).

Spinal Meningitis — Bryonia ø (5d × 4h); Bell. ø (4d × 4h); Ver. Vir. q (8d × 3h).

Suicidal Mania — Ignatia ø (5d × 4h); Cimicifuga ø (8d × 4h); Lillium Tig. ø (10d × 4h); Aurum Met. 3x (3g × 4h); Ars. Alb. 3x (4g × 4h).

Scalet Fever — Acon. Radix (10d × 4h); Amon Carb. (5d × 4h); Arm Triphyllum (3d × 4h); Ferr. Phos. 6x (4g × 4h); Ailanthus Glandulosus ø(8d × 3h); Spigelia 200 (6h).

T

Tonsilitis — Baryta Carb. 3x (3g × 4h); Kali Mur. 3x (3g × 4h); Lac. Can. 30 (1d × 4h); Phytolacca (8d × 4h); Baryta Mur 200 (4h).

Trembling Limbs — Lolium Temulentum ø (5d × 4h).

Tetanus — Angustura ø (5d × 1h); Hypericum ø (10d × 2h); Gels ø (10d × 3h); Passiflora ø (10d × 4h). Oenantha Croc. 30 (8h).

Typhus Fever — Baptisia q (8d × 4h); Hyoscymus q (8d × 3h); Echinacea ø (10d × 3h); Merg. Viv. 200 (6h).

U

Urticaria — Urticaria Urens ø (10d × 4h); Apis q (10d × 4h); Antim Crude 3x (3g × 4h); Astacus Flub. 30 (6h).

Ulceration of the Cornea — Calc. Sulph. 2x (3g ×4h); Bell q (5d × 3h); Potash Bi-cromate ø (3d × 4h); Corydalis ø (10d × 4h).

Ulcers in Mouth — Zinc Sulph 1x (Local).

V

Vaginismus — Plantina Met. 6x (3g × 4h); Cacaine Hydrochlorate ø (Local); Alumen 30 (6h).

Vomiting (Pregnant) — Cerium Oxalicum 1x (5d × 3h); Ingluvin 6x (5g × 3h).

Vomiting — Ipecac ø (5d × 4h); Bismath Met. 3x (3g × 4h); Ver. Alb. ø (4d × 3h); Amygldalis Pesica ø (10d × 4h); Sepia (5d × 3h); Colchicum (10d × 3h). Ferr. Mur. 200 (8h).

Varicocele — Puls. ø (5d × 4h); Hamamelis ø (Local).

Varicose Ulcers — Lobelia (Local); Zinc Sulph 1x (Local).

Valvular Disease of Heart — Calc. Flour 3x (3g ×4h); Spongia ø (5d × 4h).

Vertigo — Acon ø (5d × 4h); Ammonium Iodatum 3x (2g × 4h); Secale Cor ø (10d × 3h); Kali Phos. 3x (3g × 4h); Degitalis ø (5d × 3h); Iodine ø (5d × 4h).

Vaccinosis — Thuja (4d × 3h); Gunpowder 200 (4h).

W

Worms — Santonin 3x (3g × 4h); Podophyllin 3x (4g × 4h); Acid Sulph (50d × 2h); Chelone. 30 (3h).

Warts — Thuja ø (4d × 3h); Mag. Sulph 3x (2g × 3h); Acid Nit ø (Local); Chromic Acid ø (Local); Sabina ø (Local).

Weak Heart — Digitalin 6x (3g × 4h); Glonoin ø (2d × 4h); Phaseolus Nana ø (10d × 3h).

Writer's Cramp — Nat. Phos. 3x (3g × 4) ; Conium Mac. ø (5d × 4h); Mag. Phos. 6x (4g × 3h); Physostig. 200 (8h).

Y

Yellow Fever — Camphor ø(10d × 2h); Cadmium Sulph 3x (3g × 4h); Crotalus Horridus (5d × 3h); Cadmium Sulph 200 (6h).

Z

Zoster, hertis — Alnus Rubra ø (30d x 5h) ; Nat. Sulph. 1X (Local) ; Taraxacum ø (30d x 6h)

EXTERNAL ORGANOTHERAPY

Chapter - 14
EXTERNAL DEFINITE PRESCRIPTION

Alnus ø –
Apply locally to the effected parts in chornic herpes, eczema and prurigo, mixing with little bit of water.

Acid Boracicum 1x –
For styes, rub with sterilised cotton, or dusling powder on ulcerated surfaces.

Amyl Nitrosum ø –
Inhalation of mother tincutre will give immediate relief in paroxysms of asthma.

Acitic Acid ø –
Locally, for warts.

Argemone Mexicana ø –
Its lotion and ointment is very beneficial in ulcers and warts.

Alstonia Scholaris ø –
Use locally in ulcers and rheumatic pains.

Agaricus Muscarius ø –
Apply ointment or lotion in chilblains.

Badiaga ø –
Use ointment or Oil, in swelling of glands.

Bellis Perenis ø –
When applied, affords great relief in wounds and ulcers due to injury. Also in naevi. Use its oil on moles.

Balsam Peru ø –
Locally, in indolent ulcers, scabies, cracked nipples, rhagades, itch. Promotes granulations and removes fetor.

Benzoic Acid ø –
Rub its lotion on ganglion. Apply ointment for wens.

Chrysarobinum 3x –
Its external use in the form of ointment is very efficacious in ringworm, psoriasis, herpes and acne rosacea. Locally, in ringworm of the scalp 10% in glycerine & alcohol.

Chloralum 1x –
In offensive foot-sweat, apply its ointment.

Calotropis Gig. ø –
Use locally for leprosy.

Cromic Acid ø –
Apply ointment in warts.

Castor Oil ø –
Apply oil in herpes zoster.

Chlorum ø –
Useful locally for gangrene.

Citric Acid 1x –
Rub its ointment in freckles.
Chrysophanic Acid ø –
For ringworms, apply ointment.
Cochlearia Armoracia ø –
Cures dandruff, apply the losion on scalp. Use as a gargle in scorbutic gums and sore-throat. Hoarseness and in relaxed condition of fauces.
Citric Acid ø –
Use as mouthwash for bad odor. Relieves cancer pain when applied its ointment.
Ceanothus Americana ø –
Use as gargle with a glass of worm water.
Caulophyllum ø –
For thrush (fungus infections of skin-folds, mouth and vagina), apply local ointment.
Cistus Canadensis ø –
Apply its lotion, as a wash to arrest fetid discharges.
Dioscorea Villosa ø –
Its lolion and ointment are very beneficial for whitlow.
Eupatorium Aromaticum ø –
Its ointment is used in sore-mouth and sore-nipples.
Gaultheria Oil –
Locally, for pruritus & epididymitis.
Geranium Mac. ø –
Inject high-up inside vagina, tincture with 9 parts of water, for metrorrhagia and leucorrhoea. Apply its ointment, in ulcers.
Galium Aparine ø –
Use ointment, in open ulcers of cancer.
Hydrocotyle ø –
For lupus, use its ointment locally.
Iodoform 1x –
Apply ointment for soft chancre.
Iodum ø –
A great skin disinfectant. Use its lotion in bites of insects, reptiles.
Ichthyolum 1x –
Externally very effective for chronic eczema, psoriasis, acne and scabies.
Iris Versicolor ø –
For felon, use its liniment.
Jequirity ø –
Lotion and ointment of this drug are very beneficial in lupus and ulcers.
Kali Permanganicum 1x –
Used locally to correct fetor in cancer, ulcers and ozaena.
Lupulin 1x –
Use ointment, in painful cancer.
Methylene Blue 1x –
Locally for chronic otitis with foul smelling discharge.
Menthol 1x –
It affords great relief when used as ointment for itching, esp., for pruritus vulvae.

Mentha Piperita ø –
For pruritus vulvae, use externally in the form of lotion.
Mag. Sulph. 1x –
Locally, mixing with water, for septic conditions, erysipelas, orchitis and boils.
Natrum Hyposulph 3x –
Apply ointment, in liverspots.
Oleum Jecoris Aselli ø –
Is specific local remedy for ringworm. Rub oil on the whole body in dwarfish, emaciated babies.
Oil of Cinnamon –
In aquaous sol., it is best local disinfectant. Three drops of Oil on sugar promptly relievers paroxysms of hiccough.
Plumeria Cellinus ø –
Apply locally, for snake-poisoning.
Paeonia ø –
Use ointment, for piles & ulcers.
Protargol ø –
Use tincture twice daily in gonorrhoea and syphilitic chancres.
Picric Acid 2x –
Ointment of this drug is best for burns.
Ricinus Communis ø –
Massage on breast to induce secration and increase of milk.
Rumex Acetosa ø –
For epithelioma of face, rub gently on face of its ointment.
Ratanhia ø –
locally tincture is very efficacious in reatal complaints.
Rananculus Bulb. ø –
Apply tincture to heal of affected leg in chronic sciatica.
Rhus Glabra ø –
Locally to soft spongy gums, aphthae, pharynagitis.
Sabina ø –
Its tinature is very beneficial for warts.
Sabadilla ø –
Apply on the scalp for head-lice.
Sulphurous Acid ø –
Wash the whole face for acne, with lotion. Use also for pastular eruptions in beard.
Stellaria Medis ø –
Apply its lotion for chronic rheumatic pains, stiffness of joints, gout.
Saxonite 1x ø –
For eczema, burns and scalds, sores and bleeding piles, use its ointment.
Sempervivum Tectorum ø –
Locally, use its tincture for bites of insects, stings of bees and for poisoned wounds and warts.
Selaginella ø –
Tincture externally for bites of snakes and spiders.
Teucrium Marum (dry powder) –
Locally, for polypi.

Tanic Acid ø –
Checks haemorrhages, apply with tincture.
Thiosinamine 1x –
Great success has been gained for dissolving scar tissue, tumor, enlarged glands, lupus, by applying the ointment.
Ustilago maydis ø –
Very efficacious for psoriasis.
Vinca Minor ø –
For eczema, use its ointment.
Vanila Planifolia ø –
Apply tincture on scalp with water for hair-wash.
Viola Odorata ø –
Magically reliaves pains for bee-stings.
Veratrum Viride ø –
Use its lotion in rheumatic swelling and corn inflammation & erysipelas.

Chapter - 15
BIOCHEMIC MEDICINE

Schüsslerism comprises twelve tissue remedies. The most preferable potencies according to the gradation are :
1. Calcarea Fluorica — 12X, 200X, 30X, 6X.
2. Calcarea Phosphorica — 6X, 12X, 30X, 3X.
3. Calcarea Sulphurica — 6X, 12X, 200X.
4. Ferrum Phosphoricum — 12X, 6X.
5. Kali Mutiaticum — 6X, 3X, 12X.
6. Kali Phosphoricum — 6X, 3X, 12X.
7. Kali Sulphuricum — 6X, 12X, 30X.
8. Magnesia Phosphorica — 3X, 6X, 12X.
9. Natrum Muriaticum — 12X, 30X, 200X.
10. Natrum Phosphoricum — 3X, 6X, 12X, 30X.
11. Natrum Sulphuricum — 6X, 12X, 30X, 3X.
12. Silicea — 12X, 6X, 30X, 200X.

Frequency of Doses
A dose every hour or two, in acute cases ; in severe painful affections, a dose every fifteen minutes ; in chronic affections, one to four doses daily.
The external use of the remedies in suitable cuases is indicated and has been found efficacious. Only the lower triturations are used for this purpose.

Maxim of Combinations
All phosphates may be adminstered in a single combined prescription and likewise all muriates and all sulphates. The combination of sulphates with muriates or of muriates with phosphates is not justified. Only silicea can be mixed will all other tissue remedies.

Materia Medica of Twelve Tissue Remedies

CALCAREA FLUORICA (CF)
Characteristic Indiations — Affections of surface of bones, enamel of the teeth, and the part of all elastic fibres. Indurations. Knots, kernels and hardened gland in the female breasts. Fissure of rectum. Aching in the lumber region. Nodes on the legs.
Guiding Symptoms — Large indurated tonsils.
The chief remedy in true croup.
The useful remedy for varicose veins.
Fissures or cracks in the palms of the hands.
Indurated glands of stony hardness.
Swelling or indurated enlargements, having their seat in the fasciae and capsular ligaments of joints or in the tendons.
Adminstration — The higher potencies give the best results, especially in affections of the bones. It can be used externally in such diseases as fissura ani, bony growths, haemorrhoids,

varicose veins and whitlow. It is applied by dissolving about 20 grains of the desired potency in half a glass of water and applying it on cotton.

CALCAREA PHOSPHORICA (CP)

Characteristic Indications — The sphere of action of the remedy includes all bone diseases. Is of use in defective nutrition. Is also of use during dentition, in convulsions and spasms occuring in weak. Has restorative power after acute diseases. Pains where bones form sutures or symphyses and numb, crawling pains with chilliness, due to anaemic symptoms, worse from wet, tendency to perspiration and glandular enlargement. Glands inflamed and swollen. Pains worse at night. Retarded dentition.

Guiding symptoms — Headaches before and during the second dentition ; worse near the region of the sutures.

Crawling as if ice water were on upper part of occiput.
Fontanelles remain open too long, skull is soft and thin.
Complaints during teelhing ; too rapid decay of teeth.
Sore aching in the throat, with much pain in every direction on swallowing.
Chronic enlargement of the tonsils.
Craves salted or smoked meats. Much flatulence. Abdomen sunken and flabby.
Colic with green slimy undigested diarrhoea with foetid flatus. Choera infantum.

FERRUM PHOSPHORICUM (FP)

Characteristic Indications — Useful in all febrile disturbances and inflammations at their onset, especially before exudation commences.

Guiding Symptoms — Eyes inflamed, red with burning sensation, sore and redlooking and retinal congestion. Sensation as if grains of sand were under eyelids.

Fist stage of oitis ; rediating pains, pulsation in the ear.
Epistaxis, especially in children.
Ulcerated sore throat, dry, red, inflamed, with much pain. First stage of diptheria.
Vomiting of undigested food.
Vomiting of bright-red-blood.
Inflammatory stomach-ache in children from chill with loose evacuations.
Haemorrhoids, bright-red blood with a tendency to coagulate.
Incontinence of urine from weakness of the sphincter.
Acute, febrile or initiatory stage of all inflammatory affections of the respiratory tract. Rhinitis, laryngitis, trachitis, pneumonia, pleurisy. Bronchitis of young children.
Croup, for the febrile symptoms. Whooping cough with vomiting of food ; loss of voice, hoarseness.
Articular Rheumatism.
All catarrhal and inflammatory fevers during the chilly stage, rigors, heat, quickened pulse and pain.
Hyperaemia, from mechanical injuries, fresh wounds. not yet suppurating. Abscesses, boils, carbuncles and felons. Erysipelas. Measles, scarlet fevers. Suppurative processes on the skin with febrile symptoms.
Anaemia, blood-poverty want of red blood. Pre-exudative stage of inflammation.

Adminstration — Triturations of 6X and 12X are recommended by schiissler. 1X or 2X are used for anaemia. Its external application is also effective in sprains, wounds, haemorrhages and haemorrhoids.

Stool is hot, watery, profuse, offensive, noisy and sputtering.

Fistula is ano, atternating with chest symptoms, or in persons who have pain in all the joints from any change of weather.

uterine displacements with rheumatic pains.

Involuntary sighing.

Rheumatism of the joints with cold or numb feeling sensation as if parts were asleep.

Copious night sweats in phthisis.

Senile itching of the skin.

Flabby, shrunken, emaciated children. Rickets. Non-union of fractured bones.

Nasal, rectal and uterine polypi.

Symptoms worse from cold, change of weather, sensitive to cold, from getting wet.

Adminstration — The lower triturations, 3X and 6X are the potencies usually employed. Large doses ae useless and even injurious. For the aged, this remedy should not be given in the lower potencies.

CALCAREA SULPHURICA (CS)

Characteristic Indications — Cures purulent discharges from the mucous membranes and purulent exudations in serous sacs. The presence of pus with a vent is the general indication. Hastens suppuration.

Guiding Symptoms — Pimples and pustules on the face.

Gum-boils.

Painless abscesses about the anus in cases of fistula.

Burning itching of soles of feet.

Herpetic eruptions all over.

Yellow thick and lumpy mucous discharge in cough, leucorrhoea, gonorrhoea etc.

Administration — The most common potencis for internal use are the 6X and 12X. Low potencies are very efficacious in purulent eye troubles. Also useful externally in such affections as felons, ulcers and abscesses.

KALI MURIATICUM (KM)

Characteristic Indications — For the second stage of inflammation of serous membranes with fibrinous exudations in the interstitial connective tissues. White or gray coating at the base of the tongue, white or gray exudations, glandular swellings, discharges or expectorations of a thick, white fibrinous phlegm.

Guiding Symptoms — Chronic catarrhal conditions of the middle ear. Closed Eustachian tubes. Snapping and noises in the ear.

The sole remedy in most cases of diptheria.

Constipation where fat food disagree.

Diarrhoea after fatty food.

Chief remedy in chronic cystitis and puerperal fever. Useful in glandular swellings, follicular infiltrations.

Watery discharge from the nostrils.

Small ulcers in mouth, inflammed gums.

All the stomach and abdominal symptoms are worse after taking fatty food, pastry or any rich food.

The rheumatic and other pains are increased by motion.

Adminstration — Triturations like 6X and 12X are schissler's preference. Recommended in burns, boils, carbuncles, skin affections, warts etc. to be externally applied on lint dressing.

KALI PHOSPHORICUM (KP)

Characteristic Indications — Conditions arising from want of nerve power, as prostration, exertion, loss of mental vigor, dipression. Neurasthenia. Is restorative in mascular debility following acute diseases.

Guiding Symptoms — Hysteria from sudden emotions. Brain-fag from overwork. Depressed spirits, general irritability. Loss of memory. Nervous dread without any special cause.

Cerebral anaemia. Pains in weight in the back of the head, better while eating.

Ulceration of membrana tympani and middle ear suppurations when discharges are foul, inchrous and offensive.

Thick yellow discharge from the nose.

Excessive dryness of tongue in the morning.

Noisy, offensive flatus.

Amenorrhoea with depression of spirits, lassitude and general nervous debility.

Leucorrhoea scalding and orange-coloured.

Intense sexual desire after menses.

Enuresis in larger children. Urine quite yellow like saffron.

Puerperal mania, childbed fever.

Paralytic or rheumatic lameness, with wtiffness after rest, yet becoming better by gentle motion.

Itching of palms and soles.

Neuralgic pains occurring in any organ, with depression, failure of strength, sensitiveness to noise and light, improved during pleasant excitement, and by gentle motion, but most felt when quite or alone.

Paralysis of any part of the body. Paroxysms of pain with subsequent exhaustion. Spinal anaemia from exhausting diseases.

Alopecia areata. Itching of the inside of hands and feet.

Atrophy, wasting diseases with putrid stools. Gangrenous conditions. Septic haemorrhages.

Cold air aggravates all pains.

Administration — Both the lower and higher potencies seem to work best.

KALI SULPHURICUM (KS)

Characteristic Indications — Yellow mucous discharges. Rise in temperature at night producing an evening aggravation. Another guiding indication is amelioration in the cool, open air. Chronic rheumatism of joints. Yellow coating on tongue.

Bloated, full sensaton in abdomen ; must loosen clothing, walk about and constantly pass flatus.

Menstrual colic. Membranous dysmenorrhoea.

Chorea, involuntary movements and contortions of the limbs.

Febrile symptoms, chills run up and down the back with shivering.

Pains < on the right side, from cold and > by warmth and bending double.

Administration — Most recommended potency is 6X trituration, which acts best when given in hot water. In colic, the 30X potency in water with frequent doses is very efficacious.

NATRUM MURIATICUM (NM)

Characteristic Indications — Used in chronic scrofulous ailments affecting the glands, bowels and skin. It acts upon he blood, lymphatic system, the mucous lining of the digestive tract and upon liver and spleen. Cures malnutrition, anaemia and emaciation. Mucous membrane everywhere are affected, with secretions of transparent, watery, coarse, forthy mucus. The tongue has a clean, shiny appearance, or bubbles of frothy saliva extend along its sides or is broad, pallid, puffy, with a pasty coat.

Guiding Symptoms — Melancholia at puberty. Brain-fag.

Hypochondriacal mood, readiness to shed tears, consolation aggravates. Depression with tendency to swell on disaggreeable and depressing subjects.

Hammering headache, generally worse in the morning. Itching eruptions on margin of hair at the nape of the neck.

Useful in blephritis, sunstroke and for muscular asthenopia.

Cracking of ears when chewing.

Old nasal and phryngeal catarrhs with loss of smell and taste.

Chronic sore-throat, with feeling of lump and great dryness of the throat.

Guiding Symptoms — Patient is very irritable but timid.

Yellow crusts on the eyelids, yellowish or greenish purulent discharge from the eyes.

Earache, with discharge of watery or yellow matter.

Great rattling in the chest, ratting of mucus with cough.

Neuralgic or rheumatic pains are shifting, wandering and flitting in nature.

Great aggravation in the evening and in a heated room. Amelioration in the cool air.

Adminisstration — The best results are obtained by 6X and 12X potencies. In febrile conditions it must be given frequently. It is applied externally in dandruff and diseases of the scalp.

MAGNESIA PHOSPHORICA (MP)

Characteristic Indications — Is best adapted to lean, thin, emaciated persons of the highly nervous organization, and prefers light complexion and the right side of the body. Pains are relieved by warmth and pressure. Antispasmodic, hence is curative in cramps, spasms, tetanus, epilepsy and paralysis agitans.

Guiding Symptoms— Headache, after mental labour, always relieved by the application of wormth.

Orbital and supraorbital neuralgias, worse on the right side and relieved by warmth.

Neuralgic pain, made worse bywashing face and neck in cold water.

Toothache > by heat and hot liquids.

Severe pains in decayed teeth. Complaints of teething children.

Hiccough. Regurgitation of food.

Enteralgia. Flatulent colic forcing patient of bend double, > by rubbing, warmth, pressure, accompanied with belching of gas which given no relief.

Flatulent colic of children and the newborn.

Waterbrash, water coming up into the throat, not acid. Violent thirst for large quantities. Ravenous hunger. Heartburn after eating. Aversion to bread.

Haemorrhoidal constipation. Torn, bleeding, smarting feeling after stool, which is hard, difficult and crumbling, with stitches in the rectum.

Uterine troubles > by lying on back, on a pillow.

Backache relieved by lying on something hard.

Emaciation while living well.

Intermittent fever after abuse of quinine, living in damp regions.

All skin affections with watery blisters or vesicles and thin whitish scales. Effects of insect-bites. Nettlerash and itching appears after bodily exertion.

Adminstration — Sixth potency is of great choice. The homoeopathic school recommends the higher potencies. It may be externally applied in such disseases as the stings of insects.

NATRUM PHOSPHORICUM (NP)

Characteristic Indications — Diseases of infants suffering from overfeeding with milk and sugar. Ailments with excess of acidity. Thin and moist coating on the gontue. The soft palate also has a yellowish, creamy look. Sour eructions, sour vomiting and greenish diarrhoea. Acts upon the bones and scrofulous glands, lungs and abdominal organs.

Guiding Symptoms — Acid taste in the mouth. Yellow, creamy coating at the back part of the roof of the mouth.

Difficult speech. Moist, creamy or golden-yellow coating at the back part of the tongue.

Nausea and vomiting of acid fluids and curdled masses. Stomachache from presence of works.

Habitual constipation with occasional attacks of diarrhoea in young children.

Intestinal thread-worms with symptoms of acidity or picking of the nose. Itching at the anus from worms.

Sweling of glands of neck. Goitre.

Itching all over body, like insect bites.

Jaundice (Use 1X trit). Marasmus of children. Exudations and secretions yellow, honey-coloured.

Adminstration — Schiissler recommends the 6X potency. though the higher and highest potencies have also been employed with success. It may be used as an injection in worm troubles.

NATRUM SULPHURICUM (NS)

Characteristic Indications — Is of great use in liver affections, sand in the urine, diabetes, gout, figwarts. Its complaints are those that are brought on by living in damp houses, basements and cellers. Asthmatic complaints are worse in wet weather. The chief characteristic is a dirty greenish-gray or greenish brown coating on the root of the tongue and aggravation from lying on the left side.

Guiding Symptoms — Mental troubles arising from a fall or other injuries to the head. Suicidal tendency, must exercise restraint.

Bitter taste in the mouth, full of slim, thick and tenacious, white, must hawk up constantly.

Liver engorged, worse lying on left side.

Flatulent colic, with cutting pains in abdomen.

Chronic gonorrhoea and sycosis.

Humid asthma, rattling of mucus, developing from bronchial catarrh. Spinal meningitis, with drawing back of the neck and spasms in the back.

Tendency to warts around eyes, scalp, face, chest, anus, etc.

Ailments of hydrogenoid constitution. General aggravation from lying on the left side.
Adminstration — 6X trituration.

SILICEA (SIL)

Characteristic Indications — Acts prominently upon bones, joints, glands, skin and mucus surfaces, producing malnutrition. Suited to imperfectly nourished constitutions, owing to deficient assimilation. It is the remedy for ailments attended with pus-formation and is closely related to all fistulous burrowings. Silicea ripens abscess, since it promotes suppuration. Ailments affecting the periosteum. Cures chronic gouty rheumatic affections.

Guiding Symptoms — Headache from nape to vertex, more on right side, < by noise, exertion, light, study and relieved by warmth.

Lachrymal fistula. Styes, Boils and cystic tumorr around eyes and lids.

Itching of nostrils. Sneezing ; coryza, nasal catarrh.

Toothache : at night, when neither heat nor cold gives relief.

Large abdomen in children, constipation, if stool recede after having been partly expelled.

Menses are associated with icy coldness over whole body and constipation and foetid foot sweat.

Whitlow. Habitual foetid perspiration of the feet. Nails crippled and brittle. Tonic spasm of the hand when writing. Painful tonic spasm in the feet and toes during a long walk.

Exhaustion with erethism.

Febrile symptoms consist of chilliness all day, heat in afternoon and all night with burning in feet. Sweat at night, with loss of apptite and prostration. Offensive sweat of feet.

Skin heals with difficulty and suppurates easily.

Amelioration by heat and warm room and in the summer.

Adminstration — Schüssler recommends the 6X and the 12X potencies, but in the homoeopathic school the most brilliant results have followed the use of the higher attenuations. Apply externally in carbuncles, ulcers, bascess and ozaena as a spray.

BIOCHEMIC THERAPEUTICS

Abscess — FP, KM, NS, SIL., CS, KP, CF.
Addison's Disease — NM.
Amenorrhoea — KM, KP, KS, NK, CP.
Anaemia — FF, KM, KP, CP, NM, NP, SIL., NS.
Aneurism — FP, CF.
Angina Pectoris— KP, MP, FP.
Aphonia— FP.
Arthiritis— NM, FP, KM, KS. MP, SIL., NS.
Asthma— SIL., NS, KS, KM.
Atrophy (Marasmus)— NM, CP, SIL.
Backache— NM, KP, CP, MP.
Bites of Insects— NM.
Bronchial Catarrh— NM, FP, SIL., CS.
Burns— KM, NP. CS.
Chicken Pox— FP.

Cholera— FP, KP, CP, MP.
Chorea— MP, SIL., NM, CP.
Colic— MP, NS.
Constipation— NM, KM, FP, NP, SIL.
Cough— KM, MP, KS, NM.
Croup— CS, CP, KM.
Delirium— NM, KP.
Dentition— CP, CF, FP, MP.
Diabetes Mellitus— NM, NS, KP.
Diarrhoea— FP, KP, NP, NM, SIL., NS.
Diphtheria— KM.
Disentery— KP, KM, MP.
Dysmenorrhoea— MP, NM.
Earache— FP, KM.
Epilepsy— KM
Erysipelas— NP, FP.
Exophthalmic Goitre — NM
Fever— FP, KM, KS, NM, KP.
Fistula in Ano— CP, CS.
Gall-Stones— NS, CP, MP.
Glandular Affections— SIL., KM, CF.
Gonorrhoea — NP, FP, NM
Haemorrhage — FP, KP, CF, SIL.
Headache — KP, FP, SIL., NM.
Hiccough — MP, NM.
Hoarseness — KS, FP, KM.
Hydrocele — CP, CF, SIL.
Hydrocephalus — CP
Hysteria — KP, NM.
Influenza — NS, KP.
Intermittent Fever— NS, NM.
Leucorrhoea— CS, SIL., NM, KM.
Mechanical Injuries — FP, KM, SIL.
Measles — KM, KS, FP.
Meningitis — CP, NS, FP.
Mouth Affections — KM, KP, NP.
Mumps — FP, KP, MP.
Orchitis— CF, FP.
Paralysis — KP, MP.
Phthisis — CS, CP, NM, SIL., FP.
Pleaurisy — CS.
Pneumonia — FP, KM, SIL.
Rheumatism — KM, FP, KP, NP, KS, CP.
Rickets — SIL., CP.
Sciatica — KP, NM, SIL.
Speticaemia — KS.

Sore Throat — KM, FP, NM.
Spermatorrhoea — NP, KP.
Sunstroke — NM
Syphilis — KM, SIL., NK.
Tonsillitis — FP, MP, SIL., KP.
Tumors — CF, KS, SIL.
Thyphoid Fever — KP, FP.
Ulcers — SIL., KM.
Urinary Disorders — FP, KP, NP.
Vertigo — KP, NS.
Vomiting — FP, NM, NS. CP.
Writter's Cramp — NP, KM.
Whooping Cough — FP, MP, KM.
Worms — CF, FP, KM.

BIOCHEMIC REPRETORY

MENTAL AFFECTIONS
Anxiety : CP, NP, KP.
Consolation, aggravated by : NM.
Delirium tremens : FP, KP.
Emotions, sudden hysteria from : KP.
Forgetfulness : MP, CP.
Hallucinations : KP.
Impaired memory : CP
Insanity : FP, SIL.
Loss of consciousness, sudden : CS.
Loss of memory : KP.
Night terrors, in children : KP.
Sighing : NM, KP.
Somnambulism : KP.
Talk while asleep : KP.
Weeping, disposition to : KP.

HEAD, SCALP AND SENSORIUM
Bald spots : KS, CP.
Brain, Violent pains at base of : NM.
    Water in : KP.
Congestive Headache : SIL., NM, FP.
Dandruff : KM, KS, NM, MP.
Effects of falls or injuries to head : NS.
Eruptions on scalp, itching : NM
Falling out of hair : KS, NM, SIL.
Hair, painful on combing it : FP, NS.
Headache, accompanied by, vomiting of bile : NS.
    constipation : NM

colicky pains : NS.
    nausea : CF.
    flatulence : CP.
Headache, before and after menses : NP.
    after menses : NM.
Headache, aggrevated by, cold : CP
    heat : CP.
    reading : NS.
Headache, ameliorated by, gentle motion : KP.
    nosebleed : FP
    wrapping up head wormly : SIL.
    Headache, catarrhal : NM
    chronic : CP, SIL.
    during, dentition : CP.
    menses : NM, NS.
    from sun heat : FP.
    on awaking in morning : NP.
Migraine : NM, SIL.
Mouth full of saliva : NM
Open fontanelles : SIL., CP.
Sweat of head in children : CP, SIL.
Trobbing in the head : FP.
Vertigo : CP, FP, NS, SIL.
Vomiting, of sour froth : NP.
    of undigested food : FP.
Yellow crusts on scalp : CS.

EYES
Abscess of cornea : CS, SIL., KM.
After injuries to eye : CS.
Agglutination of lids : NP, SIL.
Black spots before eyes : KP.
Blepharitis : NM, SIL.
Boils around lids : SIL.
Conjuctivitis, acute : CF, FP, NM, NP, KS,
    chronic : NS.
Cystic tumors around lids : SIL.
Diplopia : MP, KP.
Drooping of eye-lids : KP.
Eyes, itching : MP.
    styes on : SIL.
Glucoma : NM.
Hemiopia : CS.
Iritis : KM, NM.
Keratitis : CP, NM.
Lachrymation, acrid : NM

burning : NP
Nystagmus : MP.
Obstruction of tear-duct : NM.
Onyx : KM.
Ophthalmia, discharge creamy : NP.
    neonatorum : KS.
Photophobia : CS, KM, MP, NS.
Purulent discharge from eyes : CS, KS.
Redness of eyes : FP, NM.
Soreness of eye-balls : KP.
Trochoma : KM.
White, mucus discharge from eyes : KM.

EARS

Discharges from ear, yellow : KP.
    foetid : Kp
Earache, with sharp, stiching pain : FP
    worse in damp weather : NS.
Excessive flow of blood to ear : FP.
Inflammation, of external ear : FP, KM.
    middle ear : Km.
Itching in auditory canal : KP, NM.
Muco-purulent discharges : FP.
Otalgia : FP.
Otorrhoea : KS, SIL., KP, CP.
Otaitis, suppurative : CS, KP, SIL.
Polypoid excrescence closing meatus : KS.
Tinnitis Aurium : KP, FP, KM, NS, NM.

NOSE

Acrid discharge from nose : SIL.
Catarrh, acute : FP, KM.
    chronic : NM, SIL.
Catarrhal fever : NS, FP.
Coryza, Chronic : SIL.
    clear watery : NM.
    dry : CF, NM.
Discharges, tinged with blood : CS.
Edges of nostrils sore : CS.
Epitaxis, bright red blood : FP.
    during menses : NS.
    from coughing : NM.
Hawking of mucous from posterior nares : KP.
Ineffectual desire to sneeze : CF.
Nasal polypi : CP.
Obstruction of nose : KS, KM.

Ozaena : CF, CP, KP, SIL.
Perverted sense of smell : MP.
Predisposition to catch cold : FP, SIL.
Syphilitic ozaena : NS.
ulcerated nose in scrofulous children : CP.
White around nose : NP.
Acne : KS, KM, CS, SIL.
Cheeks, swelling of : CS.
    sore : FP.
Chin, eruptions on : NM
Cutting pains in face : MP
Epilhelioma : KS.
Face, pimples on : KP, CS.
Forehead, pustular eruptions : NM.
Itching of face : NM, KP.
Loss of power of facial muscles : KP.
Lupus : CP, SIL.
Prosopalgia : NP, MP.
Spasmodic neuralgia : MP.
Tic Douloureux : FP.

MOUTH

Acid taste : NM, NP, SIL.
Aphthae : KM.
    with much salivation : NM.
Blisters, pearl-like, at corners : NM.
Breath offensive : KP, NM.
Children, white ulcers in mouth of : KM
Desquamation of lips : KS.
Gum-boils : CF, SIL., KM, NM.
Lockjaw : MP.
Noma : KP.
Perforating ulcer of palate : SIL.
Salivation : NM, KP.
Stomatitis : KP.
Trismus : MP.
Uvulitis : NM.

TONGUE AND TASTE

Acid Taste : NP.
Bitter taste in morning : CP
Coating on tongue, brownish : KP, NS.
    cracked : CF.
    white-furred : KM.
Dry tongue : KP, NM
Glossitis : FP.

Loss of taste : NM.
Mapped tongue : NM, KM.
Speech difficult : NP.
Ulcers on tongue : SIL.

TEETH AND GUMS
Bleeding of gums : KP, NM.
Complaints during teething : CP.
Decay of teeth, pain in : KP.
Dental fistulae : SIL.
Gums, Blisters on : NS.
    inflamed : CP.
Spongy : KP.
painful : KS, Cp.
Looseness of teeth : CF, SIL.
Ranula : NM.
Teething ailments during pregnancy : CP.
Toothache, after warm food : FP.
   alternates with frontal headache : KP.
   ameliorated by, cold : FP.
      hot liquids : MP.
Toothache, changes place rapidly : MP.inflammatory : FP.
   neuralgic : MP.
   rheumatic : CS.
Ulceration of gums : NM

THROAT
Burning of throat : FP, CP.
Chronic sore throat : NM.
Deglution painful : FP.
Diptheria, first stage : FP.
Dry throat : FP, NM, NS.
Fillicular Pharyngitis : KM, NM.
Goitre : CP, CF, SIL., NP.
Laryngismus stridulus : MP.
Mumps : NM.
Suffocative feeling in throat : MP.
Throat, covered with tough mucus : KS.
   feeling of lump in : NM, NS, NP.
   sore, of singer : CP, FP.
   ulceraled : FP, KM, NM.
Tonsils, enlarged : CP, KP.
   inflamed : FP, KP.
Voice : Loss of : KP.

GASTRIC

Acidity : NP
After eating, regurgitation of food : MP.
Aversion, to bread : NM.
    fat food : NP, KM.
    meat : SIL., FP.   milk : FP.
    sour food : FP.
    sweets : KP.
Bilious colic : NS.
Colicky pains : KS.
Cavings, bitter : NM.
    eggs : CP.
    salt : NM
    sweets : SIL.
Dyspepsia, acid : NP.
    flatulent : MP.
Eructations, bitter : KP
    sour : NS, KP.
Flatulence, excessive accumulation of gas in stomach : CP.
Gastritis : FP, KM.
Gastralgia, relieved by warmth and bending double : MP.
Haemorrhage from stomach : KM, FP.
Heartburn, after eating : NM, SIL.
Hiccough : MP, CF, NM.
Infant vomits as soon as it nurses : SIL.
Loss of appetite : FP, KM, NP, KP.
Nausea : KS, NP.
    and vomiting : MP.
Stomach, haemorrhage from : KM.
Ulceration of stomach : NP.
Waterbrash : NP, NM, KP.

ABDOMEN AND STOOL

Abdomen, colic : MP.
    gas accumulation : NS.
    swollen : KP, MP.
Anus, fissured : SIL., NM.
    fistula in : CS, SIL.
    itching at : CP, NP.
painless : KP.
Dysentery, bloody : KP.
    very painful : MP.
Enteritis : FP, KP.
Haemorrhoids, bleeding : CF, KM.
    Chronic : CP.
Hernia : CP.
Ineffectual urging to stool : KS.

Intestinal ulcer : CS.
Large abdomen in children : SIL.
Noisy offensive flatus : KP, CP.
Proctalgia : NM.
Prolapus ani : CS, KP, FP.
Stool, black : KS.
Clay-coloured : KM.
    green : NS.
    knotty : NS
    painful : FP.
    rice-watery : KP.
    scanty : NP.
Tenesmus : KP.
Undigested stools : FP
Ulcers, intestinal : CS.
Worms : NP, FP, KM.

URINARY
Albuminuria : KM, KS.
Bleeding from urethra : KP.
Burning, during urination : NS.
    after urination : NM.
Cystitis : FP, KM.
Enuresis, nocturnal : MP, KP.
Gravel : CP, NS
Haematuria : FP.
Incontinence of urine : CP.
Ischuria : FP.
Kidneys, pan in : FP
Retention of urine : MP
Supression of urine : FP.
Urine, brick duct sediment : NS, SIL.
    bloody : NM.
    copious : CF, CP.
    emits pungent odor : CF.
    pus and muscus : NS.
    uric acid, excess of : KM, SIL.
Vesical neuralgia : MP.

MALE SEXUAL ORGANS
Balanitis : KS.
Bubo : CS, FP
Chordee : MP, NP
Chronic Syphilis : SIL., NM.
Desire, sexual, gone : NP.
Discharge of prostatic fluid : NM.

Emissions, during stool : NM
Erethism, sexual : SIL., NP.
Genitals, itching of : NS.
Gleet : KS
Gonorrhoea : NP.
discharge bloody : KP.
Purulent : CS.
Hydrocele : SIL., CF.
Impotence : KP, NM.
Induration of testicles : CF.
Loss of pubic hair : NM
Masturbation : CP.
Orchitis : CP, FP.
Spermatorrhoea : CS, NP, KP, SIL.

FEMALE SEXUAL ORGANS
Amerrhoea : KP.
Breast, hard knots in : CF.
Displacement of the uterus : CF.
Dryness of the vagina : NM, FP.
During mense, headache : NM.
Dysmenorrhoea, membranous : MP.
Itching of vulva : NM, SIL.
Leucorrhoea, corroding : NM, NS.
like white of eggs : CP.
profuse : SIL.
scalding : KP.
watery : NM, NP.
Masturbation in children : CP.
Menses, black : KM.
    last too long : CS
    strong odor : KP.
    every two weeks : CP.
    sacnty : KP, KS.
Metrorrhagia : KS, SIL.
Nymphomania : CF, SIL., CP.
Oophortis : FP, MP.
Prolapsus uteri : CF, KP.
Vaginismus : FP, MP.

PREGNANCY AND LABOR
Childbed fever : KP.
Convulsions, puerperal : MP.
Loss of hair during childbirth and lactation : NM.
Morning sickness, vomiting of undigested food : FP.
Nipples crack and ulcerate easily : SIL.

Phlegmasia alba dolens : NS.

RESPIRATORY
Asthma, bronchial : KS, KM.
Bronchitis : FP, CS.
    chronic : NM, SIL.
Catches cold easily : FP, NM.
Chest, rattling of mucus in : KS, NS, KM.
Congestion of lungs : FP.
Cough, acute : KM, FP.
    causes headache : NM.
    chronic : CP.
    dry : FP.
    spasmodic : MP, KM.
whooping : KS, FP.
Croupy Hoarseness : KS.
Dyspnoea : FP, NM, KS, CP.
Empyema : CS, SIL.
Expectoration, copious : KS.
    coughed up with difficulty : NM.
    frothy : KP.
    purulent : NS, CS.
    yellowish : CF.
Frequent hawking : CP.
Intercostal muscles sore : NP.
Involuntary urination when coughing : FP, NM.
Laryngitis : FP, KM.
Phthisis : CS, SIL., FP, NP.
Pleurisy : FP, NM, KM.
Pneumonia : KM, CS, SIL., FP.
Spasmodic closure of windpipe : MP.
Suffocative cough, in children : CP.
Voice, loss of : KM, FP.

CIRCULATORY
Angina pectoris : MP, KP.
Chronic heart disease : SIL.
Endocarditis : FP.
Lymphangitis : FP.
Pains at base of heart : NP.
Palpitation, with anxiety : CP, NM.
    feels pulse in different parts of the body : NP.
Pulse, irregular : KP.
    rapid : NM, SIL.

BACK AND EXTREMITIES

Arthritic rheumatism : NP.
Back, pain in, low down : CF.
    between scapulae : CP
Backache, aggravated by motion : SIL.
    ameliorated by lying on something hard : NM
Bruised feeling all over : KP.
Chilblains : KM, KP.
Chronic swelling of legs : KM.
Coccyx hurts after riding : SIL.
Emaciation of neck in children : NM.
Excruciating pains in joints : MP.
Extremities numb : NM, CP.
Felon : CS, FP.
Hamstrings, painful contractions of : NM.
Hangnails : NM.
Involuntary jerking during sleep : NM.
Joints, chronic rheumatism of : CP, NM.
Knees, inflamed : CF.
Locomotor ataxia : NS, SIL.
Muscular weakness : KP.
Neuralgic pains in limbs : KS, MP.
Panaritium : CS, FP.
Rheumatism, aggravated by motion : FP
        change of weather : CP.
    ameliorated by gentle motion : KP
Sciatica : KP, NS, MP.
Slow in learning to walk : CP.
Stiffness of body : KP.
Strans of ligaments on tendons : FP.
Sweat of axillae or feet offensive : SIL.
Tonic spasms of hands and feet : SIL.
Wounds suppurating : CS, SIL.

Nervous

Adynamia : KP.
Chorea : NM, MP.
Depression, nervous : KP.
Facial paralysis : KP.
Globus Hystericus : KP.
Involuntary movements : MP.
Lockjaw : MP.
Neuralgia, inflammatory : FP.
    like electric shocks : CP, MP.
Night terrors of children : KP.
Shooting along nerves : NM, MP.
Spasm, titanic : CP, MP.
Tic Douloureux : FP.

Trembling of the body : CP, KP, NS.
Writer's cramps : CP, MP, NP.
Sleep and dreams
Children cry out during sleep : CP.
Dreams, lascivious : KP.
Excessive sleep : NM.
Insomnia : NM.
sleeplessness, after exhaustion : MP.
    from nervous irritation : NM.
Somnambulism : KP, NM.
Unrefreshing sleep : NM.

FEVER
Catarrhal fever : FP, KM.
Fever, entric : KS, FP, KM.
    inflammatory : FP.
    puerperal : KM.
    rheumatic : KM, NM.
    typhoid : KS, KM, NM, FP.
Perspiration, about head : SIL.
    profuse : KP.
    while eating : KP.
Rigors : FP.
Yellow fever : NS, FP, KP.
Abscess : SIL., KM, CF.
Acne rosacea : CP, NP.
Alopecia areata : KP.
Boils : MP, CS, KM
    tendency to : SIL.
Chicken-pox : FP, NS.
Dandruff : NM, KS, KM.
Eczema, with yellow-greenish watery vesicles : NS.
    white scabs : CP.
Eruptions, herpetic : CS
Erysipelas, phlegmonous : SIL.
    vesicular : KM.
Freckles : CP.
Hair Falls out : KS, NM.
Hang-nails : NM
Insect-bites : NM
Itching of skin all over body : NP, MP.
Jaundiced skin : NS, KM.
Measles : FP, KM.
Naevus : FP.
Prurigo : CP.
Pustules, malignant : KP, SIL.

Skin, bleeds when scratched : CS.
    dirty : NM.
    scales on : NS, KM.
    watery vesicles : NM.
Tubercles on skin : CP.
Vaginal pruritus : CP, NS.
Warts on palms : KM, NM.
Wrinkled skin : CP.

TISSUES
Abscess, of gums : CF, SIL.
Anasarca : NM.
Bedsores : KP.
Breasts, tumors in : CP.
Burns : CS, KM.
Cancer : KP, CP.
Dropsy : SIL., NM.
Ecchymoses : KM.
Indurations : CF.
Marusmus : CP, NP.
Onychia : SIL., CF.
Scurvy : KM, KP.
Septicaemia : KP.
Tuberculosis : NP, SIL., CP.
Ulcerations, fistulous : SIL., CF.
    purulent : SIL.
Wounds suppurating : CS.
Modalities
Aggravation, night : SIL.
    motion : KM, FP, CP.
    morning : NS.
    from change of weather : CP.
        eating rich food : KM.
        getting wet : CP.
        suppressed foot-sweat : SIL.
    damp weather : NS
    heated room : KS.
    when alone : KP.
Alelioration, by bending double : MP
    cold : FP
    eating : KP.
    gentle motion : KP.
    lying down : CP
        on something hard : NM.
    pressure : MP.
    rubbing : CF.

in cold open air : KS.
    dry weather : NS.
      worm room : SIL.

MENTAL ORGANOTHERAPY

Chapter - 16
PSYCHIATRY : THEORY & PRACTICE

Module - I

THE CLINICAL EXAMINATION

Psychiatric Examination : The examination of the informal mental status should begin immediately and includes an evaluation of the patient's use of language, content of discussion, appearance, mood and affect and manner of relating. During the interview, the physician should make observations about the following : i) Appearance ii) Attitude iii) Behaviour and phychomotor activity iv) Emotional state of the outward expression of the patients internal emotional state.

v) Speech, i.e. Tone of speech, amount of speech, speech impairments and aphasia vi) Perception vii) Judgement viii) Content of Thought ix) Cognition and Sensorium x) Thinking Process

The clinical laboratory tests has become increasingly important in the diagnosis and treatment of psychiatric illness. *Screening tests for organic illness are :*

L. F. T., SGOT, SGPT.
Blood urea nitrogen.
Thyroid function tests.
Vitamin B12 and folate levels.
Arterial blood gas analysis.
Electroencephalography (EEG).
Dexamethasone suppression test.
TRH Stimulation Test.
Sleep Polysomnography
Positron Emission Tomography.
Intelligence and personality have to be measured by psychological tests :
a) Intelligence tests. (IQ)
b) Minnesota Multiphasic Personality Inventory. (MMPI)
c) Thematic Apperception Test. (TAT)

Module - II

SCHIZOPHRENIC DISORDERS

Men tend to suffer schizophrenia earlier than women. Women tend to have a better prognosis for schizophrenic disorders in many parts of the world. Onset usually occurs in late adolescence or early adulthood, although cases continue to appear with decreasing frequency throughout adult life. Return to independent living and social and occupational functioning is often more common than complete remission of symptoms. Socio-economic status is correlated with the prevalence and incidence of schizophrenia as well as its course.

Diagnostic Subtypes of Schizophrenia

1. Catatonic - Catatonic negativism which is an apparently motiveless resistance to all instructions or attempts to be moved.

2. Disorganized - This does not involve organised delusions or catatonic features, marked by the following features : i) Grossly disorganized behaviour,

ii) Incoherent speech and marked loosening of associations.

iii) Flat inappropriate affect.

3. Residual - Patients who have experienced at least one psychotic episode, continue to experience disability from symptoms.

i) Odd beliefs or magical thinking.

ii) Overelaborative speech,

iii) Marked lack of initiative, interest or energy.

iv) Marked impairment of role functioning,

v) Unusual perceptual experiences.

4. Paranoid - Delusional and hallucinatory synptoms are often organized around a single theme. Social and occupational functioning may be well preserved. Diagnostic criteria are as follows : a) Absence of incoherence. b) Absence of marked loosening of associations.

5. Undifferentiated - Criteria for diagnosis are as follows :

i) Grossly disorganised behavior.

ii) Prominent delusions and hallucinations.

6. Others - These categories were not included in the general types for a variety of reasons, including overlapping catagories and lack of diagnostic reliability.

I. Schizoaffective disorder.

II. Hebephrenic.

III. Paraphrenia.

IV. Oneiroid.

V. Pseudoneurotic.

Complications :

1. Many schizophrenics are unable to complete educational plans after the onset of illness despite normal or high intelligence.

2. Due to impaired work performance, schizophrenics may have significant difficulties finding employment, particularly during economic depressions.

3. They may enter the criminal justice system, referred to as the criminalization of the mentally ill.

Treatment :

Group therapy has long been a mainstay of the treatment of schizophrenic patients in both inpatient and outpatient settings. Psychosocial rehabilitation has become a significant part of treatment programs of schizophrenia because raturning patients to productive lives in the community has become a priority. However, neuroleptic medications have revolutionized the treatment of schizophrenia.

Module - III

ORGANIC MENTAL SYNDROMES

An organic mental syndrome is the manifestation of transient or permanent brain tissue dysfunction. Behavioral and psychological abnormalities vary due to variability in the area of the brain that is affected the mode of onset, the progression, the duration and the nature of the pathophysiologic processes.

There is a failure of normal metabolic processes, cerebral insufficiency in all cases of organic mental syndrome. Derangement of cerebral functioning may result from a number of following pathophysiologic or biochemical processes :

1. Interference with macromolecular synthesis.
2. Deficiency of fuels for oxidative metabolism.
3. Impaired mechanisms of release, conservation, and use of chemical energy.
4. Disruption of the process of synaptic transmission.
5. Significant alterations in electrolyte content, hydration, pH and osmolarity.
6. Disruptions of brain anatomy or disequilibrium in functionally related systems.

Module - IV

MOOD DISORDERS

Instead of remaining angry with the lost individual, the anger is turned inward by the depressed person. Sigmund Freud emphasized the importance of loss in depression. He felt that this phenomenon accounted for the typical findings of guilt, lowered self-esteem, self-reproach and suicidal ideation. He did not explain all depression in this manner. He clearly stated that some depression is psychogenic in origin and in other cases biologically determined.

Diagnosis :
The diagnostic categories of major depression and bipolar disorder
Symptoms of a manic syndrome

a) Hyperactivity - Some manic individuals accost strangers and attempt to engage them in conversation or in unrealistic schemes. Affected individuals make elaborate plans and engage in numerous endeavors. They are always doing something or anticipating what they will do next.

b) Elevated or intensified mood - Some patients are euphoric, extremely cheerful or happy. They have little ability to lolerate frustration and irritability may progress to hostility, belligerence and assaultiveness.

c) Rapid shifts in mood - When depressed, they may act on sudden suicidal impulses. This mingling of manic and depressive syndromes is referred to as bipolar disorder, in which aspects of each syndrome become part of an ongoing clinical picture.

Treatment :
1. Lithium Carbonate.   2. Tricyclic antidepressants.
3. Monoamine Oxidase (MAO) inhibitors.
4. Electro -Convulsive Therapy. (ECT).

Laboratory Tests :
1. Dexamethasone suppression test.
2. Thyrotropin-releasing hormone (TRH) stimulation test.
3. Sleep polysomnography.

Module - V

ANXIETY DISORDERS

Anxiety was viewed primarily as a psychological response to internal or external stress. However, biologic factors are thought to play a role in some types of anxiety.

Endogenous anxiety occurs spontaneously without any indentifiable precipitating stress. Eight stages of endogenous anxiety include :

i) Generalized phobic avoidance.
ii) Depression.
iii) Spontaneous and sudden subclinical anxiety attacks.
iv) Gradual progression to full-blown panic attacks.
v) Hypochondriacal fears of occult disease,
vi) Development of anticipatory anxiety that unpredictable anxiety will result,
vii) Abuse of drugs or alcohol to control anxiety.
viii) Phobic avoidance of situations in which panic attacks occur or from which escape might be impossible if panic did occur.

Psychological components of anxiety :
1. Situational anxiety.
2. Anxiety about death.
3. Separation anxiety.
4. Stranger anxiety.
5. Anxiety about mutilation, loss of prowess and loss of attractiveness.
6. Anxiety about dependency.
7. Anxiety about loss of control.
8. Anxiety about loss of self-esteem.
9. Signal anxiety.
10. Anxiety about intimacy.
11. Anxiety about being punished.
12. Anxiety about the emergency of another effect.

Treatment :
Supportive psychotherapy.
Expressive psychotherapy,
Systematic desensitization.
Biofeedback.
Antidepressant drugs,
MAO inhibitors,
Beta-blocking agents

Module - VI

PERSONALITY DISORDERS

Personality - the set of characteristics that defines the behavior, thoughts and emotions of an individual.

Ego-syntonic symptoms, whereby patients do not recognize that anything is wrong with them that needs to be changed. They view existing disturbances as being the result of the world being out of step with them. Ego-dystonic symptoms, whereby patients may be experiencing internally distressing symptoms, which are self-induced, but they are still unable to alter their behavior.

Clinical Picture :

In general, patients with personality disorders tolerate stress poorly, and they do not seek help to change their characters but to alleviate the outside stress. If stress is great, as it can be in physical illness, patients may regress even more and can develop transient psychotic reactions in which they loss touch with reality and become unable to function for brief periods of time. These patients may seek help as a result of a concurrent medical or surgical problems or because of a primary emotional distress ; in any case, these patients may elicit strong negative reactions in the physicians and other health care personnel who take care of them.

Social relationships are disrupted or absent altogether. Because indiduals with personality disorders can be irritating and infuriating to those involved with them, the reactions to personality disorders by these involved
individuals are often more pronounced than the disorder itself in the affected person.

Module - VII

SUBSTANCE USE DISORDERS

Substance use disorders must be carefully defined at the outset because terms such as drug abuse, addiction, and dependence evoke social disapproval and are variously defined within different cultures. Pathologic use of centrally acting substances is divided into the categories of psychoactive substance dependence and abuse.

Categories of substance abuse and dependence :
1. Cocaine
2. Alcohol.
3. Narcotics.
4. Anxiolytics.
5. Nicotine.
6. Sympathomimetics.
7. Cannabis.
8. Inhalants.
9. Hallucinogens.

Module - VIII

CHILD PSYCHIATRY

Child psychiatry is the study and treatment of the mental and behavioral problems of childhood. As such it overlaps with a variety of pediatric subspecialities. An understanding of standard childhood development is essential to the understanding of childhood psychopathology, since seeming major difficulties may be normal at certain ages.

Childhood psychosis
A. Autistic disorder :
1. Language abnormalities include echolalia.
2. Have a great need for consistency in their environment.
3. Social development is usually abnormal.
4. Decreased nystagmus in response to vesti-bular stimulation.

B. Childhood Schizophrenia :
1. Propensity to disgrace with poor attention span.

2. Preoccupation with grotesque fantasies.
3. Unusual mannerisms.
4. Possible abnormal motor movements.

C. Symbiotic Psychosis :
1. Parents misperceive themselves as their child.
2. Loss of ego boundaries.
3. Great anxiety at the threat of separation of the child from the parent is seen in both.

Childhood Depression :
1. Child between the ages of 7 and 30 months demonstrate anaclitic depression.
2. Preschool children who are depressed often show depressive equivalents.
3. Biologic vulnerabilities and a sense of helplessness or incompetence may play role at the age of school-going children.
4. Adolescents also demonstrate the usual signs of depression, especially a pervasive sense of boredom and lack of future orientation.

Sleep Disorders :
1. Somnambulism.
2. Night terrors.
3. Nocturnal enuresis.
4. Cataplexy.
5. Hypnagogic hallucinations.

Eneuresis :
1. Diurnal enuresis occurs during the waking hours.
2. Nocturnal enuresis is a parasomnia occuring during stages 3 and 4 of sleep.

School Phobies :
1. Vulnerable child syndrome.
2. Homosexual panic in an older child.
3. Malingering.
4. Separation anxiety suffered by the child.

Attention-deficit Hyperactive Disorder (ADHD) :
1. Excitability.
2. Impulsivity.
3. Short attention span.
4. Distractibility.
5. Difficulty concentrating.

Learning Disorders :
1. Interfere with the child's ability to perform certain intellectual functions.
2. Language disabilities.
3. Developmental dyslexia.

Child Abuse :
This occurs when the individuals in a child's environment retard his or her development by hurting the child.

PSYCHIATRIC ORGANOTHERAPY

Chapter - 17
MENTAL PHILOSOPHY

MENTAL DISEASES
Almost all the so-called mental and emotional diseases are nothing more than corporeal diseases in which the symptom of derangement of the mind and disposition peculiar to each of them is increased, whilst the corporeal symptoms decline (more or less rapidly), till it at length attains the most striking one-sidedness, almost as though it were a local disease in the irrisible subtle organ of the mind or disposition. (Organon of Medicine, Aphorism : 215, Samuel Hahneman).

Mental diseases are one-sided psychic deviations affecting the entire psycho-somatic architecture where the symptoms of derangement of mind and disposition are increased while the physical symptoms aggravate.

CLASSIFICATION OF MENTAL DISEASES

I. Somato-psychic : Mental diseases aggravating with the decline of corporeal diseases which threatens to be fatal :
The cases are not rare in which a so-called corporeal disease that threatens to be fatal - a suppuration of the lungs, or the deterioration of some of the other important viscus, or some other disease of acute character, e.g., in childbed etc. becomes transformed into insanity, into a kind of melancholia or into mania by a rapid increase of the physical symptoms that were previously present, whereupon the corporeal symptoms lose all their danger.

TREATMENT

1. Construction of the complete picture of the disease.
a) Collection of all the symptoms of the previous corporeal diseases before it become a disease of psychy and disposition, taking help from the report of the patients' friend.
b) Accurate collection of present symptoms of disposition and psychy, observed by the patients' friend and by the physician himself.
2. Selection of medicine.
A medicine having antipsoric miasm should be sought for which is capable of producing striking similar symptoms on psychosomatic sphere.

II. Suddenly appearing mental diseases :
If, however, insanity or mania (caused by fright, vexation, the abuse of spirituous liquors) have suddenly broken out as an acute disease in the patients' ordinary calm state, although it almost always arises from internal prora, like the flame burning forth from it, yet when it occurs in this acute manner it should not be immediately treated with antipsorics, but in the first place

with remedies indicated for it out of the other class of proved medicaments (e.g., aconite, belladonna, stramonium, hyoscyamus, mercury etc.) in highly potentized, minute, homoeopathic doses, in order to subdue it so far that the psora shall for the time revert to its former latent state, wherein the patient appears as if quite well.

TREATMENT

1. These cases should be treated by admins-tering highly potentized, minute homoeopathic doses of proved acute medicines (e.g., aconite, belladonna, stramonium, hyoscyamus etc.) having similar psychic state in their pathogenisity.
2. Antipsoric treatment of prolonged time should be continued for the prevention of recurrance.

III. Doubtful origin mental diseases :
If the mental disease be not quite developed and if it be still somewhat doubtful wheather it really arose from a corporeal affection, or did not rather result from faults of education, bad practices, corrupt morals, neglect of the mind superstition or ignorance, the mode of deciding this point will be, that if it proceed from one or other of the latter causes it will diminish and be improved by sensible friendly exhortations, consolatory arguments, serious representations and sensible advice.

TREATMENT

1. Identification of the cause
Mental affection of psychic aetiology will be improved by sensible exhortations, consolatory arguments and sensible advice.
2. Selection of medicine.
  a) Psychotheraphy
     i) Free-Association
     ii) Dream-Analysis
     iii) Cathersis
     iv) Abbreaction
  b) Anti-psoric medications
  c) Appropriate diet and regimen.

IV. Psycho-somatic : Mental diseases aggravating from prolonged emotional causes :
There are, however, as has just been stated, certainly a few emotional diseases which have not merely been developed into that form out of corporeal diseases, but which, in an inverse manner, the body being but slightly indisposed, originate and are kept up by emotional causes, such as continued anxiety, worry, vexation, wrongs and the frequent occurrence of great fear and fright. This kind of emotional diseases in time destroys the corporeal health, often to a great degree.

TREATMENT

1. Treatment by means of psychical homoeopathic remedies will be of great help.
2. Reestablishment of health will be obtained by suitable diet and regimen.
3. Radical anti-psoric treatment should be continued in order to prevent recurrance.

APHORISM

If the antipsoric remedies selected for each particular case of mental or emotional disease be quite homoeo-pathically suited for the faithfully traced picture of the morbid state, which, if there be a sufficient number of this kind of medicines known in respect of their pure effects, is ascertained by an indefetigable search for the most appropriate homoeopathic remedy all the more easily, as the emotional and mental state, constituting the principal symptom of such a patient, is so unmistakably perceptible,then the most striking improvement in no very long time.

Mental Symptom Materia Medica

PSYCHIATRIC DIAGNOSIS

1. Great fear and anxiety of mind, with great nervous excitability ; afraid to go out, to go into a crowd where there is any excitement or many people ; to cross the street. - **Phobic Anxiety Disorder.**

2. Sensation of a cloud enveloping her. Great depression, with dream of impending evil. Fears riding in a closed carriage, of being obliged to jump out. - **Claustrophobic Obsessional Psychoneurosis.**

3. Loss of memory ; cannot remember names of books, persons or places, arithmetical calculation difficult. - **Psychogenic Amnesia.**

4. Constantly dwelling on suicide. Profound melan-choly : feels hateful and quarrelsome ; desire to commit suicide ; life is a constant burden. - **Psychotic Depression.**

5. Mental delusions, as if everything about her were small ; all persons physically and mentally inferior but she is physically large and superior. - **Passive-aggressive Delusional Grandeur Personality.**

6. In writing uses too many words or not the right ones ; omits final letter or letters in a word ; cannot concentrate the mind to read or study. - **Psycho Somatic Verbal Amnesia.**

7. Mental excitability ; ecstasy, with almost prophetic perceptions ; with a vivid imagination ; great loquacity wants to talk all the time ; jumps from one idea to another one word often leads into another story. - **Catatonic Excitement with Schizophreniform Disorder.**

8. Imagines he sees ghosts, hideous faces and various insects ; black animals, dogs, wolves. Fear of imaginary things, wants to run away from them. - **Acute Hallucinatory Paranoia.**

9. Fixed ideas : as if a strange person were at his side : as if soul and body were separated, as if a living animal were in abdomen ; of being under the influence of a superior power. - **Psychogenic Paranoid Delusion.**

10. Incessant and violent fidgety feeling in feet or lower extremities ; must move them constantly. - **Ideokinetic Hyper-apraxia.**

11. Changeable humor ; one moment laughing, the next crying ; "sudden change from grave to gay, from lively to serene". - **Cyclothymic Personality Disorder.**

12. Illusion of a mouse running from under her chair. - **Illusory Psycho Neurosis.**

13. Strange temper, laughs at serious matters and is serious over laughable things. Thinks herself a demon; curses and swears. - **Schizophrenic cyclothymia.**

14. Irritable ; peevish and cross on walking ; ugly kick and scream ; easily angered ; cannot endure opposition or contradiction ; seeks disputes ; is beside himself. Weeps all day, can't calm herself; very sensitive, even cries when thanked. - **Maniac Depressive Psychoses.**

15. Lascivious mania : immodesty, will not be covered, kicks off the clothes, exposes the person ; sings obscene songs ; lies naked in the bed and chatters. - **Obsessional Depressive Psycho Neurosis.**

16. Faints easily ; after getting wet ; from extremes of heat or cold ; riding in a carriage; while kneeling at church. - **Neurasthenic Hysteria.**

17. Oversensitiveness ; all the senses more acute, light, hearing, smell, taste, touch unusual activity of mind and body. - **Organic Ideomotor Apraxia.**

18. Profound depression of spirits, can hardly avoid weeping ; is very timid, fearful and weeps much ; indifferent about what is being done for her. - **Implicit Depressive Psychosis.**

19. After continued loss of sleep, long-lasting anxiety, over-exertion or mind and body from nursing the sick ; anguish from the loss of his dearest friend : indifference ; tired of life ; sadness before menses. - **Anxiety Neurosis.**

20. Weakness of memory , cannot remember names, words or initial letters ; has to ask name of most intimate friend ; even forgets his own name. - **Organic Retrograde Amnesia.**

21. Great sadness and weeping. Dread of being alone ; of men ; of meeting friends ; with uterine troubles, Indifferent: even to one's family ; to one's occupation to those whom she loves best. - **Psychogenic Hypochondriasis.**

22. Melancholy mood ; sad, hopeless, from care, grief, sorrow ; with weeping, "the least thing makes the boy cry." - **Functional Mental Involutional Melancholia.**

23. Restless, anxious, does everything in great haste ; must change position often ; everything startles him. The countenance is expressive of fear; the life is rendered miserable by fear; is sure his disease will prove fatal ; predicts the day he will die ; fear of death during pregnancy. - **Phobic Implicit Anxiety Syndrome.**

24. Lack of confidence in himself and others ; feels as though he had two wills, one commanding him to do what the other forbids.- **Asthenic Personality Disorder.**

25. Amiable in disposition if feeling well, but easily disturbed by very slight emotion ; easily offended. Mental conditions rapidly, in an almost incredibly short time, change from joy to sorrow, from laughing to weeping. - **Obsessive Cyclothymic Personality Disorder.**

THERAPEUTIC INDEX
of
Homoeopathic Medicines for Psychiatric Diseases

A
Abarognosis - Cimex ; Kali Oxalicum ; Scutellaria Lat. Acanthesthesia - Can. Sat. ; Stannum ; Merc. Cyanide.
Sycotic Co.
Adrenal Virilism - Atrop. Sulph. ; Bufo. ; Elaps Cor. ; Zinc. Mur.
Agoraphobia - Boletus Laricis ; Formica Rufa ; Sil. Ahypnia- Calc. Iod. ; Helonias ; Lyssin ; Ustilago.
Alethia - Corydalin ; Juncus Eff. ; Sedum Acre.
Alzheimer's Disease - Botulin ; Daphne Ind.; Lithum Phos. Lupulus ; Merc. Dul. ; Ova Tosta ; Phloridzin; Pinus Rubra ; Rosa Centi. Sapo Dome ; Stilling in ; Typha Lat.
Amaurosis - Kali Chloricum ; Myricin ; Sticta Pul.; Thymol.
AmentiaCarduus Cryspus ; Gum Oliban ; Plumb. Iod. ; Urea Pura.
Anxiety - Canna Glauca ; Cuprum Ass. ; Ephedrin.; Ferrum. Pyrophos. ; Gelsemin ; Hura Brasil.; Iris Florentina ; Irisin ; Kali Carb. ; Ononis Spinosa; Phos. Piper Nig. ; Silica Marina.
Aztec **Idiot** - Croton Tig. ; Geum Urban. ; Matico ; Sepia.

B
Beard's Disease - Apocynin. ; Myrrhae Gummi ; Psorinum.
Bell's Mania - Abies Excelsa ; Pix Liquida ; Titanium.
Bradyphrenia - Pavia Ohioensis ; Rhodium ; Senega ;
Ulmas Fulva.
Bruxomania - Bromoform ; Galium Aparine ; Sulph ; Tilia Europoea.
Bulimia - Cuprum Cyanide ; Ergotin : Ledum ; Nupher Advena.

C
Cacopathia - Actaea Spicata ; Haematin ; Senecio Aureus.
Cataplexy - Acid Hydrocyan ; Bebeerine ; Quercus Alba ; Selenium.

Cephalalgia - Kali Benz.; Syphil. ; Tuberculinum Rosen. **Claustrophobia** - Arg. Oxydat. ; Baryta Mur. ; Ingluvin ; Yerba Reuma.
Compensation Neurosis - Barbus Fluviat. ; Cimicifuga ; Oxalis Acetosa
Cotard's Syndrome - Eupat. Perf. ; Gossypin. ; Merc. Cyanat.
Creutzfelitt-Jakob Disease - Adonidim ; Dirca Pal. ; Salix Alba.
Cyclothymia - Acid Mur. ; Aurum Iod. ; Dam.ana ; Gelsemin ; Iridium Chloride ; Koch's Lymph ; Magnesia Carb. ; Myrtus Chekan.; Niccolum Sulph. ; Quassin. ; Trional.
Cynophobia - Filix Mas. ; Granatum. ; Petroleum ; Rumex Acetosa.

D

Dacnomania - Apocynum Can. ; Carboneum Sulph. ; Pancreatin.
Demensia - Aluminia Oxide.; Anthemis Nobilis.; Bapticin ;
Cactus G.; Calc. Formate ; Coffea Tosta ; Escoba Amergo ; Fel Touri; Lippa Mexicana ; Repens' Zinc. Carb.
Demonophobia - Cicuta Vir. ; Kali Nit. ; Natrum Iod. ; Pyrocarbon.
Down's Syndrome - Radium Chloride ; Scirrhinum ; Vanila.
Dysthymia - Arg. Cyanatum ; Coffea Tosta ; Nux Mos. ; Tabacum.
Dystrophoneurosis - Chin. Phos. ; Grindelia Rob. ; Moschus ; Zinc. Brom.

E

Emetomania - Bismuth Subnit. ; Corydalin ; Kali Benz ; Pepsin.
Epileptic Furor - Cornus Florida ; Iodoform ; Myricin ; Plat. Mur.
Erotomania - Carboneum. ; Chin. Ars. ; Natrum Acet. Exhaustion **Psychosis** - Agraphis Nutans ; Ferr. Brom ; Meloe Majaslis.

F

Free-floating Anxiety - Morgan Compound ; Passiflora ; Pinus Rubra.
Furor Uterinus - Caffeinum. ; Hedera Helix ; Inula. ; Phos. Iod.

G

Galactosaemia - Abies Nigra ; Calc. Lactophos. ; Nicotinum ; Slag.
Gelineau's Syndrome - Boletus Satanas ; Desmodium Gan. Indigo.
Geromorphism - Chin. Bi-sulph. ; Kali Phos. ; Opuntia Vulgaris.
Guilt-neurosis - Bufo Vulgaris ; Elas Cor; Malva Sylvestris; Thymol.
Gynaephobia - Coffeine Citrate ; Ferr. Val. ; Lathyrus Cicera ; Vitrum. Alb.

H

Hallucination - Aeon Ferox ; Cuprum Ars.; Lachesis ; Oleum Ricinis.
Hebephrenic Dementia - Juncus Eff. ; Kali Nit. ; Psrorinum. **Hurler's Disease** - Myricin. ; Nuphar Lat. ; Odonte Necrosin.
Hydrocephalic Imbecile - Croton Tig. ; Myrrhae Gummi; Petrol.
Hyperthymia - Abeis Excelsa ; Carya Alba ; Nat. Iod. ; Sepia.
Hypokinesia - Bromoform ; Filix Mas. ; Radium Chloride
Idiocy - Ammom. Brom.; Digitalin ; Medorrhin. ; Stannum Iod.

I

Imbecile - Acid Oxalicum ; Quercus Alba ;   Trional ; Zinc Carb.
Insanity - Aurum Iod. ; Cactus G. ;   Fel Tauri ; Radium Chloride.
Insomnia - Coffea C. ; Cyprip.; Daphne Indica; Passiflora ; Sumbul.
Involutional Psychosis - Acid Tart. ; Barosma   Crenata ;
Duboisia Myop. ; Ingluvin ; Lithium ; Cltricum ; Nigella Sativa ; Ozaenin ; Pinus Sylvestris ; Rous Sarcoma.
Jargon Aphasia - Kalmia Lat.; Pituitrin. ; Ranan. Repens.
Jocasta Complex - Cydonia Vulg. ; Escoba Amargo. ; Titanium.

J

Juvenile Chorea - Melilotus Alba ; Phos. Amor. ; Rubia Tinctoria.

K

Kainophobia - Carduus Cryspus ; Ephedrin. ; Sfachys Betonica.
Kinaesthetic Aura - Amyl. Nit. ; Calc. Silicata ; GumOliban ; Sepia.
Kleptomania - Curare ; Plumb. Carb. ; Rhus Radicans ; Zinc. Iod.
Korsacoff's Syndrome - Glechonia Hedera ; Kali Brom,
; Picrotoxin.

L

Lagneia Furor - Cadmium Brom. ; Doryphora ;   Pastinaca Sat.
Lasegue's Syndrome - Antipyrin ; Gadus Morrhua ; Pareira Brava.
Libido-damning - Bismuth Carb. ; Ephedra Vulg. , Usnea Barbata.
Lypemania - Euonymin.; Mimosa Humulis; Rubus Villosa.; Squilla.

M

Mai Du Siecle - Baryta Phos. ; Myrtus Chekan ; Yerba Reuma.
Mania - Adonidin ; Ingluvin ; Trit. Repens ; Vanila
Marchiafava's Disease - Carboneum Sulph ; Radium Chloride
Melancholia - Angelica Atrop. ; Canna Angust. ; Erythrinus ;
Eserinum Sulph ; Grind. Squar. ; Marmorak ; Nux Mos. ; Pimp. Saxif. ; Raphanus Sat. ;Ulmus Fulva.
Micropsychia - Cornus Circinata; Saponin ; Stan. Mur. Tongo.
Motor Alexia - Carboneum Oxy. ; Duboisine ; Geum Urban; Myricin.

N

Narcomania - Arg. Cyanat. ; Kali Benz, ; Meloe Majalis , Wyethia.
Neumann-Pick's Disease - Boletus Sot. ;   Typha Lat. ; Zinc. Mur.
Neurotic Anxiety - Bufo Vulg. ; Odonte Nercosin ; Piper Nig.
Nymphomania - Murex Perp. ; Robinia ; Stan. Mur. ; Trichos. Dioica

O

Obsessional Psychoneurosis - Angop. Lance. ;   Epilob. Pal. ;Stan. Iod.
Oneirodynia - Apocynin. ; Dioscorea Vil. ; Indium Met.

Organic Amnesia - Cerium Oxal.; Ocim. Grst,; Stramonium.
Osmolagnia - Bismuth Val. ; Mag. Met; Thyroidin ; Typha Lat.
Oxygusia - Asparagus ; Kali Hypophos ; Phenacitin ; Urtica Dioica.

P

Pantaphobia - Coccus Cacti; Homarus ; Luffa Amara ; Ruta G.
Paralytic Dementia - Ephedrin. ; Ferrum Pysophos ; Sedum Acre.
Paranoia - Baryta Nit. ; Cadmium lod.; Juglandin; Kali Caust.; Lobelia Erinus; Millefolium ; Natrumi Lact. ; Oleum Gaul.; Petrol.; Ptelea Trif. ; Rosa Damascena ; Vipera Torva.
Parkinson's Disease - Boletus Laricis ; Helonias ; Nupher Lut.
Pica - Helonin ; Kali Brom., Lycopus Virg. ; Pix-Liquida.
Pituitary Cachexia - Alumina Oxide ; Kali Nit.
Post-hypnotic Psychosis - Acid Mur. ; Barbus Fluviat. ; Quassin.
Presbyophrenia - Calc. Formate ; Elatrin ; Rhus Ven ; Salix Alba.
Presenile Dementia - Bapticin. ; Koch's Lymph ; Zinc.Carb ; Iris Florentina ; Lyco. ; Mag. lod. ; Niccolum Met. ; Rumex Acetosa ; Stillingin ; Xanthium Spin.
Psychalgia - Kali Nit. ; Oxalis Acetosa ; Stan lod. ; Selenium.
Psyclampsia - Abies Excelsa; Haematin. ; Quercus Alba ; Piperin.
Psychogenic Nocturnal Polydipsia - Ingluvin ; Oxalis Acetosa.
Psychoparesis - Ambra Grisea ; Carduus Cryspus ; Micromeria.
Psychoprophylaxis - Apis Virus ; Asclepin ; Caffeinum ; Cornin ; Diphtheria Antitoxin ; Hepa-tica.; Lithium Phos.;
Titanium; Uranium Met. ; Zinc. Met.
Pubertas Praecox - Digitalin; Escoba Amargo ; Pyrocarbon
Pykno-epilepsy - Cuprum Phos. ; Iris Germ ; Nasturt Off.

Q

Quasi-psychotic State - Kali Oxal. ; Nuphar Lut. ; Silica Marina.
Quiescence - Acid Butyric. ; Marmorek ; Phloridzin.

R

Raptus Maniacus - Acid Tart. ; Daphne Indica ; Rous Sarcoma.
Rendu's Tremor - Curare ; Gadus Morrhua ; Usnea Babata
Retrograde Amnesia - Cadmium Brom. ; Nat. Murbit. ; Rubus Villosa.
Rhypophobia - Antipyrin;MelilolusAlba; Mimosa Humulis ; Squilla.

S

Saint Mathurin's Disease - Arg. Cyanat. ; Juncus Eff ; Tongo.
Schizo-affective Psychosis - Hyos. Hydro.; Nigella Dam. ; Typha Lat.
Schrizophrania - Baryta Phos. ; Galium Aparine ; Ulmus Fulva.
School-phobia - Cuprum Cyanide ; Gossypin. ; Yerba Reuma.
Semantic Aphasia - Boletus Sat.; Geum Urban. ; Sedum Acre.
Senium Praecox - Adonidin. Myrtus Cheken ; Syphil. ; Varatrin.
Sexual Neurasthenia - Acon Radix. ; Caffeine Cit. ; Upas Tieute.

Simmond's Disease - Alumina Oxide ; Fel Tauri; Nat. rod.
Somnambulism - Ammon Brom. ; Lobelia ; Thea Sinensis ; Trional.
Status Choreicus - Plumb. Carb.; Rhus Radicans ; Zinc. Iod.
Stewart - Moral Syndrome -Ceanothus Amer. ; Equiset. Arv. ; Homarus ; Kali Cyanatum ; Lithium Hipp.; Methylene Blue ; Ononis Spinosa ; Phytolaccin ; Taxus Baccara.
Stupor - Angust. Spuria ; Grind. Squar.; Saponin. ; Urtica Dioica.
Syncopal. Attack - Cornus Circin. ; Kali Nit. ; Vinca Minor.

T

Tachyphrenia - Merc. Dulc.; Pinus Rubra ; Stachys Betonica.
Tay-Sach's Disease - Atrop. Sulph.; Formica Rufa ; Hura Brasil.
Thanatophobia - Acetic Acid ; Canna Glauca ; Matico ; Uva Ursi.
Tonaphasia - Abies Exceisa ; Pavia Ohioensis ; Tuber. Rosen.
Torsion Neurosis - Damiana ; Mag. Carb. ; Rumex Acetosa.
Tremor Opiophagorum - Apocyn. Can. ; Cicuta Vir. ; Fel Tauri.
Tyrannism - Arg. Oxydat. ; Carya Alba ; Thea Sinensis.

U

Uncinate Epilepsy - Acid Oxalic. ; Quercus Alba ; RhusVen.
Urolagnia - Kali Benz ; Mag. Iod.; Piperin ; Triticum Repens.

V

Vagabond Neurosis - Filix Mas. ; Lippa Mexicana ; Pituitrin.
Verbal Agraphia - Duboisia Myop. ; Nigella Sativa ; Squilla.
Visual Alexia - Plumb. Carb. ; Stachys Betonica ; Rhodium.

W

Wernicke's Aphasia - Kali Brom. ; Rubia Tinct.; Titanium.
Wilson's Disease - Amyl Nit. ; Barosma Crenata ; Koch's Lymph.
Windigo Psychosis - Aurum Iod.; Digitalin. ; Yerba Reuma.
Writer's Tremor - Cuprum Cyanide ; Escoba Amargo. ; Zinc. Iod.
Xenophobia - Aralia Spinosa ; Nat. Acet. ; Psorin. ; Sycotic Co.
Xerophobia - Ilex Opaca ; Myricin ; Zinc. Mur.

Z

Zelophobia - Acid Uricum ; Coffea Tosta ; Tabacum ; Zinc. Phos.
Zonaesthesia - Croton Tig. ; Ergotin. ; Passiflora ; Pinus Rubra.
Zooerastia - Aeon. Ferox. ; Calc. Brom. ; Kali Carb. ; Elaps Cor.
Zoophobia - Bufo Vulg. ; Merc. Cyanide; Oleum Ricinus.
Zoosadism - Abeis Excelsa ; Natrum Iod. ; Radium Chloride.

BEDSIDE ORGANOTHERAPY

Chapter - 18
BEDSIDE PRESCRIBER (POTENCY)

1. **Influenza Fever** = Bapt., Acon, Eupat Perf., Gels, R.T., China, Chin Sulph.
2. **Typhoid** = Bell, Bept, Gels, Terebinth, Bryo, Ac. Nit., Phos, RT.
3. **Hyper-acidity** = C.V., Arg. Nit, Iris.V., Puls, N.V., Ac. Sulph, Robin, Ant. C., Lob. Inf., Chamo.
4. **Indigestion** = Ancard, Lyco, N.V., Robin, Iris V., China, Puls, C.V., Ant. C., Chelid.
5. **Appendicitis** = Bell, Lach, Dios.V., N.V., Plumb. M., R.T., Colocyth, Ars., Iris Tenex, Merc. Cor., MP.
6. **Asphyxia** = Am. Carb., Ant. T.
7. **Asphyxia neonatorum** = Ant. T.
8. **Asthma** = Ars., Ant. T., Acon, Lob. Inf., Passiflora, Nat. Sulph, Sambucus N., Ipecac, Kali Carb.
9. **Inflamation (Burning) of Urinary System** = Apis, Ars., Berb. V., Canth, Dulc, Equsetu Hy., Tereb., Benz Acid.
10. **Heartburn phyrosis** = Arg. Nit., C.V., Lyco, N.M., N.V., Puls, Acid Sulph.
11. **Bronchitis** = Phos., Ant. T., Caust, Rumex, H.S., Sulph, Bryo, M.S., Dulc, R.T., Kali Bich.
12. **Bruises** = Arn., Bellis, Calendula, Hamamelis, Hypericum, Led, R.T., Ruta, Cicuta V.
13. **Burns, Scalds** = Ars, Apis, Canth, Caust, H.S., U.U., Kali Bich., Picric Acid.
14. **Boils, Curbancles** = Bellis, Bell, Sil, H.S., Aes. Hip., Lach, Taran, C. Pyroyen, Anthraxinum.
15. **Chicken-pox** = Acon, Dule, Led, R.T., Apis, Bryo, K. Mur.
    Prophylaxis = Variolinum, Vaccininin, Maladrinum.
16. **Chilblains** = Abrot, Agar, Canth, H.S., Ac. Mur., Ac. Nit, R.T., Tereb, Sil, Sulph, M.S., Apis.
17. **Cholera Infantum** = Aethusa Cyn., Podo, Cuprum Ars., Calc. P., Ver Alb., Ipecac.
18. **Colic Pain** = Acon, Arg. Nit, Bell, Chamo, China, Colo, Dios., M.P., N.V., Plumb. Met., Rheum., Ver Alb.
19. **Conjunctivitis** = Apis, Bell, Ars, Canth, Euphrasia, Heper, M.S, Puls., Arg. Nit.
20. **Constipation** = Alumina, Aesc Hip., Bryo, Calc. C., Caust., Hydrestin, N.M., N.V., Graph, Ac. Nit, Psor, Syphil, Sil.
21. **Cough** = (A) Dry = Acon, Bryo, Calc. C., Rumex, Cina, Heper., Phos, Caust, Ars. Ant Tart, Drosera, Kali Carb.
    (B) Loose = Ant Tart, C.C., Hep., Ipec, Puls, M.S., Sulph, Dulc, Nat Sulph.
22. **Dandruff** = Baryta C., Fluor Acid, Kali S., Sepia.
23. **Diarrhoea** = Aloe, Ant. C., Ars., C.V., Chamo, MS., Podo, Phos, Sulph, N.V., Acid Phos, Puls., Sep., Bryo.
24. **Dysentry** = Aloe Soc, Podo, MS, Merc Cor, China, NV., Phos, Arg Nit, Colch.

25. **Dysmenorrhoea** = Bell, Cinic, Coff., Gels, Ver Alb., MP., Puls, Gnaph, Vil Op., Colo., Ham.
26. **Dyspnoea** = Am. Carb., Ant T., Aralia R., Kali C., Nat. S., Ipec., Spongia, Samb. Nig., Hep., MS., Lob. Inf., Ars.
27. **Earache** = Acon, Bell, Chamo, Puls, MS., Plantago, Kali Bich.
28. **Eczema** = Ant. C., Ars., Crot Tig., Petrol, R.T., Kali Ars., Vinca Minor, Cic, Sepia, Merc C., Psor, Heper, Graph.
29. **Nocturnel Eneuresis** = Ac. Benz, Caust, Equisetum, Medo, Apis, Sarsa, Puls, Kreosote.
30. **Eructations, belching** = Anac, Ant. C., Lyco, Phos, N.V., Robin, Puls, C.V., China, Sulph, Graph. Nat Carb.
31. **Eye-lids agglutinated** = Ant C., MS, Puls Sulph, Graph, Euphrasia.
32. **Acne** = Kreo, Ledum, NV., Bell, Breb Aq., Psor, Kali Carb.
33. **Boils** = Arn, Bell, Bellis, HS, MS, Sil, Tar.C, Lach, Fer Iod., Sulph, Phyto.
34. **Ganglion** = Ac. Benz, Ruta, Sulph, Sil, Thuja, Calc. Flour.
35. **Stomach Pain (gastralgia)** = Ars. Arg. Nit, C.V., Chamo, Coccus, Colo, Dios, Graph, MP, NV., Plumb, Met, Ver Alb., Ox. Acid.
36. **Gastritis** = Bell, Ars, Hydras, Ipecec, Kali Bich, Phos, N.V.
37. **Gleet** = Agnus, Canth, Kali Sulph, Thuja, NM, Ac. Nit, Sabal. S., Hydras, Can Sat.

38. **Arthritis** = Led, Ac. Benz, R.T., MS, Bryo, Caust, Cimicifiza, Kali Iod.
39. **Gout** = Benz. Acid, Lith. Carb., Urtica U., Guaiacum, Ac. Uric.
40. **Gum-boil** = Calc. flour, Hekla L., M.S., Sil., Bell.
41. **Hematemesis** = Cactus., Millifol., Ham, Ipec., Geran, Phos, Sec. Cor.
42. **Haemorrhoids** = Aesc. Hip, N.V., Acid Nit, Phos., Lyco, Ars., Aloe. S., Acid Mur., Ratan., Millefol.
43. **Hair Falling out (Alopecia)** = Ars, Flouric Acid, N.M., Phos, Sepia, Selen, Graph., Acid Nit.
44. **Headache** = Gels, Glon, Bryo, Sep., Acon, Bell, Coffea C.
45. **Heartburn** = Arg. Nit., C.V., Lyco, N.V., N.M., Puls, Acid Sulph.
46. **Hiccough** = Cic, Cuprum Met., Ign, Mosch, Sul. Acid.
47. **Urticaria** = Apis, Ant. C., Urt. U., Dalc, N.M., R.T., Bovista.
48. **Hoarseness** = Acon, Bell., Phos, Rumex, Samb., H.S., Spon., M.S., Kali Bich., Arg. Met.
49. **Hydrocele** = Apis, Con, Rhodo, Puls, Spong., Sil., Flour Acid.

50. **Influenza** = Acon, Bapt, Allium Cepa, Eupat Perf., Bell., R.T., Phos.
51. **Insommia** = Coff., Passiflora, Sumb., Gels, Chamo., Can. Ind.
52. **Jaundice** = Chelid, Myrica, China, Chionanth, Podo, Taraxacum, Bryo, Lyco, Nat Phos., Phos.
53. **Infantile Jaundice** = Chamo, Myrica.
54. **Kidney Inflamation (Nephritis)** = Berb. V., Canth, Apis, Cupr. Ars., Phos, Sabad.
55. **Lachrymation** = Cepa, N.M., Euphrasia, Kali Iod., Puls.
56. **Laryngitis** = Acon, Caust, M.S., R.T., Spongia, Rumex, H.S., Bell.
57. **Lentigo** = Kali Carb., Lyco, Sepia, Sulph, Ac. Nit.
58. **Leucorrhoea** = Graph, Sep, Syphil, Kreo, Thuja, Bov., Alumina, Kali Bich, Ova Tosta, Phos, N.M., M.S.
59. **Liver Enlargement** = Chlid, China, Chionanth, N.V., Mag. Mur., Tarax.

60. **Corns** = Ant. C., Graph, Sil, Petrol, Thuja, Ac. Nit.
61. **Bromidosis (offensive sweat)** = Sil, Bapt, Psor, H.S., Nit Acid, Tellur.
62. **Liver Spots** = Arg. Nit, Caulo., Sepia., Lyco.

63. **Lumbago** = Aesc. Hip, Kali Carb., Gnaph, R.T., Sulph, Eupat Perf, Sabal Ser., Ruta.
64. **Marasmus** = Abrot, Calc. Phos., Sil.
65. **Pain in breasts (mastodynia)** = Bell., Murex., Lac. Acid., Con.
66. **Measles** = Acon, Kali Bich., Puls., Bryo., Euphrasia.
67. **Mumps** = Acon., Baryta Carb., Phyto., Sil., Bell., Merc. Cor.
68. **Nausea** = Ars., Arg. Nit, Ipec., N.V., Kreo., Puls., Ferr. Met., Kali Bich.
69. **Nipples ulcerated** = Sep., Con, Graph, Phyto.
70. **Nyphomania** = Murex., Plat., Lil Tig., Hyos. Nig.
71. **Obesity** = Calc. C., Fucus., Phyto, Phos., Thyroidin.
72. **Ophthalmia** = Acon, Euphresia., Puls., Kali Bich.
73. **Nephritis** = Berb. V., Canth, Apis., Phos., Caust.

74. **Otorrhoea** = Heper., Kali Sulph., Sil, Puls., Tellur., C.C., Bell, Chamo.
75. **Otitis Media** = Acon, Bell., K.M., M.S., Puls., Baryta Mur. Merc. Pulcis.
76. **Orchitis** = Rhodo., M.S., Bell., Spongia., Ham.
77. **Panaritium (felon)** = Bryo., Dios., H.S., Sil., Acid Flour.
78. **Whooping Cough** = Dros., Justicia, Ipec., Lob. Inf., Heper., Cuprum Met., Kali Mur.
79. **Pharyngitis** = Bell., Arg. Nit., Kali Bich., Phyto, M.S. H.B., Wyethia, Sang. Can., Baryta Carb.
80. **Nasal Polyp** = Thuja, Phos, Lemna Minor., Sang. Nit., C.C.
81. **Pruritis** = Dolicos., Anac., Crot. Tig., Rumex, U.U., R.T., Mez. Kreo., Graph.
82. **Gumboil** = Hekla L., Sil, Calc. Flour.
83. **Pyorrhoea** = Merc. Cor., Nit Acid., Sil, Staphis., Bapt.
84. **Ringworm** = Tub., Ars., Graph., Tellur., Mez.
85. **Scabies** = Crot. Tig., Psor, Sulph. H.S., Sepia.
86. **Sciatica** = Col., Plumb. Met., Gnaph., Ignatia, Phyto, R.T., Ruta.

87. **Scurvy** = Ars., Mur. Acid, M.S., Phos., Fer. Phos.
88. **Sebaceous Cyst** = Acid Benz, Con, Kali Iod., Bar. Carb.
89. **Insomnia** = Can. Ind., Coff., China., Passif., Ign. Sumbucus., Sulph.
90. **Sneezing** = Allium Cepa, Kali Iod., Sebad, Sang. Nit.
91. **Spermatorrhoea** = Agnus., Arg. Nit, Calad, Staphis., Selen, N.V., Phos., Acid Phos., Salix Nigra.
92. **Stomatitis** = Borax, Nit Acid, M.S., Acid Sulph.
93. **Ptyalism (saliva)** = Iris. V., Iod, Ipec, Nit Acid., Acetic Acid, Kali Iod.
94. **Sty** = Puls, Sil, Staphi, Graph, H.S., Sep.
95. **Tonsillitis** = Baryta Carb., Bapt, Phyto, M.S., Sil., Bell. Kali Mur, Sang.
96. **Torticollis** = Cimicifuga, Lachanthis.

97. **Urticaria** = Apis, U.U., Bov., Dulc., N.M., R.T., Ars., Ant. Crude., Nat. Phos.
98. **Vertigo** = Glon, Con, Sep., Tab., Alum, Bryo, N.V., Phos.
99. **Vomiting** = Ipec, N.V., Ars., Puls., Phos., Bismuth. Kali Bich., Iris V., Cupr. Met.

100. **Car-sickness** = Cocculus, Kreo, N.V., Petrol.
101. **Warts** = Thuja, Dulc, N.M., Caust, Ant Crude., Nit Acid, Nat Carb.
102. **Worms** = Filix Mas., Cina, Teucr., Spig., Stan, Chelone.
103. **Amenorrhoea** = Puls, Graph, Nat Mur.
104. **Angina Pectoris** = Spig, Bryo, Cactus.
105. **Anorexia** = N.V., Hydrastis, China.
106. **Aphonia** = Arg. Met, Caust, Acid Nit., Spong.
107. **Leucoderma** = Ars. Sulph Flavum.
108. **Toothache** = Bell, Chamo, Puls. Plantago., Kreo., Spigel.

Chapter - 19
BEDSIDE PRESCRIBER (TINCTURE)

1. **Hepatomegaly** = Carduus Marianus q (5d'3).
2. **Jaundice** = Myrica Cerifera q (10d '3); Chionanthus Virg q (10d'3).
3. **Dyspepsia** = Robinia q (5d'3); N.V. q (5d '3); Gentiana L q (25d '3), Pepsinum q (30d '3)
4. **Acute Gastritis** = Acon q (3d '4)
5. **Nausea** = N.V. q (5d '4).
6. **Constipation** = Hydrastis q (10d'2); Bryo q (3d'2).
7. **Worms** = Chelone q (20d'2); Filix Mas q (15d '3); T.M.V q (3d '3). (Pin worm)
8. **Anaemia** = Helonias Dioica q (5d '3).
9. **Rheumatism** = Guiacum q (20d'3); R.T. q (5d'3); Rhodo q (5d'3).
10. **Pharyngitis** = Phyto q (10d '3).
11. **Tonsillitis** = Phyto q (10d' 3).
12. **Laryngitis** = Caust q (5d'3).
13. **Asthma** = Aspidos q (25d'3); Senega q (5d '3); Lobelia q (10d'3).
14. **Whooping Cough** = Dros. q (8d '4); Corallium Rubrum q (5d'4).
15. **Menses delayed** = Puls q (5d'3).
16. **Menses irregular** = Trillium P. q (20d '2).
17. **Menses profuse** = Sabina q (10d '3).
18. **Menses painful** = Vib op q (10d '3); Dios q (10d'3);19.
19. **Leucorrhoea** = Sec Cor q (5d'3); Hamemelis q (10d '3);
20. **Diarrhoea** = Acid Phos q (10d'4); Aloe q (5d'3).
21. **Vomiting** = Vir Alb q (5d'3); Ipec q (5d'4).
22. **Conjunctivities** = Euphrasia q (5d '3); Bell q (5d'3);
23. **Headache** = Gels q (5d'3); Glonoin q (5d '3); Bryo q (5d'3);
24. **Gout** = U.U. q (10d'3);
25. **Sciatica** = Gnaphalium q (10d'3);
26. **Hiccough** = Caulo q (10d'1h).
27. **Neuralgia** = Spigalia q (5d '3); Bryo q (5d'3);
28. **Fever** = Acon q (5d'3); Gels q (5d'3); R.T. q (5d'4);
29. **Acidity** = Carica P. q (25d'3);
30. **Amenorrhoea** = Jonasia Asoka q (10d '3); Puls q (2d'3); Aleteris Farinosa q (2d'3);
31. **Spinal irritation** = Actea Rece q (5d'3).
32. **Stiffness of neck** = Lachnanthis q (3d'3); Actea R. q (5d'3);
33. **Vertigo** = Cocculus Ind q (3d '4); Gels q (5d'3);
34. **Aphonia** = Rhus Glabra q (5d'3);
35. **Colic** = Dios q (10d'4); Colo q (5d'3);
36. **Pain in liver region** = Chelidonium q (10d'3);
37. **Bed wetting** = Cina q (5d'3);
38. **Otitis** = Acon q (5d'3);
39. **Dysentry** = H. Anti-Dysenterica q (10d'3); Aloe q (5d'3);
40. **Urticaria** = U.U.q (10d'3); Apis q (10d'3);

TINCTURE (External Application)

1. Acetic Acid q – Worts, Leucoderma
2. Balsam Peru q – Scabies, Craked Nipple, Eczema.
3. Chrysophanic Acid q – Rigworm.
4. Cochleria Armoracia q – Dandruff.
5. Oleum Jacoris Aselli q – Ringworm.
6. Cinnamon Oil q – 5 drops oil with sugar relieves hiccough.
7. Rhus Glabra q – Soft spongy gum, Aphthac.
8. Sabina q – Warts.
9. Sabadilla q – Head-lice.
10. Vinca Minor q – Enzema.
11. Acs. Hip q – Piles.
12. Apis Mel q – Stings of bees & wasps.
13. Arn q – Cuts, abrasions, bruises, sprains & strains.
14. Calend q – Ulcer, wound, injury, cuts, burns, Inject vagina in Leucorrhoea.
15. Canth q – Burns, Ulcers caused by burns, Eczema.
16. Mullen Oil q – Earache, Anal fissure.
17. Plantago q – Toothache, Piles.
18. Kreosote q – Toothache, Naevus.
19. Skookum Chuck q – Eczema.
20. Echinacea q – Antiseptic wash
21. Lappa Major q – Carbuncle
22. Berb. Aqui q – Acne.
23. Hydrastis q – Corns.
24. Thuja q – Wort, Naevus.
25. Staphis q – Head-lice.
26. Lyco q – Prickly-heat.
27. Iodine q – Ringworm.
28. U.U. q – blister due to burns.
29. Ruta q – sprains & strains, bruises.
30. Ledum q – punctured wound.
31. Pytolecca q – gurgles in pharyngitis.
32. Gaultheria Oil q – Rheunatism, Gout, Scitica.
33. Hail Loss q – Jaborandi q.
34. RT. q = Sprain & Strain.

Chapter - 20
BEDSIDE PRESCRIBER
(Biochemic Remedies)

1. Indigestion = KM, FP, Sil.
2. Insomnia = KP, FP.
3. Headache = CP, FP, KP, Sil.
4. Wart = NM, NS.
5. Sty = FP, Sil.
6. Anemia = CP, NM.
7. Diarrhoea = CS, NP, MP.
8. Rheumatism = CF, NS, KP.
9. Croup = NM, MP.
10. Dysmenorrhoea = KP, MP, CP.
11. Worms = NP, KM.
12. Constipation = CS, KS., Sil.
13. Scrofuloderma = MP, CF, NM.
14. Tonsillitis = KM, CF, CP.
15. Ringworm = KS, NP.
16. Toothache = KP, NP, NS, CP.
17. Chilblain = FP, Sil.
18. Sleeplessness = KS, NS, CF.
19. Colic = MP.
20. Pruritus = CP.
21. Vomiting = FP, KM, NP, NM.
22. Rheumatism = CP, KS, MP, CS, NS.
23. Bloody Dysentry = CP, NM, FP.
24. Ricket = CP, NP, Sil.
25. Nocturnal Eneuresis = KP, NP.
26. Laryngitis = FP, KS.
27. Leucorrhoea = CP, KM, NP.
28. Acne = CS, KS, Sil.
29. Asthma = CF, FP, KM, NS.
30. Measles = KM, NM.
31. Hiccough = KM, NP.
32. Wooping-cough = CP, KM.
33. Backache = CS, NP.
34. Dyspepsia = FP, CP, MP.
35. Fever = FP, KM, MP.
36. Headache = NS, NM, CP.

Chapter - 21
FIRST-AID MEDICINE

Contused Wounds
Injury caused by the impact of some hard blunt object resulting damage to the soft tissues beneath the skin.
Give ARNICA 30 thrice daily. If it seems to be delay in the disappearance of the bruise, use LEDUM 6 three times a day after ARNICA. Also apply ARNICA lotion with ten drops of tincture to the half pint of cold water.

Incised Wounds
Skin cut by a sharp instument.
If the cut is superficial, a dressing of gauze with HYPERICUM lotion containing 10 drops of mother tincture to the half pint of water should be placed over the cut. A few doses of STAPHISAGRIA 30 can be given if the wound is causing pain.
CALENDULA 30 may be given internally twice daily in addition to the local dressing to assist healing.

Punctured Wounds
Wound caused by the needle, nail, thorn, knife, splinter etc.
Internally LEDUM 30 thrice daily. After this HYPERICUM 6 may be given if the wound is painful.

Bites and Stings
LEDUM is of very wide use in this connection. A few doses of LEDUM 30 is needed to reduce swelling, alliviate pain and counter the effects of the poison.
For a severe allergic reaction to bee stings CARBOLIC ACID 30 is advised every one hourly. If the part affected is burning and stinging with rapid swelling give APIS 30; if there is redness and burning give CANTHARIS 30; if the part is burning and blue in colour TARANTULA CUBENSIS 30 will give relief.
Apply externally a few drops of mother tincture :
for bee sting— LEDUM
for wasp sting— ARNICA
for snake-bite— HYPERICUM

Burns and Scalds
CANTHARIS 30, a dose every 10 minutes should be given to allay pain. HYPERICUM lotion with 10 drops of q to the half pint of water may be used. URTICA URENS ointment is an excellent dressing for small burns or scalds. Also URTICA URENS 30 may be taken internally as an alternative to CANTHARIS for relief of pain.

Eye Injuries
Adminster HYPERICUM 6 in hourly doses if there is much pain in the eye. For persisting pain after removal of dust or other foreign body, the affected eye should be bathed with EUPHRASIA lotion and EUPHRASIA 6 given internally.

Sprains
Give ARNICA 30 every hour for six doses. This should be followed by RHUS TOX 6 thrice daily till better. If the injury is close to bone and the periosteum is damaged RUTA 6 is to be indicated. ARINCA lotion containing 5 drops of tinctue to the half pint of water may be applied locally as a moist compress.

Asphyxia
A condition of oxygen lack due to interference with respiration.
When the patient is full of sticky phlegm with the face blue, cold and covered with clammy sweat, use ANTIMONIUM TARTARICUM 30 every fifteen minutes.
Give CARBO VEG 200 a single dose and then 30 for further doses, when the face is pale, puffy, bluish, covered with cold sweat and there is very specific symptoms of air hunger and collapse.

Shock or Collapse
When there is great hunger for air, coldness and desire to be fanned, give CARBO VEG 200 a single dose.
If the skin is cold and beads of cold sweat on the forehead, use VERATRUM ALBUM 30 a few doses.

Convulsions
BELLADONNA 200 for sudden onset of fit accompanied by violent movements.
CUPRUM MET 30 for violent convulsions with fingers flexed, thumbs clenched, jaws clenched and violent jerks and spasms.
HYOSCYAMUS 200 when fit is caused by fright accompanied by frothing at mouth.

Fainting
For the fainting attack from anger— VERATRUM ALBUM 30
from emotional upset— IGNATIA 200
from excitement— COFFEA 200
from fright— ACONITUM NAP 30
from loss of blood— CHINA 30
from sight of blood — NUX VOM 200
from sever pain— ACON NAP 200
from strong odours— NUX VOM 30, PHOS 30

Nose Bleed
VIPERA 200 a single dose is of special value in epistaxis. For profuse flow of bright red blood FERRUM PHOS 30 may be given for afew doses.

Cholera
VERATRUM ALBUM 6 for drenching cold sweats, diarrhoea and vomiting. CAMPHORA 30 complaints of burning in abdomen and extreme degree of prostration, surface icy cold with desire to be uncovered. CUPRUM MET 200 is indicated for cramps very marked, icy cold all over, wants to be covered, not sweating.

Travel Sickness

BORAX 30 is indicated for fear of downward motion, of value in air travel.
LAC DEFLORATUM 30 is a remedy used during emergencies, of value in car sickness.
All symptoms are worse riding in a carriage or on shipboard having nausea associated with loathing indicates COCCULUS 6, to be taken thrice daily before starting and during the journey.

COMPOUND ORGANOTHERAPY

Chapter - 22
COMPOUND REMEDY

A healthy organ cannot be diseased, so every effort should be made to tone and balance the affected area. Allways pay special attention to the affected organ, for it may be anticipated that the correct organ remedy or group of remedies will also eliminate the disease affecting that organ.

The dose should be twice daily for chronic states if 30-th potency are employed. When 200C remedies are adminstered the dose will be once daily. Potencies used for the acute conditions may be given hourly or even more frequently if needed.

THERAPEUTIC INDEX
Abortion (threatened)
Aletris F. 30, Calc. Flour 30 ,Caulophyl 30, Lil. Tig. 30
or
Calc. Carb. 200, Helonias 200, Nux. Vom. 200, Secale Cor. 200, Terebinth 200, Thuja Occ. 200
Alopicia
Acid Mur. 30, Zinc Met. 30, Anacard. 30, Puls. 30, Sulphur 30
or
Lyco. 30, Ceanothus 30, Artemisia Abrot. 30, Rosmarinus 30
Abscess
Bell 30 , Echinacea 30, Calc. Sulph 30, Sil 30
Acidity
Bismuth 30, Nat. Phos. 30, Robin 30, Spirea Ulm. 30, Berb. V. 30, Pimpinella 30
Amenrrhoea
Absinth 30, Mentha 30, Lil. Tig. 30Mag. Phos. 30, Murex 30
Aphonia
Polygonum 30, Lachesis 30, Ferr. Phos. 30, Borax 30
Arthritis
Rhus Tox 30, Crotal. H. 30, Colch. 30, Medo. 30, Sil 30, Cimic. 30
or
Ferr. Iod. 30, Morphin 30, Ruta G. 30, Iodium 30, Cuprum Met. 30, Kali Brom. 30
Asthma
Ratanhia 200, Thuja 200, Terebinth 200, Stannum Met. 200, Drosera 200, Kali Carb. 200
or
Bell 30, Drosera 30, Oleand. 30, Kali Phos. 30, Rumex 30, Grindel 30
Blood Pressure (High)
Glono. 30, Sumbul 30, Calc. Flour. 30, Aur. Mur. 30, Viscum. 30
Blood Pressure (low)
Gels 30, Ars. 30, Xanthox. 30
Bronchitis
Bell. 30, Drosera 30, Tussilago 30, Nat. Mur. 30, Ferr. Phos. 30

Burns
Urtica U. 30, Ferr. Phos. 30, Nat. Mur. 30, Kali Mur. 30
Cancer
Kali Ars. 200, Morphin 200, Lyco. 200, Ars. Iod. 200, Carbo. Animalis 200, Cuprum Acet. 200
Cholera
Camphora 12, Ver. Alb. 12, Phos. 12, Cuprum Ars. 12, Carbo Veg. 12, Ars. Alb 12
One dose after every motion.
or
Ars. Alb. 30, Verat. 30, Cuprum 30, Xanthox 30, Plumb. 30, Anacard. 30
Colic
Acid Mur 6, Rheum 6, Carbo Veg. 6, Ambra Grisea 6, Aethusa Cyn. 6, Helonias 6
Frequently repeat doses.
Collapse
Verat. Alb. 3X
or
Carbo Veg. 6, Acid Mur. 6, Nat. Mur. 6, Helonias 6, Ignatia 6, Sec. Cor. 6
Doses should be repeated frequently.
Common Cold
Rheum 12, Ipecac. 12, Bell 12, Kali Brom. 12, Mag. Carb. 12, Carbo Veg. 12
Conjunctivitis
Euprasia 30, Bellis 30, Acon. Nap. 30, Puls. Nig. 30, Ferr. Phos. 30
Constipation
Podo. 30, Nat. Mur 30, Berb. Vul. 30, Opuim 30
or
Ratanhia 200, Kali Brom. 200, Mag. Carb. 200, Bryo. Alb. 200, Cocculus 200
Convulsion
Chamom 30, Mag. Phos. 30, Absinth 30, Sambucus Nig. 30
Cough
Bell 30, Eupat. Perf. 30, Antim Tart. 30, Nat. Mur. 30, Conium 30
Ammon Carb. 30, Senega 30
or
Rumex 3X, Bryo. 3X, Drosera 3X, Ipecac. 3X, Bell 3X, Nat. Mur. 3X
Dandruff
Rosmarinus 30, Lyco. 30, Ceanothus 30, Calc. Sulph. 30, Pilocarpus 30, Kali Mur. 30
Deafness
Agraphis N. 30, Chenopod. 30, Quin. Sulp 30, Nat. Mur. 30, Calc. Flour 30
Debility
Chinin. Ars. 2X
Five grains of trituration three times daily.
or
China q, Agrimonia q, Xanthox q
Ten drops in water twice daily.
Diabetes M.
Lecithin 200, Morphin 200, Pineal 200, Ars. Iod. 200, Aurum. Mur. 200, Arg. Nit 200
or
Taraxacum 30, Uva Ursi 30, Nat. Phos. 30, Syzygguim 30, Berb. Vul. 30, Lyco. 30

Diarrhoea
Myrica C. 3X, Sulph. 3X, Podo 3X, Ipecac 3X, Erigeron 3X
Use after every motion.
   or
Ver. Alb. 12, Puls. Nig. 12, Thuja 12, Terebinth 12, Zinc. Met. 12, Sulph 12
Use after every motion
Diarrhoea (Chronic)
Arn. Mont. 200, Chininum Ars. 200, Cuprum Ars. 200, Ricinus 200
Phos. 200, Puls. Nig. 200, Sec. Cor. 200
Dysentery
Phos. 30, Morphin 30, Cuprum Acet. 30, Colchicum 30, Ars. Alb. 30
Dyspepsia
Nat. Phos. 30, Agrimonia 30, Bismuth 30, Ipecac 3X, Erigeron 3X
Use after every motion.
   or
Ver. Alb. 12, Puls. Nig. 12, Thuja 12, Terebinth 12, Zinc. Met. 12, Sulph 12
Use after every motion
Diarrhoea (Chronic)
Arn. Mont. 200, Chininum Ars. 200, Cuprum Ars. 200, Ricinus 200, Phos. 200, Puls. Nig. 200, Sec. Cor. 200
Dysentery
Phos. 30, Morphin 30, Cuprum Acet. 30, Colchicum 30, Ars. Alb. 30
Dyspepsia
Nat. Phos. 30, Agrimonia 30, Bismuth 30, Hyos. N. 200, Stramo. 200, Cuprum Ars. 200, Ammon Brom. 200
   or
Pilocarpus 30, Cicuta V. 30, Absinth 30, Lobelia 30, Kali Brom. 30
Arg. Nit. 30, Fucus 30
Fever
Bell 3X, Bapt Tinc. 3X, Ferr. Phos. 3X, Kali Mur. 3X
   or
Ipecac. 6, Bryo. 6, Rhus. Tox. 6, Bapt. Tinc. 6, Eupat. Perf. 6, Gels. 6
Fistula
Acid Fluor. 30, Aur. Mur. 30, Caust. 30, Calend. 30, Calc. Fluor. 30
Flatulence
Carbo Veg. 3X, Asaf. 3X, Gels 3X, Mag. Phos 3X, Colocynth 3X
Use every four hourly.
Fractures
Symphytum 3X, Eupatorium 2X, Caland. 2X, Calc. Phos. 3X, Calc. Iod. 3X, Calc. Fluor. 3X
Gastric Ulcer
Symphytum 30, Ornithog. 30, Arg. Nit. 30, Condur. 30, Kali Mur 30, Calc. Sulph 30
Gastritis
Symphytum 30, Bismuth 30, Calend. 30, Ferr. Phos. 30, Kali Mur. 30
Goitre
Acid Sulph 200, Sec. Cor. 200, Iodium 200, Kali Brom. 200, Ammon Carb. 200, Ammon Mur. 200, Sanguinaria 200

or

Iris. V. 30, Calc. Fluor. 30, Agrimonia 30, Iodium 30, Lycopus. Virg. 30

Gonorrhoea

Echinacea 30, Canth 30, Tussilago F. 30, Thuja 30, Iris Verr. 30, Kali Mur. 30, Nat. Sulph 30

Gout

Ferr. Iod. 30, Aur. Mur. Nat. 30, Ammon. Caust. 30, Ruta G. 30, Cuprum Met. 30, Phyto 30

or

Urtica U. 30, Lyco. 30, Formica 30, Ferr. Phos. 30, Menyanthes 30

Haemorrhages

Phos. 30, Acid Sulph. 30, Melilotus 30

(Take 5 drops every 15 minute intervals.)

or

Gels 6, Ambra Grisea 6, Sanguinaria 6

(Use every two hourly.)

Hernia

Cuprum Met 30, Morphin 30, Theridion 30, Ammon Carb 30, Murex 30, Lyco. 30, Baryta Carb. 30

Hiccough

Discorea 3X, Ignatia 3X, Passiflora 3X, Scutell 3X

or

Camphora q

(Take 5 drops every two hourly.)

Hydrocele

Act. Rac. 30, Apis Mel. 30, Puls. Nig. 30, Rhodod. 30, Samarium 30

Impotency

Hycrocot. 30, Kali Phos. 30, Salen. 30, Staphis 30, Xanthox 30

or

Arg. Nit. 200, Kali Carb. 200, Platina 200, Lyco. 200, Ignatia 200 Sec. Cor. 200

Indegestion

Bismuth 12, China 12, Puls. 12, Mag. Carb 12, Ambra Grisea 12, Arg. Nit. 12, Carbo. Veg. 12

Influenza

Cad. Sulph. 6X, Cinnam. 6X, Ferr. Phos. 6X, Bell. 6x, Nat. Sulph 6x, Kali Mur 6X

Insomnia

Coffea 30, Daphne 30, Absinth. 30

Jaundice

Podo. 30, Terebinth 30, Zinc. Met. 30, Sulph. 30

or

Carduus M. 3X, Chelid. 3X, Colest. 3X, Berb. Vulg. 3X, Nat. Sulph 3X

(If 3X potency fails, try items above in 30.)

Leprosy

Mezerium 200, Thuja 200, Anacard. 200, Zinc. Mt. 200, Symphytum 200

Leucoderma

Acid Picric 200, Carbolic Acid 200, Phosphoric Acid 200, Bismuth Met. 200, Zinc. Met. 200, Anacard 200, Arg. Nit. 200

Leucorrhoea

Agrimonia 30, Absinth 30, Graph 20, Lil. Tig. 30, Kali Mur. 30, Calc. Phos. 30
Low Blood Pressure
Crocus Sat. 30, Phytolacca 30, Helonias 30, Croton Tig. 30
Lumbago
Rhus. Tox. 6X, Cimic. 6X, Erigeron 6X, Nat. Phos. 6X, Ferr. Phos. 6X
(Every three hourly.)
Malaria
Antim Ars. 12, Cuprum Ars. 12, Spirea 12, Cedron 12, Sambucus 12, Acid 12, Morphin 12
    or
China 30, Pupulus T. 30, Sambucus. Nig. 30, Anacard. 30, Baptis. 30, Ferr. Phos. 30
Marsmus
Kali Iod. 30, Ars. Iod. 30, Antim Iod. 30, Aurum Iod. 30, Ferr. Met. 30, Silicea 30
Measles
Bell 3X, Euphorbium 3X, Puls. 3X, Gelsem. 3X, Ferr. Phos. 3X, Kali Mur. 3X
    or
Antim Tart. 6, Terabinth 6, Ferr. Met. 6, Carbo Veg. 6, Sulph. 6
Migraine
Coffea 30, Absinth 30, Juglans R. 30, Berb. Vul. 30, Passiflora 30, Sepia 30, Podo. 30
Meningitis
Bell. 30, Fucus 30, Latrod. 30, Bacil 30
Menorrhagia
Cocculus 30, Caulophul. 30, Ratanhia 30, Ignatia 30, Ammon. Mur. 30
    or
Aletris F. 30, Sepia 30, Mag. Phos. 30, Sabina 30, Chamom. 30, Murex 30, Lil. Tig. 30
Morning Sickness
Nux. Vom. 12, Nat. Mur 12, Ipecac. 12, Mentha V. 12, Aletris F. 12
Mumps
Salvia 30, Bell. 30, Tarantula 30, Kali Mur. 30
Neuralgia
Passiflora 30, Colocynth 30, Acon. 30, Plantago. 30, Coffea 30, Kalmia 30, Scutell. 30
Obesity
Graph. 6X, Thyroid. 6X
    or
Graph 30, Fucus 30, Junglans R. 30, Iod. 30, Thyroid 30
Otitis Media
Chenopod. 30, Pilocarpus 30, Bell. 30, Kali Mur. 30, Ferr. Phos. 30, Merc. Sol. 30
(The above potencies are for the chronic. Give the same remedies in 3X for the acute.)
Pharyngitis
Salvia 3X, Cinnam 3X, Bell. 3X, Bryonia 3X, Asclepias T. 3X, Ferr. Phos. 3X, Kali Mur. 3X
Pruritus
Urtica U. 30, Iris F. 30, Dirca 30, Rad. Brom. 30
Psoriasis
Petrol. 30, Zinc. Met. 30, Ars. Alb. 30, Echincea 30, Kali Sulph. 30
Pyorrhoea
Cuprum Iod. 30, Morphin 30, Sepia 30, Acid Sulph. 30, Acid Sulph. 30, Kresote 30, Silicea 30
Rickets

Ver. Alb. 30, Calc. Iod. 30, Chamo. 30, Iod. 30, Kali Phos. 30, Scutell 30
Rheumatism
Sil. 30, Rhus. T. 30, Arctium L. 30, Xanthox. 30, Cimic. 30, Taraxacum. 30
    or
Auram Mur. Nat. 200, Ferr. Iod. 200, Ammon Caust. 200, Ruta G. 200, Phytolacca 200, Iodium 200, Morphin 200
Ringworm
Sepia 3X, Sulph 3X
    or
Sanguinaria C. q
Apply locally thrice a day.
Scabies
Echinacea 30, Euphorbium 30, Sepia 30, Sulph 30
    or
Psorinum 200
Use once weekly.
Scitica
Phytolacca 200, Kali Iod. 200, Guiacum 200, Morphin 200, Colocynth 200, Ruta 200
Septicaemia
Echinacea 30, Anacard. 20, Calc. Sulph. 30, Rosemarinus 30, Kali Mur. 30
Sinusitis
Lachesis 30, Kali Bich 30, Ars. 30, Drosear 30, Bell. 30
Sore Throat
Cinnam. 3X, Bell. 3X, Origanum. 3X, Baryta C. 3X, Phytolac. 3X
Spermatorrhoea
Salix Nig. 30, Sabal Ser. 30, Cichona 30, Selen. 30, Xanthox. 30, Staphys. 30
Stillbirth
Thuja 200, Cocculus 200, Ferr. Met. 200, Ignatia 200
Styes
Heper Sulph 6X, Puls. 6X, Thuja 6X
Suppuration (Promotes)
Silicea 12X
Suppuration (restrains)
Heper Sulph. 3X, Calc. Sulph 3X
Sweat (offensive)
Sulph 30, Silicea 30
Synovitis
Sumphytum 3X, Apis Mel. 3X, Calc. Fluor. 3X, Kali Mur. 3X, Ferr. Phos. 3X
Try 30c potency in cases slow to respond.
Syphilis
Kali Iod. 30, Aur. Met. 30, Merc. 30, Thuja 30
Tetanus
Hypericum 6, Bell. 6, Ambra Grisea 6, Sulph. 6
    or
Mephitis 30, Passiflora 30, Dioscorea 30, Mag. Phos. 30, Pothus Foetidus 30, Anacard. 30
Tonsilitis

Salvia 6X, Baryta. 6X, Bell. 6X, Ferr. Phos. 6X
(Every four hourly.)
Toothache
Bryo. 30, Plantago 30, China 30, Coffea 30, Puls. Nig. 30
Typhoid
Anacard. 30, Lachesis 30, Bell. 30, Baptis T. 30, Ferr. Phos. 30, Nat. Sulph 30
Urticaria
Helleb. Nig. 3X, Urtica U. 3X, Euphorbium 3X, Apis Mel. 3X, Nat Phos. 3X, Kali Phos. 3X
The above in 30c may prove effective.
Vertigo
Arg. Nit 12, Gels. 12, Morphis 12, Antim Curde 12, Baptisia 12, Bryo. Alb. 12, Ambra Grisea 12
Vomiting
Camphor. 12, Ipecac. 12, Nat Mur. 12, Ammon Carb. 12, Ammon Mur 12
    or
Ipecac 3X, Mentha 3X, Nux Vom. 3X, Ver. Alb. 3X
(Give every 15 minutes until vomiting ceases, then thrice daily.)
Warts
Thuja 30, Castoreum 30, Echinacea 30, Euphorbium 30
    or
Castor Oil, Chelidonim q, Thuja q, Strong Acetic Acid
(Apply externally any one of the above.)
Whooping Cough
Sec. Cor. 30, Sambucus 30, Drosera 30, Kali Brom. 30, Mag. Carb. 30, Zinc Met. 30, Arg. Nit 30
    or
Drosera 30, Ambra. Gris. 30, Bell. 30, Ipecac. 30, Kali Mur. 30
Worms
Chelone 30, Teucrium 30, Ambrosia 30, Filix Mas 30, Ferr. Mur. 30
Writer's Cramp
Colocynth 30, Passiflora 30, Mag. Phos. 30, Loblia I 30, Discorea V. 30

Chapter - 23
DRUG INDEX

Anthrkokali 3 —Skin affections like scabies, prurigo, chronic herpes and ulceration.
Geranium Mac.ø — Half-dram dose gastric ulcers.
Solidago Oil or Solidago Virgo ø —25 drop dose to promote expectoration in bronchitis & bronchial asthma.
Crataegus ø — Increases B. P. a heart tonic.
Yahombinum ø, 3 — Sexual stimulent (3, 1 drop, once.)
Kali Arsenicum 30 — Numerous small nodules under the skin.
Podo ø + Santonin 3X — For worms.
Guaiacum ø — Acute rheumatism & artiritis.
Gentiana Lutea ø — Increases appetite.
Lycopus Virg ø — Lowers high B.P. and reduces heart rate.
Adrenalin (200 - 10M) — For high B.P.
Narcissus ø — Nausea followed by violent vomiting and diarrhoea.
Rhamnus Purshiana ø (Cascara Sagrada) — For prompt paliation in constipation.
Calcaria Calcinata 3X, 30 — For warts. (8 grains dose)
Pituitary ø, 30 — For high B.P.
Testis 3X — Increases male sexual power.
Placenta 3X — Helps to formation of milk after delivery.
Corpus Luteum 3X — Menarche not at time. Increases the power of uterus. Underdeveloped female sex characters.
Ovyry 3X — Used in retarded womanhood. Promotes balanced development of female organs. Pregnancy does not take place even coition with husband, with regular menses.
Parotidinum 30 — Preventive for mumps.
Dios. Vill q + Iris Tenax q — Appendicitis.
Myrica q — Jaundice.
Napthaline 6X — for whooping cough.
Formica Rufa q, 30 — For bedwetting.
Eryngium Aquaticum q, 30 — For emission of sperms without erection.
Gratiola 30 — For nymphomania, and masturbation.
Scutellaria q — for hiccough.
Borax 3X — Acts magically in restoring the voice in case of sudden hoarseness brought on by cold if dissolved in the mouth.
Gingeng q, 30 — in lumbago, scitica and chronic rheumatism.
Rosemary Oil — for baldness.
Senega q — For bronchiectesis.
Silica Marina q, 3X. trit — for Constipation of all ages.
Cinnamon q + Viburnum Prunifol 6x + Bapt Tinc. q — For abortion.
Lach 30 + Tarentula 30 — For abscess.
Cicuta V. 30 + Cuprun Met. 30 + Oenanthe Crocata 30 — for convulsions.
Phloriyin 6 + Cephalendra Indica q + Abroma Augusta q — Diabetes.
Titanium 6 — of sexual weakness too early ejaculation of semen during coitus.
Myristica Sebifera q + Hydrocotyle Asiatica q + Strychnine Ars. 30 — For elephanthis.
Ferrum Picric 30 + Millefol 30 — for epistaxis.
Iris Vers 30 — to abort paronichia. constipation (30-th)

Morgan Gaertner 30 + Cholesterinum 30 + Cardus Marianus q — Gall-stones.
Fluoric Acid 6 — Fistula in ano.
Ficus Vesiculosus q — For exopthalmic goitre.
Urtica Urens 30 — for gout.
Ampelopsis ø, 30 — For hydrocele.
Borax 30 — Sterility.
Anacard ø — In elephantiasis, give 1 drop thrice daily.
Aloe ø — In dysentry, 2 drops 4 times.
Ars 3X — In suppression of urine in cholera with delirium and restlessness. Dose — 1 drop, hourly.
Aletris Farinosa ø — Uterine tonic.
Aralia Racemosa ø — Asthma, hay-fever and leucorrhoea.
Baryta Iod 1X — One grain thrice daily for indurated glands, esp. tonsil & breasts.
Bellis Perenis ø — 5 drops twice a day for nocturnal emissions, spermatorrhoea, discharge of prostatic fluid in the urine, vertigo consequent on masturbation.
Baptisia ø — for malaria & typhoid fever.
Castor Oil (Ricinus ø) — One drop thrice for dysentery of children.
Cenic Cio ø — 5 drops thrice, for all kinds of menstrual disorders.
Croton Tig. ø — for obstinate constipation.
Cantharis ø — 5 drops thrice excites sexual organs in both sexes.
China ø — for fever, derangement of stomach & bowels, epilepsy, titanic spasm & convulsions.
Caulophyllum ø — for false labor pain, habitual abortion, spasmodic dysmenorrhoea and prolapsus uteri.
Damiana ø — Invigorates the nervous system and increases the tone of the body. For chronic prostatic dischage, spermatorrhoea, impotency.
Hymosa ø — For rheymatism & lumbago.
Lobelia Inflata ø — Vomiting of pregnancy with nausea and morning sickness.
Mullen Oil ø — For incontinence of urine, bed-wetting at night, constant dribbling of urine or frequent urging to urinate.
Origanum q — Voluptuous dreams, nocturnal emissions, excessive strong desire for sexual intercourse.
Secale Cor q — For amenorrhoea, 10 drops thrice a day.
Thlapsi B. P. ø — 5 drops thrice, haematuria, renal colic and dropsy due to kidney affections.
Viburnum Opulus q — Spasmodic dysmenorrhoea, post-partum pains, habitual abortion, leucorrhoea with violent uterine pains.
Piscidia q — A nerve sedative, insomnia, pains of irregular menses ; regulates of flow.
Vibernum Preunifolium q — for obstinate hiccough.
Merc Dule. 1X + Sulph q — For paliative in constipation. (2 grain dose)
Malandrinum 30 — for the ill-effects of vaccination ; chronic eczema following vaccination.
Thymus Gland Extract — High potencies very efficient in exophthalmic goitre.
Thyroidinum 2X — For fibroid tumour of the breasts.
Terebene 1X, 30 — for chronic bronchitis and winter coughs. Loosens secretion, relieves tightened feeling, make expectoration easy. Huskiness of public speakers and singers.
Choline (1dram fluid extract) — for cancer.
Tarentula Cubensis 30 — for pruritus, esp. about genitals. As a curative and preventive during the period of invasion.

Stillingia q, 30 — Valuable for intercurrent use.
Pilocarpus (Jaborandi) — In limiting the duration of mumps.
Natrum Phos 1X — For jaundice.
Naphthaline 1X — for pinworms, one gram dose.
Lupulin 1X — Best in seminal emissions.
Kamala q — For tape-worm, 60- drop doses.
Potassa + Iodine — 30 grains Potassa and 4 grains Iodine to 1 Oz. of water, 10 drops thrice, expels tapeworms dead.
Iodoformum 2X — 3 grains on the back of the tongue will relieve attack of asthmatic breathing.
Glycerine — Pure glycerine in t.s.f. doses, t.i.d., with lemon juice for pernicious anaemia.
Geranium Mac, q — Half-dram dose in gastric ulcers.
Fluoroform 1X — 2 per-cent. watery solution, 2-4 drops, after parxysms, for whooping-cough.
Cuprum Oxidatum Nigrum 1X — For all kinds of worms, including tape-worms.
Oil of Chenopodium — For roundworm, hookworm, 10 drops every two hours for three doses.
Bowel Nosodes should Not Be Repeated within three months. (200) (1M)
Morgan-Pure (Paterson) — Marked skin eruptions. Lever diseases. Bilious headache. Actual presence of gall-stone.
Morgan-Gaertner (Paterson) — Skin diseases. Liver Affections. Cholecystitis. Renal colic.
Proteus (Bach) — Cramp of muscles. Herpetic eruption at the mucocutaneous margins.
Bacillus No. '7' (Paterson) — Loss of sexual functions. Bronchial asthma.
Geartner (Bach) — Malnutrition. Diseases of childhood. Inability to digest fat.
Dys. Co. (Bach) — Duodenal ulcer oftern calls for this nosode.
Sycotic Co. (Paterson) — Chronic gastro-enteritis. Profuse leucorrhoea.
Mutabile (Bach) — Skin eruption alternates with asthmatic symptons.
Adrenalin 6X — Acute urticaria. Asthma.
Insulin 30 — For acne, Carbuncles, itching eczema.
Staphyloccin 30 — Acne, abscess, furuncle ; empyema.
Streptococcin 30 — For anti-febrile action.
Syphilinum (1X - 50M) — Shifting rheumatic pains. Chronic eruptions. Succession of abscesses. Ulceration of mouth, nose, genitals, skin.
Thymus Serpyllum q — For respiratory infections of children, dry asthma, whooping-cough.
Thymus Gland Extrat (10 M) — High potencies very efficient in exophthalmic goitre.
Thyroidinum 1X, 30 — In hypo-thyroidism (myxaedema & cretinism), Rickets, Psoriasis. Goitre, Improves the memory. Uterine fibroid. Nocturnal enuresis. Fibroid tumors of the breasts, 2X trit.
Pituitary Gland 30 — For development of the sexual organs.
Lac Caninum — Sore throat, Rheumatism.
Rodium Bromide 30 — Rheumatism, Gout. Acne rosacea, naevi, moles, ulcers and cancers. Lowered blood-pressure.
Uranium Nitricum 3X — Diabetes.
Morbilinum 200 — Prophitactic and curative for measles.
Influenzinum 30 — for influenza.
Scirrhinum 200 — Cancerous diathesis ; enlarged glands ; cancerof breast ; worms.
Pertussin 200 — Whooping-cough and other spasmodic coughs.
Variolinum 30 — Bachache, Aching in legs.

Tuberculinum 30 — For any renal affections. Tuberculosis, Enlarged tonsils. Acute articular rheumatism.
Carcinosin 200 — Painful mammary and uterine carcinoma.
Vaccininum 200 — for skin eruptions.
Malaria Officinalis 30 — for malaria.
Magnetis Poli Ambo 30 — For tendency of old wounds to bleed afresh.
Lac. Vaccinum 30 — For headache, rheumatic pains, constipation.
Lac Felinum 30 — For eyestrain, ciliary neuralgia, photophobia. Dysmenorrhoea.
Cholesterinum 3X — For Cancer of the liver. Opacities of the vitreous. Jaundice. Gallstone. Insomnia.
Baccillinum 30 — For tuberculosis. Attacks of suffocation at night with difficult cough.
Ustilago q — For irresistible tendency to masturbate.

Chapter - 24
DRUG MANUAL

Petroleum (Rock Oil) — Herpes : of genital organs extending to perineum and thighs; itching, redness; skin cracked, rough, bleeding; dry or moist.
Causticum (Tinctura acris sine Kali) — Disturbed functional activity of brain and spinal cord, from exhausting disease or severe mental shock resulting in paralysis.
Causticum — Hoarseness with rawness, and aphonia.
Nur Moschata — Dyspepsia of old people.
Nux Mos. — Loss of memory.
Ammonium Carb. — Antidotes stings of insects.
Ars. — Ailment from ; Chewing tabaco, alcoholism ; stings of venomous insects.
Borax — When Rhus. seems indicated, but fails to cure, in chronic urticaria.
Bromium — Hard goitre cured after Iod. failed.
Cina — In pertussis, after Drosera.
Cina — Has cured aphonia from exposure when Acon. Phos. and Spon. had failed.
Cocculus — Has cured umbilical hernia with obstinate constipation, after Nux. failed.
Collinsonia Can. — Has cured colic after col. and Nux. had failed.
Conuum Mac. — Is followed well by Psor. in tumors of mammae with threatening malignancy.
Fluoric Acid — After, Phos. Acid, in diabetes.
After, Spon., in goitre.
Graph — After, Sepia, gushing leucorrhoea.
Heper Sulph — Renders patients less susceptible to atmospheric changes, and cold air.
Ipecac — Is followed well by, Ant. tart., in foreign bodies in larynx.
Kalmia Lalifolia — Antidotes the effects of bad beers.
Psor — After, Lactic Acid, in vomiting of pregnancy.
Sabina — Follows, Thuja, in condyloma and sycotic affections.
Selenium — Itch checked by mercurials or sulphur often requires selenium.
Sulphuric Acid — In constussion and laceration of soft parts, views with Calendula.
Thuja — Cinnabaris is referable for warts on prepuce.
Naja Tripudians (Cobra Virus) — Severe stitching pain in region of heart.
Coca — Prevents caries of teeth.
Ratanhia — Constipation : Stool hard with great straining ; fissures of anus.
Sabadilla — Worm affections of all age, esp., of children.
Sabadilla — Sneezing in spasmodic paroxysms ; followed by lachrymation; copious watery coryza.
Carbo. Animalis — Is often useful after bad effects from spoiled fish and decayed vegetables.
Carbo Animalis — Glands : indurated, swollen, painful ; in neck, axillae, groin, mammae.
Cicuta Virosa — Convulsions : with frightful distortions of limgs ; lock-jaw.
Marc. Dul. — Calarrhal inflammation of middle ear ; deafness & olorrhoea.
Merc. Cyanide — For dishlheria, also effective as a prophylactic.
Abrotanum — Itching Chilblains.
Acon. — Amenorrhoea in plethoric young girls.
Actaea Racemosa — Ciliary neuralgia.
Abortion at third month.
Excessive muscular soreness after dancing, or other violent muscular exertion.
Acsculus — Fullicular Pharyngitis.

Severe dull backache in lumbo-sacral articulation.
After Collinsonia has improved piles, Aesc. often cures.
Aethusa — Cannot bear milk in any form.
Aethusa — Epilaptic spasms ; jaws locked, foam at the mouth.
Agaricus Muscarious — Delirium : in typhoid.
Pain in lumber and sacral region.
Agnus Castus — Pemature old age, from seminal losses, from abuse of the sexual powers. Complete impotence.
Allium Cepa — Nasal Polypus.
Calarrhal laryngitis.
Traumatic Chronic neuritis.
Aloe Soc. — Itch appears each year, as winter approaches. (Psor.)
Headache, alternating with Lumbago.
Haemorrhoids ; like a bunch of grapes. (Mur. Acid)
Alumina — Itching eruption, worse in winter. (Petr.)
Constipation : great straining, no ability to pass ; inactivity of rectum.
Ambra Grisea — Discharge of blood between periods, at every little accident — a long walk, after every hard stool.
Violent cough in spasmodic paroxysms, with eructations and hoarseness.
Ammon. Carb. — stopping of nose, mostly at night ; must breathe through the mouth ; snuffles of infants.
Putrid sore throat.
Emphysema, Panaritium ;
Ammon. Mur. — Obstinate constipation accompanied by much flatus.
Leucorrhoea : Like white of egg, after every urination.
Offensive sweat of the feet, (Alum., Graph, Psor., Sanic, Sil.)
Amylenum Nitrosum — Often paliative in incurative cases. Agina pectoris
Henmicrania (one-sided headache)
Anacardium — Sudden loss of memory.
Apt to choke when eating drinking. (Can. S., Nit. Ac.,)
Warts on palms & hands (Nat. M.)
Anthracinum — Gangrenous ulcers ; felon, carbuncle, erysipelas of a malignant type.
Antim Crude — Large horny Corns on soles of feet. (Ran.)
Whooping-cough.
Antim. Tart. — Relieve the death-rattle cough. (Taran)
Ant. Tart. — When seems indicated in coughs, require Heper.
Apis — Urticaria.
Open cancer.
Intermittent fever.
Incontinence of urine, can scarcely retain the urine a moment, and when passed scalds sevely.
Apocynum Can. — dropsy.
Acute hydrocephalus.
Metrorrhagia.
Amenorrhoea in young girls
Murex — Excessive sexual irritation driving to self-abuse (Orig., Zinc). Sore pain in uterus.
Kalmia Latifolia — Acute neuralgia, rheumatism, gout.

Severe stitching pain in right eye and orbit. (left eye — spig.)
Rumex — Cough remedy.
Sensation of lump in throat. Skin : itching of various part.
Calc. Phos. — Diarrhoea and great flatulence.
At puberty : acne in anaemic girls.
At every attempt to eat, colic pains in abdomen.
Fistula in ano.
Bovista — Persons who suffer from tettery eruptions, dry or moist.
Stammering children. (Stram.)
Discharge from nose and all mucous membranes very tough, tringy, tenacious. (Kali bi.)
Haemorrhage : after extraction of teeth. (Ham.)
Helonias Dioica — Diabites.
Albuminuria : acute or chronic. (Kidney disease).
Soreness and heaviness in pelvis. (Lappa.)
For the bad effects of abortions and miscarriages.
Merc. Biniod. — Glandular throat affections of left side.
Tubercular paryngitis.
Merc. Protoiod — Right-sided throat affections.
Picric Acid — Headache : from any type of overwork.
Praipism (persistenterection of the penis), with spinal disease ; erections violent, long lasting ; profuse seminal emissions ; satyriasis (male nymphomaria) (Canth., Phos.)
Kali Brom. — Loss of memory.
Acne : simplex, rosacea.
Often curative after Eugenia Jambos in acne.
Canabis Indica — Very forgetful.
Cantharis — Burning, cutting pains in urethra during micturation.
Sarsaparilla — Herpetic eruptions on all parts of body. Itch-like eruptions, becomes crusty.
Equisetum Hyemale — Burning pain in urethra while urinating.
Dulc — Urticaria over whole body.
Warts, on face or back of hands and fingers.
Drosera — Whooping-cough.
Crocus Sativa — Dysmenorrhoea (Ustilago.)
Croton Tig. — Acute eczema over whole body. (Rhus.)
Intense itching of genitals of both sexes. (Rhus)
Kreosote — Post climacteric diseases of women. (Lach.)
Haemorrhage : after the extraction of a tooth (Ham.)
Itching all over, esp., of pudenda and vagina.
Incontinence of urine. Burning during & micturation. (Sulph.)
Leucorrhoea : worse between periods (Bov., Borax.)
Rheum — Sweat of scalp. Suitable for children, during dentition.
Ranunculus Bulbosus — Most effective remedies for the bad effects of alcoholic beverages.
Spasmodic hiccough.
Herpes Zoster.
Day-blindness, pressure and smarting in eyeballs.
Rhododendron — For orchitis. Acute inflammatory swelling of joints, wandering from one joint to another.

Fluoric Acid — Old cicatrices become red around edges, & threaten to become open ulcers. (Caust. Graph.)
Naevus flat.
Fistula lachrymalis.
Rapid caries of teeth ; fistula dentalis.
Petroselinum — Gonorrhoea, Gleet.
Spongia Tosta — For goitre. Thyroid glands swollen even with chin.
Angina Pectoris.
Spermatic cord swollen.
Cina — Involuntary urine. Spasmodic cough with sneezing.
Hamamelis Virg. — Traumatic conjunctivitis.
Lobelia Inflata — Extreme nausea and vomiting ; morning sickness. Spasmodic asthma, pertussis, with dyspnoea threatening suffocation.
Glonoine — Bad effects, from having the hair cut.
Eupatorium Perfoliatum — Bone pains.
Painful soreness of eyeballs.
Sambucus Nig. — Attacks of suffocation as in last stage of croup.
Oedamatous swelling in various parts of the body, esp. in legs.
Baptisia Tinc — Painless sore throat.
Dysentery of old people.
Taraxacum — Gastric headache. Jaundice with enlargement of liver.
Tarantula — Boils, abscess, carbuncle, malignant ulcers.
Pruritus valvae becomes intolerable.
Chelidonium — Hepatic diseases : jaundice.
Spasmodic cough.
Gall-stone (Terrible attacks of gall-stone colic, card. m.)
Sabina — Tendency to miscarriage.
Ailments : following abortion.
Pain extending from sacrum to pubes.
Fig-wart with itching and burning.
Promotes expulsions of moles or foreign bodies from uterus. (canth.)
Cannabis Sativa — Obstinate constipation, causing retention of the urine ; Dyspnoea & asthma.
Acute inflammatory stage of gonorrhoea.
Dioscorea Villosa — Violent colic.
Emissions during sleep ; vivid dreams of women all night. (staph.)
Hydrastis — Hard cancer.
Broken down by excessive use of alcohol.
Hawks yellow viscid mucus from posterior nares.
Pruritus.
Calcaria Ars. — The slightest emotion causes palpitation of heart.
Caladium — Impotence : relaxed penis, with sexual desire and excitement ; no erections, no emission.
Pruritus vaginae ; induces onanism. (Orig. Zinc.)
Calc. Carb. — Acidity, diseases arising from defective dentition. Delayed dentition with head sweats.

Mag. Mur. — Continual rising of white froth into the mouth.
Enlarged liver with pressing pain
Mezereum — Toothache : in carious teeth. (Kreo.)
Visicles appear around the ulcers, hair is glued and method together.
Itching eczema.
Millefolium — Painless haemorrhage after labor or abortion, miscarriage. Leucorrhoea ; of children.
Muriatic Acid — Malignant affections of mouth.
Prolapse while urinating
Typhoid.
Freckles, eczema solaris.
Ruta — Aching in and over eyes, with blurred vision.
Prolapse of rectum.
Warts : with sore pains, on palsm of hands.
Collinsonia Canadensis — Chronic bleeding piles.
Dysmenorrhoea. Constipation.
Colchicum — Abdomen distended with gas.
Smell painfully acute ; nausea and faintness from the odor or cooking food.
Coffea Cruda — Ailments : the bad effects of sudden emotions.
alternate laughing and weeping.
Lachesis — Climacteric ailments.
Trembling in whole body.
Boils, carbuncles, ulcers with intense pain. (Tar.)
Typhoid.
Tonsillitis.
Lac Can. — In writing, omits final letter ; cannot concentrate the mind to read or study.
Sore throat, tonsillitis.
Inflamed, painful breast.
Backache.
Sexual organs easily excited, from touch, pressure on sitting or friction by walking. (Plat., Murex, Coff., Cinamon.)
Plumbum — Violent colic in abdomen.
Brights' disease.
Liver-spots.
jaundice.
Strangulated hernia, femoral, inguinal or umbilical.
Symphytum — Pain in eye after a blow of an obtuse body.
Zinc. Met. — Violent fidgety feeling in feet or lower extremities ; must move them constantly.
Automatic motions of hands and head.
Spinal affections : burning whole length of spine; backache.
Veratrum Viride — Basilar meningitis.
Titanic convulsions, opisthotonos.
Terebinth — Worms : tickling at anus ; ascarides, lumbrici, tapeworm.
Violent burning and drawing pains in kidney, bladder and urethra. Haematuria. Spasmodic retention of urine. Albuminuria.
Natrum Sulph. — Chronic brain effects of blows, falls.

Humid asthma in children, with every change of weather.
Spinal meningitis, violent crushing gnawing pains at base of brain.
Gelsemium — Trembling of entire body.
Acid Phos. — For onanism. (with irresistible tendency to masturbate, Ust.)
Lyssin — Prolapsus uleri. sensitiveness of vagina, rendering coition painful.
Hypericum — For corns.
Prevents lockjaw.
Pains, after a fall on coccyx.
Punctured, incised or lacerated wounds.
Convulsions, afterblows on head or concussion.
Cocculus — Headache, nausea or vomiting from riding in carriage, boat or rairoad car.
Nat. Mur. — Impotence ; seminal emission : soon after coition.
Hangnails. (Graph., Pet.)
Herpes about anus.
Warts on palms of hands. (sore to touch, Nat. C.)
Painful contractions of the hamstrings. (Am. m., Caust., Guiacun.)
Urticaria, acute or chronic.
Intermittent fever.
Conium Mac. — Cancerous and scrofulous persons with enlarged glands.
Breasts sore, hard and painful before & during menses. (Lac. C., Kali. C.)
Prostatic affections.
Carbolic Acid — When burns tend to ulceration and ichorous discharge.
Constipation, with horribly offensive breath.
Caulophyllum — Ailments during pregnancy, parturition, lactation. Leucorrhoea, in little girls.
Habitual abortion from uterine debility.
Syphilinum — Loss of memory. Leucorrhoea, profuse, soaking through the napkins and running down to the heals. (Alum.)
Falling of hair.
Acute ophthalmia neonatorum. Teeth : decay at edge of gum. Craving alcohol, in any form.
Obstinate constipation for years.
Chamomilla — Violent rheumatic pains.
Milk runs out in nursing women (runs out after weaning, con.)
Nux — Catarrh : snuffles of infants. (Am. C., Samb.)
Strangulated hernia, esp. umbilical.
Backache ; lumbago, from sexual weakness, from masturbation.
Fever : must be covered in every stage of fever—chill, heat or weat.
Veratrum Album — Violent vomiting with profuse diarrhoea and colic.
Constipation, of infants and children, after Lyco. & Nux.
Dysmenorrhoea, with vomiting and purging.
Staphisagria — Mechanical injuries from sharp-cutting instruments.
For the bad effects of onanism, sexual excuses. Persistently dwelling on sexual subjects; constantly thinking of sexual pleasures.
Spermatorrhoea : emission followed by backache.
Cough excited by tobacco smoke. (Spong.)
Arthritic nodosites of joints.

Eczema : Yellow, acrid moisture oozes from under crusts; new vesicles from contact of exudation.
Fig-warts.
Stramonium — Delirium, violent mania.
Stammering.
Hydrophobia.
Convulsions : with consciousness. (Nux. — without, Bell, Cicuta, Hyos., Op.)
Bryonia — Headache : from constipation, from ironing.
Cactus Grandiflorus — Haemorrhage from nose, lungs, stomach, rectum, bladder, (Crot., Mill., Phos.)
Nit. Acid — Violent cutting pains after stool.
Fissures of rectum.
Urine : strong-smelling, "like horrse's urine".
Ulcers : easily bleeding; in corners of mouth. (Nat.)
Warts, condylomata.
Physostigma — Vision dim.
Pain after using eyes ; floating black spots.
Podophylum — Prolapse of rectum before or with stool.
Prolapsus uteri.
Suppressed menses in young girls (Puls., Tub.)
Phytolacca — Sore-throat.
Mammary abscess.
Hastens suppuration.
Platina — Sexual organs sensitive, cannot bear the napkin to touch her; valva painfully sensitive during coitus ; will faint during.
Nymphomania, Vaginismus.
Constipation : While travelling stool adheres to rectum & anus like soft clay. (Alum.)
Metrorrhagia.
Pyrogen — Septic fever.
Offensive ulcers of old persons. (Psor.)
Puls — Mumps ; metastasis to mammac or testicle.
Styes.
Delayed first menses.
Psorinum — All excretion — diarrhoea, leucorrhoea, menses, perspiration — have a carrion-like odor.
Otorrhoea.
Acne : at forms, simplex, rosacia.
Tostillitis
Constipation with backache.
Chronic gonorrhoea.
Hay fever.
Cough returns every winter.
Intolerable itching.
Melilotus Alba — Infantile spasms.
Merc. Sol. — Gonorrhoea.
Otorrhoea.

Sneezing.
Crowns of teeth decay, roots remain. (reverse, Mez.)
Mumps, tonsillitis.
Dysentery, with colic.
Leucorrhoea : pruritus.
Morning sickness.
Ulcers on gum, tongue, throat, inside of the cheek.
Merc. Sulphuricus — For hydrothorax. (Ars)
Kali Bich — Prolapsus uteri. Sexual desire absent in fleshy people.
Ipecac — Colic about umbilicus. Autumnal dysentery.
Asthmatic cough. Whooping-cough, child loses breath.
Intermittent fever.
Intermittent dyspepsia.
Iodum — Empty eructations from morning to night.
Induration of glandular tissue—thyroid, mammae, ovaries, testes, uterus, prostate or other glands.
Hard goitre.
Leucorrhoea : most abundant at times of menses.
Cancerous degeneration of the cervix.
Crotalus Horridus — Tendency to carbuncles or blood boils. (Anthr.)
Sepic typhoid or malarial fever. Blood flows from eyes, ears, nose and every orifice of the body.
Blood sweat. Conjunctivitis, iritis, keratitis.
Malignant jaundice.
Dessecting wounds ; insect stngs. Prolonged metrorrhagia.
Malignant diseases of uterus.
Caprum Met. — Spasms and cramps.
Cholera morbus, with cranps in abdomen.
Stammering speech.
Epilepsy.
Whooping-cough.
Cyclamen Europaeum — Burning sore pain in heels.
Digitalis — Dropsy : with suppression of urine.
China — pains : in every joint. Periosteum, as if strained, sore all over.
Borborygmus, colic.
Unrefreshing sleep.
Intermittent fever.
Ars. — Gastric derangements : after cold fruits ; ice cream; ice water, sour beer, bad sausage, alcoholic drinks, strong cheese.
Asthmatic breathing.
Arnica — Meningitis, Hydrocephalus.
Conjunctival or ratinal haemorrhage.
Gout & rheumatism.
Tendency to small painful boils, one after another.
Calendula — Wounds penitrating articulations with loss of synovial fluids.
Camphora — All sequelae of measles.
Argentum Met. — Seminal emissions : after onanism, almost every night.

Crushed pan in the testicles. (Rhod.)
Exhausting fluent coryza with sneezing. Hoarseness ; of singers, public speakers (Alum., Arum.t.)
Arg. Nit. — Headache : from dancing; ending in bilious vomiting.
Acute conjunctivitis, ophthalmia neonatorum, agglutinated in morning. Eye-strain from sewing. Diseases due to defective accommodation.Flatulent dyspepsia.
Urine passes unconsciously day and night. (Caust.)
Coition : painful in both sexes ; followed by bleeding from vagina (Nit. Acid)
Nat. Carb. — Chronic effect of sunstroke.
Arum Triphyllum — Coryza ; acrid, fluent ; nostrils raw, sneezing.
Aphonia : after exposure to winds ; from singing. Sore-throat
Asarum Europeum — Longing for alcohol ; a popular remedy for drunkards.
Asterias Rubens — Cancer of mammae; acute lancinating pain ; drawing pain in breast.
Sexual desire increased in women. (Lil.)
Aurum Met. — Falling of the hair.
Sulph — Have worms, but the best selected remedy fails.
Menorrhagia.
Chronic alcoholism ; dropsy and other ailments of drunkards.
Sulphuric Acid — Tendency to gangrene following mechanical injuries, esp., of old people.
Heartburn. Aphthae : bleeding gum.
Tabacum — Paroxysms, asthma and sneezing.
Constipation : of year's standing ; prolapsus ani ; herpes of anus. Renal colic.
Theridion Curassavecum — In scrofulosis where the best chosen remedies fail to relieve.
Thalaspi B. P. — Metrorrhagia : with violent cramps and uterine colic.
Menses : protracted, stays even 15 days.
Trillium Pendulum — Menorrhagia.
Haemoptysis : purulent expectoration and troublesome cough.
Tuberculinun — Takes cold easily without knowing how or where.
Meningitis.
Nocturnal hallucinations.
Itching eczema.
Ringworm.
Valeriana — Child vomits : curdled milk, in large lumps.
Sanguinaria — Eruption on face of young women.
Sanicula — Scaly dandruff on scalp, eyebrows, in the beard. Incontinence of urine and faeces.
Leucorrhoea with strong odor of fish brine.
Baryta Carb. — Memory deficient.
Scrofulous dwarfish children who do not grow.
Induration of prostate and tastes.
Chronic cough.
Bell — Convulsions, with fever. (without fever, Mag. P.)
Hallucinations.
Benzoic Acid — Gout, Arthritis, Dribbling urine of old men with enlarged prostate.
Berberis Vulgaris — Renal Colic Burning & soreness in region of kidney.
Colic from gall-stone.
Bilious colic, followed by jaundice.

Bismuth — Pyrosis.
Vomiting : of water as soon as it reaches the stomach.
Borax — Hair tangled. Aphthous sore mouth.
Eyelashs : gummy exudation, agglutinated in morning.
Leucorrhoea : two weeks between the catamenia.
Bromium — Stony hard, scrofulous or tuberculous swelling of glands, thyroid, parotid, testes.
Much rattling of mucus during cough.
Membranous dysmenorrhoea.
Kali Carb. — Food easily gets into the windpipe.
Feels badly, week before menstruation; backache, before and during menses.
Measles.
Thuja — Insane women will not be touched or approached. White scaly dandruff ; hair falling out.
White scaly dandruff ; hair falling out.
Eyelids : agglutinated at night, styes.
Chronic otitis.
Anus fissured, surrounded with flat warts.
Skin : eruption only on covered parts.
Nails : deformed, brittle.
Toothache from tea-drinking.
Mag. Phos. — Colic.
Nocturnal eneuresis.
Vaginesmus.
Medorrhinum — Chronic ovaritis, salpingitis, pelvic cellulitis, fibroids, cysts and other morbid growths of uterus and ovaries.
Scirrhus, carcinoma, cancer.
Trembling all over.
Intense burning pains in brain, extends down spine.
Renal colic, painful tenesmus of bladder ; Nocturnal eneuresis.
Asthma, dyspnoea.
Swelling of all joints.
Opium — Constipation ; of children.
Phosphorus — Small wounds bleed easily. (Kreo., Lach.)
Dandruff, falls out in clouds (Lyc.) ; hair falls out in bunches ; baldness of single spots.
Regurgitation of ingesta, in mouthful.
Capsicum — Pain in distant parts of coughing. (bladder, knees, legs, ears.)
Carbo Veg. — Looseness of teeth, easily - bleeding gums.
In the last stage of disease, with copious cold sweat, voice lost, this remedy may save a life.
Colocynth — Sciatica.
Euphrasia — The eyes water all the time & are agglutinated in the morning.
Pertussis.
Amenorrhoea.
Menses : now lasting only one hour ; lasting only one day.
Ferrum Met. — Prolapsus recti of children ; itching of anus at night.
Graph — Eczema of lids.
Morning sickness during menses. Leucorrhoea : occurs in gushes day and night.

Cancer of breast.
Eruptions upon the ears.
Chronic constipation.
Decided aversion to coition of both sexes.
Helleborus Niger — Meningitis. Hydrocephalus.
Heper — Asthma.
Herpes, surrounded by little pimples.
Ignatia — Prolapsus ani.
Sexual desire with impotency. Fever no thirst.
Lac. Defloratum — Obesity; fatty degeneration.
Constipation of 15 year's standing.
Ledum — Red pimples or tubercles on forehead and cheeks.
Rheunatism & gout.
Lilium Tigrinum — Rapid heart-beat, 150 to 170 per minute.
Lyco — Snuffles, dry nose stopped at night.
Impotence of young men, from onanism or sexual excess.
Hernia : of children.
Mag. Carb. — Heartburn. Cutting Colic.
Milk passes undigested in nursing children.
Stannum — Lumbrici, passes worms.
Paroxysms of 3 coughs. (of two, Merc.)
Spigelia — Children with ascarides and lumbrici (Cina, Stan.)
Stammering children.
Secale Cor — The slightest wound causes bleeding for weeks.
Boils mature very slowly and heal in the same manner.
Unnatural ravenous appetite. Enuresis : of old people.
Continuous discharge of watery blood untit next period.
Selenium — Hair falls off, on head, eyebrows, genitals.
Constipation : requires mechanical aids.
Aphonia.
Sil — Blood boils, Ulcers of all kinds.
Sepia — Great falling of hair.
Herpes carcinatus in isolated spots. Itching of skin.
Prolaepse uterus & vagina.
Amenorrhoea, Menorrhagia. Gleet. (Kali. Iod.)

RARE DRUG ORGANOTHERAPY

Chapter - 25
RARE MEDICATION

A

Alnuin
A unique remedy for recurrent abortion.
Dose - 3x.trit.

Aether
Is a specific remedy for acute gout.
Potency - Lower potencies.

Aqua silicata
For recurrent abcess and blind boils in the skin.
Potency - 12th attenuation.

Anhalonium Lewinii
This remedy is indicated in brain-fag, occipital headache, migrane, neurasthenia and paraplegia.
Dose - 30th attenuation.

Aranearum Tela
Is a successful remedy for sleeplessness.
Dose - 10 grains of 2x trituration.

Acid Nitro-hydrochloricum
Is indicated in cases of aphthous condition of the lips, gums and buccal mucus membrane and the gums bleed easily. Use also in axaluria, in functional torpidity of the liver during the early stages of hepatic cirhossis, and in chronic hepatitis when there is no obstruction to the flow of bile.
Dose - 5 drops of well diluted fresh acid.

Acidum Sulphuricum Aromaticum
Gastric debility, diarhhoea and colliquative sweats are the cardinal indications for this remedy
Dose - 15 drops of well diluted acid.

Ampelopsin
This remedy has a specific action in chronic hoarseness, chorea, hydrocele and renal dropsis.
Dose - 3rd trituration.

Apocynin
Is one of the most efficient remedies in dropsies, ascites, anasarca and hydrothorax. Also found of frequent service in suppression of urine and strangury.
Potency - 6x trituration.

Asclepin
Acts like a magic in headache from checked sweat.
Dose - 1x trituration.

Asparagin

Coryza and nasal catarrh, with profuse secretion of whitish fluid from nostrils and frequent violent sneezing.
Potency - 2nd trituration.

Aspidospermin
An effective medicine in many cases of asthma.
Dose - 6th trituration.

Ammonium Fluoridicum
Marvellous results are obtained in multiple tumour of breasts.
Dose - 4x trituration.

Aegle Folia
Useful in all kinds of local and general dropsy, anasarca, with diarhhoea or constipation.
Dose - ø, in 5 drop doses twice a day. 200th of this drug once a week removes impotency and restores sexual strength and vitality.

Aethiops Antimonalis
Is of use in scrofulous, glandular swelling, otorrhoea and scrofulous eye affections.
Potency - 3rd trituration.

Agave Americana
Used in stomachache with poor appetite.
Potency - ø.

Aletris Farinosa
Premature and profuse menses, with labour-like pains.
Potency - Of the tincture, 5 to 20 drops.

Ambrosia Artemisiaefolia
Lachrymation and intolerable itching of the eye-lids.
Potency - ø, 5 to 10 drops. Also 3x.

Amygdalus Persica
A valuable remedy in vomiting of various kind; morning sickness.
Potency - ø, 5 drops.

Arsenicum Bromatum
Has brilliant clinical results in diabetes.
Potency - 6x, 5 drops 3 times a day in a glass of water.

Anagallis Arvensis
A skin remedy of high order, characterized by great itching and tingling everywhere; favours expulsion of splinters.
Potency - Tincture.

Aurum Sulph
Painful swelling of mammae having cracked nipples with lancilating pains.
Potency - 3rd to 30th .

Aurum Mur
Warts on tongue and genitals.
Potency - 2nd trituration.

Aconitum Neomontanum
Is of great service in eructations and rumbling in the bowels.
Potency - 30th.

Agaricus Rhalloides

One of the best remedies for Asiatic cholera, with extreme prostration, cold sweat, Hippocratic face, frequent bilious vomiting, continuous cramps in the stomach and bloody watery stools.

Dose - Lower trituration.

Alstonia Scholaris
Very effetive remedy in cases of malaria. Use also in cases of diarrhoea and dysentery when there is violent purging.

Dose - 30 drops of tincture; also 30th and higher.

Aphis Chenopodii Glauci
Has most pronounced effects in morning diarrhoea, with tenesmus and burning in the anus. Acts like a magic in severe pain at the lower angle of the left shoulder blade.

Potency - Use 6th and higher dilutions.

Apomorphinae Hydrochloras
Gives instant relief and cures nausea, with vertigo, at times heartburn and pain between the scapulae.

Dose - 6x trituration.

Arsenicum Sulphuratum Rubrum
This remedy is of service in cases of acne, psoriasis and influenza.

Dose - 1x trituration.

Arundo Mauritanica
Is chiefly useful in coryza and hay-fever with loss of smell. Also indicated in the diarhhoea of nursing children, eczema which is attended with itching, burning and oedema of the upper extremities.

Dose - 2x Potency. Use also 30th

Asclepias Cornuti
This remedy is indicated in cases of cardiac and renal dropsy. Relieves suppression of the menses and is of service in uraemia, attended with serves headache.

Dose - Of the mother tincture, 25 minims. Also 30th

Augopora
Most important remedy of universal fame in curing constipation, which are accomplished with blood and a constant inclination to stool

Dose - Use moderate potencies

Aurum Foliatum
Insures radical cure in fistula in infant.

Potency - 3rd trituration, 4 grains of dry powder on the tongue twice a day.

Aletrin
Is found useful in want of appetite, especially in connection with uterine disorders. Uterine prolapse Leucorrhoea. Obstinate vomiting of pregnancy.

Dose - 1x. trituration.

Aloin
Very useful in pain in rectum after stool. Haemorrhoids. A lot of mucus, with sense of insecurity in rectum when passing flatus.

Dose - 3rd trituration.

Arum Dracontium
A remedy for pharyngitis with sore, raw and tender throat.

Dose - First Potency .

Aquilegia Canadensis
Curative for hysteria. Sleeplessness. Dysmenorrhoea of young girls.
Dose - 3rd Potency.

Argemone Mexicana
Colicky cramp and spasm of bowels.
Dose - 6th potency. Tincture is applied to ulcers and warts.

Areca
Is of use in helminthiasis.
Dose - Higher.

Apiol
Use in dysmenorrhoea.
Dose - 3rd Potency.

Asclepias Syriaca
Acute rheumatic inflammation of large joints.
Dose - ø

Ammonium Benzoicum
Urinary incontinence in the aged.
Potency - 2x trituration.

Amyl Nitrosum
Really cures palpitation of the heart. Hiccough. Sea-sickness.
Dose - 3rd Potency.

Arsenicum Iodatum
Watery excoriating discharge from anterior and posterior nares; sneezing, influenza. Marked exfoliation of skin in large scales. Eczema of the beard.
Potency - 3rd trituration.

Aralia Racemosa
Curative in asthamatic conditions, with cough aggravated on lying down. Sneezing with copious excoriating nasal discharge.
Potency – ø

Aspidosperma
A great remedy in many cases of asthma.
Potency - ø, 10 drops twice daily.

Actea Spicata
Rheumatic pain in small joints wrist, fingers, ankles, toes.
Potency - 3rd Potency

Arctium Lappa
Special action in eruptions on the head, face and neck; pimples; acne; sties and ulcerations on edge of the eyelids.
Potency - ø to 30th

Alstonia Scholaris
A tonic after exhausting fevers. Malarial diseases with diarrhoea, dysentery, anaemia and feeble digestion.
Dose - ø to 3rd potency. Locally, for ulcers and rheumatic pains.

Aegle Marmelos
Is found useful in diarrhoea and dysentery.
Dose - Use tincture, 10 drops at intervals of 4 hours.

Frequency of doses may be variable according to the severity of the case.
Acenasia
Has proved to be great beneficial in cold perspiration on the whole body, fetid breath, ulcers in pharynx, and haemorrhage of dark blood.
Dose - Tincture.
Agnilegia
One of the best remedies for globus hystericus, sleeplessness, dysmenorrhoea of young girls.
Dose - ø, 8 drops thrice daily.
Aqua Ptychosis
Gives instant releief in dyspepsia, indigestion, flatulence, diarhhoea and heartburn.
Dose - 5 drops of tincture, thrice a day.
Aconitum Radix
For scarlet fever
Dose - ø, 10 drop doses.
Ailanthus Glandulosa
For malignant scarlet fever, severe streptoccous infections of the throat. Also in great use in typhoid fever and bloody dysentery.
Potency - ø, 30 drop doses.
Adonis Vernalis
Most valuable in cardiac dropsy. Hydrothorax, ascites, anasarca.
Dose - tincture, 10 drop doses.
Adonidin
Is an excellent tonic and diuretic, which increases arterial pressure and prolongs the diastole. Use as substitute for Digitalis.
Potency - ø
Aconitine
For tinnitus aurium.
Dose - 3x.
Aconitum Lycotonum
Diarrhoea after eating pork.
Potency - high.
Antimonium Arsenicosum
Usefulness in emphysema with excessive dyspnoea and cough, much mucous secretion.
Dose - 3rd trituration.

B

Bacae Juniperi
For any types of spleen affections.
Potency - ø.
Betula Alba
A specific remedy for ichthyosis.
Dose - tincture.
Bilirubin

Most important remedy for gallstones and organic diseases of livers, acidity and vomiting with severe bilious headaches and dyspepsia.
Potency - 6th attenuation.
Bismuth Trisnitrate
For treating gastrodynia and many types of neuralgias.
Potency - 1x Trituration.
Borax veneta
Is curative for ichthyosis.
Dose - 1x Trituration.
Brachyglottis Repens
A great remedy for nocturnal incontinence of urine in children.
Potency - 30th attenuation.
Brassica Murialis
Tones up the functions of the liver.
Dose - tincture. Also use 30th
Broomshandle
Is found useful in herpes, the after-pain of shingles.
Potency - 200th
Boletus Laricis
Profuse perspiration at night, with chills and fever.
Dose - ø, 5 drops.
Butyric Acid
Profuse offensive sweat of feet.
Potency - 3rd attenation.
Brachyglottis
Pressure in neck of bladder, urging to urinate. Soreness in urethra; feeling. as if urine could not be retained. Urine contains mucous corpuscles and epithelium, albumin and casts. Writers' cramp.
Potency - 3rd and higher. Also of the tincture, 5-20 drops.
Badiaga
Soreness of muscles, worse in motion. Stiches in scapulae, pain in small of back, hips and lower limbs, very stiff neck. Dandruff, scalp sore, dry, tetter -like.
Potency - 6th attenuation.
Balsamum Tolutanum
Chronic bronchitis with profuse expectoration
Dose - 1st attenuation.
Baryta Acetica
Produces paralysis beginning at the extremities and spreding upward.
Dose - 3rd trituration in repeated doses.
Baryta Iodata
Acts on the lymphatic system. Indurated glands, especially tonsils and breasts.
Potency - 2nd and 3rd trituration.
Benzenum
Use in leukaemia. Twitching of lids with photophobia.
Potency - 6th potency.
Benzin Nitricum

Nystagmus. Rolling of eyeballs in their vertical axis; pupils dilated.
Dose - 6th potency

Bacillus No. 7 (Paterson)
Use for mental and physical fatigue.
Potency - 32nd and 1002nd

Boerrhavia Diffusa
A great remedy for all kinds of dropsy. Retention of urine, dribbling of urine with pain in the bladder.
Dose - 5 drops of Q, thrice daily.

Boerrhavia Rep.
Cures attack of BeriBeri and dropsy in every rainy season.
Dose - 1x, give one drop dose thrice a day.

Bryophyllum Calycinum
Useful in treatment of the first stage of cholera, serious diarrhoea and dysentery with mucus or bloody stool.
Dose - tincture, 5 drops after each stool.

Bismuthum Subnitricum
In gastralgia where there is pain in the epigastrium.
Potency - 3x trituration.

Burgamont Oil
For alopecia
Dose - apply pure oil to the scalp night and morning with slight friction.

Baptisin
Has great reputation as a remedy in typhoid fever and epidemic influenza
Potency - 3rd trituration

Beta Vulgaris
Children yield very quickly to the action in chronic catarrhal stages.
Potency - 2x trituration.

Betonica Officinalis
For pains in almost all parts of the body.
Potency - Lower.

Bixa Orellana
Recommended for leprosy, eczema and elephantiasis.
Dose - tincture and lower potencies.

Boletus Satanus
Dysentery, vomiting, great debility, cold extremities, spasm of extremities and face.
Dose - 1st attenuation.

Bolus Alba
A remedy for croup and bronchitis.
Dose - lower triturations.

Bombyx
Itching of whole body.
Dose - 3rd to 30th Potency .

Boracic Acid
Used as an antiseptic disinfectant, since it arresrs fermentation and putrefaction.
Potency - 3rd trituration.

Botulinum
Eye symptoms, ptosis, double vision, blurred vision. Cramping pain in stomach.
Dose - Higher potencies. Use also 32nd potency.
Bougmancia Candida
Cannot concentrate thoughts; brain floats in thousands of problems and grand ideas.
Dose - ø, to 6th potency.
Branca Ursina
Much fatty perspiration on head and violent itching.
Dose - 3rd potency.
Bellis Perennis
A remedy often useful for sprains and bruises. Lameness due to mechanical causes. Useful in injuries in the deeper tissues after major surgical works. Boils all over. Bruised feeling in the pelvic region.
Potency - 30th. Tincture externally, in naevi.
Berberis Aquafolium
Stimulants all glands and improves nutrition.
Dose - ø, in material doses.
Bromium
Affect especially scrofulous children with enlarged glands and goitre. Left-sided mumps.
Dose - 6th potency.
Brucea Antidysenterica
Titanic spasms with undisturbed consciousness, < least touch, cries for fear of being touched.
Dose - 6th potency.
Bungarus Krait
Is of great use for poliomyelitis.
Potency - 6th

C

Cypripedin
For post-influenzal neurosis.
Dose - 6 grains of 3x trituration, 3 times a day. Also 30th.
Calcarea Cloride
Is very efficacious in menorrhagia, metrorrhagia, severe climacteric flushing.
Potency - 6x trituration, 3 times a day.
Cineraria Maritima Succus
Used externally as a specific for cataract and corneal opacities.
Dose - Extract juice of the plant, 2 drops instilled in the eyes thrice daily.
Cynosbati
Has gained high reputation in curing gonorrhoeal urethritis.
Potency - 30th attenuation.
Cenic Cio
Is indicated in all kinds of menstrual disorders.
Dose - ø, 5 drops thrice a day.
Coffea Mocha
A specific remedy for cholera.

Dose - give 10 drops of tincture in an ounce of water every half an hour.

Caffeine
Is serviceable in cases of threatening heart failure as because it is a great heart stimulant.
Dose - 1x trituration, 1 grain dose every 15 minutes.

Crysophanic Acid
Is of great use in dandruff and reeling of the skin of palms, psoriasis, ringworm and ophthalmia.
Dose - 5 drops of acid thrice daily.

Calcaria Calcinata
A remedy for all types of warts.
Dose - 3rd trituration.

Calcaria Iodata
Used in the treatment of scrofulous affections, especially enlarged glands, tonsils, etc. Thyroid enlargement about time of puberty.
Dose - 2nd trituration.

Calcaria Renalis
Arthritic nodosites. Renal calculi.
Dose - higher potencies. Also 6th trituration.

Calcarea Silicata
Very sensitive to cold. Patient is weak, emaciated, cold and chilly, but worse from being overheated.
Potency - high.

Ceanothus Amer
Splenitis; pain in all up the left side.
Dose - 1st attenuation. Locally as hair tonic.

Cenchris Contortix
Physica and mental restlessness with dyspnoea.
Dose - 6th potency.

Cephalanthus Occi
Intermittent fever, with sore throat and rheumatic symptoms.
Dose - 30th. Also of the ø, 10-30 drops.

Carya Alba
It controls blood gushed from gums, nose, ears, and other parts. Cures scurvy.
Dose - 30th and higher.

Cervus Brasilicus
For sciatica.
Potency - 6th attenuation.

China Boliviana
Is of great service in ulcerated commissures of mouth, aphthae, corns, wry-neck.
Dose - 30th attenuation.

Chromium Oxidatum
Has been used to destroy warts, in cutting pains in eyes, in angina pectoris, lumbago.
Potency- 30th attenuation.

Cichorium
Most important remedy of universal fame in curing
constipation, headache and amblyopia.

Dose - 6x, trituration.

Cinchoninum Sulphuricum
For falling off hair, bursting headache on walking, voluptuous dreams and painful erections of penis at night.
Dose - 30th and higher.

Coffeinum
Violent trembling of all the extremities.
Potency.- 3rd trituration.

Colocynthin
Is efficacious in diarhhoea and colic, > bending forward; congestion of male genital organs and pain in them; burning pains in soles of the feet
Dose - 1x trituration.

Calcarea Arsenica
Chronic malaria. Nephritis, with great sensitiveness in kedney region. Fleshy womwn at climacteric, slightest emotion causing palpitation.
Dose - 3rd trituration.
Dose - 5 grains, 3 times a day.

Calcarea Mur
Vomiting of all food and drink.
Potency - ø

Calcarea Ovorum
Bachache and leucorrhoea.
Dose - 30th and higher.

Calcarea Picrata
A remedy of prime importance in recurring or chronic boils.
Dose - use 3x trituration.

Calotropis
Used in the treatment of syphilis, leprosy, pneumonia, phthisis and acute dysentery.
Dose - 5 drops of tincture, 3 times a day.

Camphoric Acid
Cystitis.
Dose - 10 grains, 3 times a day.

Cancer Astacus
Urticaria. Itching. Liver affections with nettle-rash over whole body.
Dose - 30th

Canchalagua
A fever remedy influenza, malaria and intermittent fever.
Dose - Tincture, 5 to 30 drops.

Calcarea Lacto-phosph
Used in cyclic vomiting and migraine.
Dose - 5 grains, 3 times a day.

Carpus Luteum
For delayed menarche and undeveloped female symptoms.
Dose - 2x or 3x.

Coniinum
For paralysis of tongue, vertigo, hemiplegia.

Dose - 12th Potency.

Coniinum Bromatum
Is serviceable for mental apathy, empty sensation in head.
Potency - 3rd

Convolvulus Arvensis
Useful in colic and diarhhoea.
Dose - 30th.

Coriaria Ruscifolia
For loss of memory, vomiting and delirium tremens.
Dose - High Potency.

Croton Chloral
Cures any types of neuralgia.
Potency - Lower attenuations.

Cocaine Hydrochlorate
Is indicated for vaginismus of newly married woman.
Dose - Use ointment of hydrochlorate cocaine, 5 grains to the ounce of vaseline, the ointment to be applied to the inside of the vagina before retiring.

Calcium Iodo Bromide
Used for erysipelas
Dose - 3rd Potency, 3 times a day.

Corydalin
Is chiefly useful in syphilitic affections, ulcers of mouth and fauces.
Potency - 3x. trituration , half grain doses.

Coccinella Septempunctata
Is indicated in neuralgic headaches, in hrobbing toothache, with profuse accumulation of saliva.
Dose - 5 drops of tincture. Also 3rd potency.

Chelone
It is an enemy to every kind of worm infesting the human body. Specially for round and thread worms.
Dose - ø 5 drop dose.

Chionanthus
Is of service in many types of headaches, neurasthenic, periodical sick, menstrual and bilious. A prominent liver remedy, jaundice, diabetes mellitus.
Dose - tincture 8-10 drops.

Cuprum cyanatum
Basilar meningitis.
Dose - 30th

Cupum Oxydatum Nigrum
For all kinds of worms.
Potency - 1x.

Cuprum sulph
Burning at vertex.
Dose - 6th and higher.

Cystisus Scoparius
Reduces the blood pressure.

Dose - 3rd trituration.
Cineraria
Has reputation in the cure of cataract and corneal opacities.
Dose - is used externally, by instilling into the eye one drop 4 times a day.
Cinnamonum
For post-partum haemorhhage.
Dose - tincture. Use 5 drops of tincture or sugar for hiccough.
Cubeba Officinalis
Leucorrhoea in little girls.
Dose - 3rd attenuation.
Chenopodium
Intense pain in scapula very marked.
Dose - 3rd Potency. Oil of chenopodium for hookworm and roundworm, 10 drop doses every 4 hourly.
Citrus vulgaris
Headache with nauseaa, vomiting and vertigo. Disturbed sleep.
Dose - 30th
Convallaria Majalis
A heart remedy which increases energy of heart's action. Sensation as if heart ceased beating, then starting very suddenly. Palpitation from the least exertions. Angina pectoris. Tobacco heart, especially when due to cigarettes.
Potency - ø, 10 drop doses.
Crataegus
Acts on muscles of heart, and is a heart tonic. Reduces blood pressure and lowers pulse.
Dose - ø , 15 drop doses.
Ceasalpania Bondulosa
Used in all kinds of ague and is more efficacious than quinine.
Dose - tincture, 5 drops thrice a day.
Calotropis Lactum
Used with marked efficacy in curing syphilis in all its stages, in all kinds of putrid gangrenous ulcers. Also reputed for relieving vomiting, watery diarhhoea, toothache, and enlargement of spleen.   Dose - 2x, I grain thrice daily.
Clerodendron Infortunata
A successful remedy in worms of children. Used also in intermittent fever.
Potency - 5 drops of tincture thrice a day.
Coleus Aromaticus
One of the most valuable remedies in suppression of urine, gonorrhoea, nephritis and cystitisis with discharge of mucous membrane.
Dose - 15 drops every 6 hourly.
Cainca
Relieves polyuria while travelling. Is also of use in Bright's disease, pain in kidneys.
Potency - 30th and higher.
Calcarea Ovi Testae
In cases of simple bland leucorrhoea. Prescribe in cases of warts.
Potency - higher.
Camphora Bromata

An unique remedy in cholera infantum, chordee, neuralgia of testes and prostate, spermatorrhoea
Dose - 6x, trituration.

Cancer Fluviatilis
For nettle rash with liver complaint, revent tumours, itching of various parts.
Potency - 200th

Carboneum Sulphuratum
Very useful in patients broken down by abuse of alcohol.
Dose - 1st attenuation. Locally in facial neuralgia and sciatica.

Carcinosin
Carcinoma of the mammary glands with great pain and induration of glands.
Dose - 200th and higher.

Carduus Marianus
Indicated for hepatic affections, causing soreness, pain, jaundice.
Potency - Tincture, 15 to 20 drops.

Cascara Sagrada
Rheumatism of muscles and joints, with obstinate constipation. Used as a palliative for constipation, 20 drops of tincture twice daily.
Dose - ø

Condurango
Painful cracks in corners of mouth.
Potency - ø, 20-30 drops.

Clematis Erecta
A remedy of much importance in disturbances of sleep, and neuralgic pains in various parts. Testicles indurated with bruised feeling.
Potency - 30th. Also of the ø, 5 drops.

Chinimum Arsenicosum
Curative in diphtheria with great prostration, in mlarial affections. Athmatic attacks which recur periodically.
Dose - 3rd trituration.

Colstrum
Diarhhoea with colic in infants.whole body smells sour.
Dose - 30th

Cereus Bonplandii
Occipital headache and pain through the globe of the eyes and orbit.
Dose - 3rd attenuation.

Cheiranthus Cheiri
For deafness and ottorrhoea.
Dose - 30th Potency.

Cornus Alternifolia
Disturbed sleep, restlessness and eczyma with cracked skin.
Dose - ø, to 6th attenuation. Tincture 30 drops.

Culex
Vertigo on blowing the nose with fulness of the ears.
Dose - 3rd most often used. Also 30th and higher.

Cuphea

Cholera infantum, much acidity, frrquent watery stools. Tenesmus and great pain. Vomiting of undigested food.
Potency - tincture.
Cadmium Sulph
Violent vomiting with persistent vomiting.
Dose - 30th
Chininum Sulph
Is of use in malaria, Acute articular rheumatism and polyarticular gout.
Dose - 30th and higher. Also 3x.
Cholesterinum
Jaundice and gallstones. Obstinate hepatic engorgements and for cncer of the liver.
Dose - 3rd trituration. And higher in dilution.
Cadmium Iodat
Itching of anus and rectum felt during the day only.
Dose - 30th
Calcarea Acetica
For cancer pains.
Potency - 3rd trituration.
Colchicium
Has been employed gout, when is great soreness of the joints and muscles. Use in the management of rheumatic fever, pleurisy of rheumatic origin.
Dose - 6x trituration.
Casein
A remedy for asthma, worse evening, after midnight, in winter and rainy season. Gives instant relief in whooping cough.
Potency - 1x. Trituration.
Caulophyllin
For severe erratic pain and stiffness in small joints. Revives labor pain and furthers progress of labor.
Dose - 3x. trituration.
Collinsonin
Apocynum CannabinumIf the symptoms indicate no other remedy, whenever the ascites is the principal
Said to be of special value in chronic nasal, gastric and pharyngeal catarrh; constipation of children from intestinal atony.
Dose - 1x. trituration.
Cornin
Is indicated for chronic malaria, hepatitis and jaundice.
Potency - 3x. trituration.
Cheno-Morha Antidysenterica
It is a very efficacious remedy for all kinds of acute and chronic dysentery.
Dose - 5 drops of tincture, 4 times a day.
Calcaria Lectica Natoanata
Is chiefly useful in hay fever, asthma and chilblains.
Potency - use moderate potencies.
Chromium Kali Sulphuratum

Said to be of use in catarrh, hay asthma and hay fever.
Potency - 30th
Coqueluchinum
Is serviceable for whooping cough.
Dose - 200th and higher.

D

Digitalin
Prescribe as a cardiac tonic. Also indicated for frontal headache, loss of appetite, intestinal flatulence, borborygmi, eructations and severe abdominal pain.
Potency - 6x. trituration.
Diplaotaxis Tenuifolia
Tones upp the functions of the liver.
Dose - tincture.
Dys. Co. (Bach)
Considerable success has followed in congenital pyloric stenosis. Used in the treatment of duodenal ulcer.
Dose - 30th attenuation.
Desmodium G.
Useful in intermittent fevers.
Dose - 5 drops of tincture, thrice daily.
Datura Ferox
Is beneficial and mania.
Potency - ø
Datura Metel
Of use in convulsions, epilepsy and delirium.
Dose - ø
Duboisin
Is found useful in locomotor ataxy, presbyopia and dryness of mouth and throat.
Potency - 6th trituration.
Diphtheria Antitoxin
A graet remedy for diphtheria.
Dose - 32nd and 1002th attenuation.
Damiana
Used in sexual neurasthenia; impotency. Incontinence of old people, with chronic prostatic discharge. Frigidity of females. Aids the establishment of normal menstrual flow in young girls.
Dose - Tinctures, 20 drop doses.
Dictamnus Albus
Soothes labour pains.
Potency - 200th
Diptherinum
For diphtheria and post-diphtheritic paralysis.
Potency - higher. Must not be repeated too frequently.
Diptrix Odorata

Used in neuralgia and pertussis.
Dose - ø, and lower potencies.
Dolichos Puriens
A general itching without eruption.
Dose - 30th. Tincture, in haemorhhoids.
Duboisin Sulphate
For hystero - epilepsy.
Potency - 12th. use also 6x trit.
Dioscorin
A remedy for many kinds of pain, colic and gall-stone colic.
Potency - 2x. trit.

E

Euphorbia Pilulifera
Is a specific remedy in all kinds of asthma.
Dose —10 drops of tincture, 15 minutes apart during paroxysm and thrice a day when paroxysm is over.
Embelia Ribens
Of great service for worms in children. Is indicated for indigestion, diarrhoea, fever, shrills in sleep and grinding of teeth.
Potency— ø, 10 drops thrice a day.
Esculentine
Has proved to be great beneficial in promptly reducing fat, it strengthens the heart and improves the general health. Also controls the intolerable rheumatic pain to which the obese is subject.
Dose — Give 1 table spoonful of tincture in an ounce of hot water, twice daily before meals.
Eryngium Maritimum
Use for cough, fever, herpes and sexual weakness.
Dose — 30-th attenuation.
Echinacea
Used for symptoms of blood poisoning, septic conditions generally. Boils, Erysipelas and foul ulcers. Appendicitis. Venom infection. Snake bites and bites and stings generally.
Dose — ø, 10 drops every 4 hours. Locally as a cleansing and antiseptic wash.
Epigaea Repens
Chronic cystitis, with dysuria; tenesmus after micturition; muco-pus and uric acid deposit, gravel, renal calculi. Burning in neck of bladder whilst urinating. Pyelitis, incontinence of urine.
Dose — 5 drops of tincture every 4 hours.
Eryngium Aquaticum
Difficult and frequent micturition. Tenesmus of bladder and urethra. Renal colic.
Dose — ø to 3-rd potency.
Eucalyptus Globulus
Indicated for many kinds of fever. Use as a stimulating expectorant. Haemorrhages internally and locally.
Dose — ø in 15 drop doses.
Euphorbia Lathyris

Useful in erysipelas. Oedema of lids. Rheumatic pains during rest.
Dose — 30-th. Also tincture, 5 drops.
Euphorbia Corollata
Nausea and vomiting of food, water and mucous.
Dose — 6-th potency. Of the ø, 10 drops.
Elaps Corallinus
Right-sided paralysis. Chronic nasal catarrh, with foetid odor and greenish crusts.
Potency — 30-th. And also 6X.
Eosin
A remedy for cancer and polyarthritis.
Dose — Use 2-nd trit, and 30-th.
Equisetum
For enuresis and dysuria. Frequent urging with severe pain at the close of urination. Incontinence in children, with nightmares when passing urine. Incontinence in old women, also with involuntary stools.
Dose —Tincture.
Euonymus Atropurpurea
Migraine. Chronic rheumatism and gout.
Dose — ø, and lower attenuations.
Eupatorium Aromaticum
Sore nipples. Sore mouth in infants. Low fevers, with extreme restlessness.
Potency —Tincture. Locally in sore mouth and sore nipples.
Euphorbium
Burning pain in bones, in limbs with paralytic weakness in the joints. Pains of cancer.
Dose — 6-th potency. Also of the tincture, 2 drops.
Eupion
A remedy for uterine displacements. Backache, followed by bland leucorrhoea. Intense sweat from slightest exertion.
Potency — 30-th. Also q, 5 to 10 drops.
Erodium Cicutarium
Used for metrorrhagia and menorrhagia.
Dose — ø.
Erechthites Hieracifolia
Haemorrhage from any part of the body.
Dose— Tincture.
Ethylum Nitricum
An unique remedy for virtigo.
Potency— 30-th and higher.
Euphorbia Cyparissias
For erysipelas, miliaria, vesicles.
Dose — 12-th attnuation.
Euphorbia Heterodoxa
Is of great use in burning pains of cancer.
Potency — Higher.
Euphorbia Ipecacuanhae
useful in gastritis and vomiting.

Dose — Lower potencies.
Euphorbia Peplus
Is employed in the treatment of erysipelas and sore-throat.
Potency — 30-th and higher.
Echafolta
For septicemia.
Dose — Tincture, apply externally to the wounds.
Elaterin
An invaluable remedy in violent vomiting and purging, especially if the evacuations are copious and watery.
Potency — 5X. trit.
Ephedrin
Is a successful remedy for exophthalmic goitre and headache.
Dose — 4-th attenuation.
Euphorbin
Burning pains in the bones is an indictation. A remedy for
the pains of cancer.
Potency — 6X. trit.
Emetine Hydrochloride
Valuable in treatment of amoebic dysentery. Pyorrhoea.
Dost — 200-th. For pyrrhoea, ½ grain. daily for 3 days.
Epilobium Palustre
For chronic diarrhoea with tenesmus and mucous discharges.
Potency— 30-th.
Egg Vaccine
For any types of asthma.
Dose—30-th. and higher.
Electricitas
Useful in anxiety, restlessness, palpitation and nervous tremors.
Dose — Higher.
Eel Serum
In kidnes affections, during the corse of heart-disease, characterised by oliguria, anuria and albuminuria.
Potency — 30-th.
Eranthis Hymnalis
Pain in occiput and neck.
Dose — Higher.
Epihysterin
Is found useful for menorrhagia and metrorrhagia.
Dose — 30-th and upwards, giving two doses weekly.

F
Fagus Cup
Coppery eruptions on the scalp. Chronic insomnia, and failing memory.
Dose — Tincture.

Fluor Albus
For neuralgia of eyes.
Potency—30-th.

Fluor. Aurant. Amar.
Insures radical cure in displacement of uterus with long-standing neuralgia.
Dose — ø, 5 drops in water night and morning.

Faecalis (Bach)
Most pronounced action in any uterine affections of brunettes, all pains are from below up; tendency to abortion.
Potency — 202-th and 1002-th attenuation.

Fluid Carefolius
Is of service in nephritis, cystitis and enlargement of the prostatic gland. Also efficacious in sexual debility especially of neurasthenic origin.
Dose — Give half tea-spoonful of tincture in an ounce of water every 6 hourly.

Ferrum Phos. Hydricum
Cures conjunctivitis and writer's cramp.
Potency — Lower trit.

Franzensbad
Of use in constipation, dyspepsia and in chronic derangement of the digestion.
Dose — Thirtieth and higher.

Ferrum Protoxalatum
For all types of anaemia.
Dose — Use 1X trit.

Fragaria Vesca
Useful for lack of mammary secretion. Prevents formaton of calculi, removes tartar from teeth and prevents attacks of gout. Chilblains.
Potency — Higher.

Franciscea Uniflora
Chronic stiffness of the muscles.
Dose — ø, rather material doses.

Formalin
In hot water as vapor most valuable therpeutic agent in pertussis, phthisis, in cattrrhal affections of upper air passages.
Dose — As vapor in hot water in respiratory affections; otherwise 3X potency.

Formica Rufa
Chronic gout and stiffness in joints. Gout and articular rheumatism; pains worse, motion; better, pressure. Complaints from overlifting.
Dose — 30-th attenuation. Also of the ø, 3-5 drops.

Ferrum Citricum
For acid dyspepsia in chlorosis
Dose — 3-rd trit.

Fluoroform
Considered specific for whooping-cough.
Dose — 2% watery solution, 4 dtops, after paroxysms.

Ferrum Maruaticum
For arrested menstruation. Pain in right shoulder.

Dose — 6-th. For anaemia, use 3X, after meals.

Fuchsina
Valuable in swollen gums.
Potency — 30-th.

Ferrum Picricum
A great remedy when the voice fails after public speaking. Warts and epithelial growths; corns with yellowish discolouration.
Dose—3-rd trit.

Fuligo Ligni
Acts on glandular system, obstinate ulcers, eczema. Cancer of womb with metrorrhagia.
Dose — Sixth trituration.

Ferula Glauca
In violent sexual excitement in women.
Potency — 6-th.

Ferrum Bromatum
For sticky excoriating leucorrhoea.
Potency —T hird. trit.

Ferrum Cyanatum
Constipation alternating with diarrhoea. Epilepsy.
Dose — 6-th potency.

Ferrum Magneticum
Small warts on hands.
Dose —Third attenuation.

Ferrum Sulphuricum
For menorrhagia, toothache, acidity with eructations of food in mouthfuls. Watery and painless diarrhoea.
Dose — 3-rd.

Ferrum Arsenicum
Skin dry. Eczema, proriasis and impetigo.
Potency — Use 3X trit.

Ficus Religiosa
Cures haemorrhages of many kinds. Haematemesis, menorrhagia, haemoptysis, haematuria etc.
Dose — First potency.

Formic Acid
Chronic myalgia. Muscular Paint and soreness. Gout and articular rheumatism.
Dose — 30-th attenuation.

Fraxinus Americana
Fever sores on lips. Uterine tumors, with bearing-down sensations. Fibrous growth, subinvolution and prolapse of the uterus.
Dose —10 drops of tincture thrice daily.

Fucus Vericulosus
A remedy for obesity and non-toxic goitre.
Dose — 30 drops of tincture three times a day before meals.

Fabiana Imbricata
Useful in the uric acid diathesis, cystitis, gonorrhoea and prostatitis.

Dose— 15 drops of tincture.
Fel Tauri
Increases the peristaltic action of the intenstines, and acts as a puragative and cholagogue. Obstruction of gall ducts. Biliary calculi. Jaundice.

Potency — Lower triturations.
Ferrum Aceticum
Pain in right detoid. Asthma with copious expectoration of greenish pus ; constant cough.

Dose — 6-th potency.
Ferri Et. Strychniae Citras
In cases of anaemia and chlorosis when attended with debility, dyspepsia and amenorrhoea.

Dose — 2X
Ferri Valerianicum
This remedy is indicated in cases of hysteria, chorea and nervous disorders in those suffering from chlorosis and anaemia.

Potency — 3X. trit.
Fraxinus Excelsior
Has been employed as a specific for gout and rheumatic artiritis.

Dose — Of the tincture, 30 drops.
Fagopyrum Esculentum
Pruritus senilis. Vehement itching in arms and legs. Preritus vulvae, with yellow leucorrhoea.

Dose — 3-rd. Also 10 drops of tincture.
Fagus Sylvatica
For headache and salivation. Dread of water.

Dose—Thirteeth.
Ferrum Idodatum
Acute nephritis following eruptive diseases. Crops of boils. Scrofulous affections, glandular enlargements, and tumors call for this remedy.

Potency — 3X.

G

Galiopsis Grandiflora
For any degree of spleen affections.

Potency — Higher.
Geranium Robertianum
A great remedy for headache, with inflammation of the nerve of the right. Arrested development of teeth.

Dose — 3-rd attenuation.
Gichtwasser
Gout and gouty nodes in several parts of the body.

Dose — ø, rather material doses.
Geartner (Bach)
The keynote of this nosode is 'malnutrition' and found to be of value in the extreme of life associated with malignancy. Marked emaciation may be taken as an indication for the use of this bowel nosode. Efficacious for coeliac diseases, ketosis, intestinal infantilism ; also for

chronic gastro-enteritis, tabes mesenterica, thread worms. (The clearing of thread worms is difficult and usually requires prolonged treatment.)
Potency — 30-th.

Gynocardia Odorata
Is very beneficial remedy in leprosy, secondary syphilis, psoriasis, eczema, scabies and other cutaneous eruptions.
Dose — Give tincture 1 drop thrice daily. Use also 5-th attenuation.

Galvanismus
Has gained high reputation in curing hydrocephalus, haemorrhoids and toothache.
Potency — 200-th and higher.

Glycerinum
Use for building up tissue, hence of great use in marasmus, debility, mental and physical.
Dose — Higher potencies. Pure Glycerine in teaspoonful doses, t.i.d., with lemon juice for pernicious anaemia.

Gun-Powder
For blood poisoning, spetic suppuration and protective against wound infection.
Potency — 2X trit.

Gentiana Lutea
Acts as a tonic, increasing appetite.
Dose — Tincture.

Guaiacum
Very valuable in acute rheumatism. Is adapted to the artiritic diathesis, rheumatic and tonsillitis. Unclean odor form whole body. Syphilitic sore throad.
Dose — ø.

Gnaphalium
A remedy of unquestioned benefit in sciatica.
Dose — 30-th. Also of the tincture, 10 drops.

Gossypium Herb.
Intermittent pains in ovaries, Suppressed menstruation. A powerful emmenagugue, used in physiological doses.
Potency — Tincture, 15 to 30 drops.

Gratiola Officinalis
Nux symptoms in females often met by Gratiola. Dsypepsia, with much distention of the stomach. Obstinate ulcers. Leucorrhoea.
Dose — 30-th

Gaertner
Pessimistic, lack of confidence. Also use for utricaria.
Dose — 200-th

Ginseng
For lumbago, sciatica and rheumatism.
Dose — ø.

Gastein
One of the best remedies for amenorrhoea, membranous dysmenrrhoea and haemorrhoids.
Dose — Higher.

Guaiacolum
Has been employed in the treatment of malaria and tuberculosis during its early stages.

Potency — Tincture.
Gelsemin
Is found useful in paralysis of various groups of muscle; influenza, measles.
Dose — 6X. trit.
Gossypin
For intermittent pain in ovaries ; acts as a powerful enomenagogue, relieves tardy menses.
Dose — 3-rd triturations.
Gaultheria Oil
In gastralgia, when there are cramping pains in the stomach.
Dose —Tincture, 20 drop doses. Also use 30-th and higher.
Gaultheria Procumbens
The sphere of this remedy covers inflammatory rheumatism, pleurodynia, sciatica and other neuralgias.
Dose — Tincture, 25 to 30 drops.
Geranium Maculatum
Ulceration of stomach, vomiting of blood.
Dose —Tincture, half dram doses in gastric ulcer.
Geranin
Constant hawking and spitting in elderly people.
Potency — 6X.
Grindelia Robusta
Raises the blood pressure. Also for burns, blisters & herpes zoster.
Dose — Tinture.
Glanderine
Useful in the treatment of ozaena, scrofulous swelling, pyaemia, erysipelas. Chronic rhinitis. Bronchitis in the aged.
Potency — 30-th.
Golondrina
A antidote to snake-poison.
Dose — High.
Guarea Trichiloides
Eye symptoms alternate with diminished hearing.
Dose — High.
Chemosis
and pterygium have been cured with it.
Dose — Tincture.
Granatum
Use for the expulsion of tapeworm.
Dose — Tincture.
Gallic Acid
A remedy in phthisis. Pain in lungs, pulmonary haemorrhage and excessive expectoration.
Potency — Frist trit.

H

Hazeline
For menorrhagia, the periods occuring about every 3 weeks.
Dose — Lower potencies.

Helianthus Annus
Very useful in fistula-in-ano; tumour of epigastrium region, throbbing swelling in the pit of the stomach involving the left side of the liver and the spleen. Also of great use in sore-throat and epistaxis.
Dose — ø, and 30-th attenuation.

Helonin
Is amazingly curative for uterine fibriod ; small tumor on the breasts, cracked nipples.
Potency — 3X. trit.

Hymosa
Is the most effective remedy in the treatment of rheumatism and rheumatic fever. It also rapidly cures lumbago.
Dose — 30 drops of tincture trice daily.

Hygrophilla Spinosa
Very beneficial remedy in leprosy and deep ulcers. Relieves paroxysms of intermittent fever at10-11 a.m., removes urticarial rashes with intense itching during heat.
Dose — Tincure, 5 drops thrice daily.

Hemidesmus Indica
Is of great service in curing all diseases depentent on blood poisoning. Also cures eruptions due to abuse of mercury.
Potency — 5 drops of q, thrice a day.

Hydrophobinum
For aching in bones. Complaints from abnormal sexual desire. Priapism with frequent emissions.
Dose — 30-th.

Hekla Lava
Of great use in exostosis, gum abscess, difficult teething and cries of bones.
Potency — 6X and higher in dilutions.

Haematoxylon Campechianum
Angina pectoris. Convulsive pain in heart region with oppression. Sensation as if a bar lay across chest.
Dose —Third potency.

Helix Tosta
Use in haemoptysis.
Dose — ø.

Hydrocyanic Acid
For hysterical and epileptic convulsions. Tetanus narcolepsy.
Dose — Sixth and higher.

Hura
A remedy for leprosy and painful stiff neck.
Dose — 6-th. Also q, 5 drops.

Hydrastin Sulph.
Haemorrhage of bowels in typhoid.
Dose — 1X

Hydrastinum Muriaticum
In dilatations of the stomach and for chronic digestive disorders.
Dose — 3-rd trituration. Locally, in aphthous sore mouth, ulcers, ulcerated sore-throat, ozaena.
Helleborus Faetidus
For falling of hair and nails ; skin peeling.
Potency— ø. Use also 30-th.
Hall
Use in exopthalmic goitre.
Potency — Higher dilutions.
Helleborus Viridis
Has most pronounced effects in diarrhoea, colic and sore-throat.
Dose — 30-th attenuation.
Homeria
Is a successful remedy for constipation, vimiting and collapse.
Dose — ø.
Hura Crepitans
Employed in the treatment of vomiting, diarrhoea, sore-throat and blindness.
Potency — 30-th.
Hydrastininum Muriaticum
For fibroma and metrorrhagia.
Dose — 6-th trit.
Hyoscyamin
Of use in ciliary neuralgia, sleeplessness and spinal sclerosis.
Dose — 6X trituration.
Hydrastin. Hydrochlorate
Is of service in epistaxis, gastric and intestinal haemorrhages and haematemesis.
Potency — 3-rd trit.
Haematin
Convulsive pain in heart region with oppression; Angina pectoris.
Dose — 4X. trit.
Hamamelin
Valuable for painful wounds. Cures haemorrhoids.
Potency — 3X. trit.
Heliotropium Peru
Is of great use in membranous dysmenorrhaea. Uterine displacement, with bearing-down sensation and loss of voice.
Dose — 3-rd attenuation.
Helmintochortos
Acts very powerfully on intestinal worms, espicially the lumbricoid.
Dose — 3-rd trit.
Henchera
Gastroenteritis, nausea, vomiting of bile and frothy mucus; stools watery, profuse, tenesmus and never get done feeling.
Dose — ø, 10 drop doses.
Hepatica Triloba

Induces free and easy expectoration. Pharyngeal catarrh, with profuse, serous sputa and hoarseness. Tenacious viscid phlegm causes continued hawking.

Dose — 2-nd potency. Also of the ø, 25-30 drops.

Hyoscin Hydrobrom
A remedy for shock.
Dose — 3-rd trit.

Hedera Helix
For delirium and chronic convulsions. Chronic hydrocephalus.
Dose — 3-rd potency.

Hydrocotyle
Curative in leprosy and lupus, when there is no ulceration.
Dose —1-st to 6-th potency.

Hagenia Abyssinica
Use to expel tape-worm
Dose — Tincture, 20 drop doses.

Hydrastin
Most important remedy of universal fame in curing fistula-in-ano.
Potency — 6X. trit.

Hedeoma Pulegioides
For leucorrhoea, with itching and burning. Bearing-down pains with much backache. Pain in thumb-joint and Tendo-Achilles.
Dose — 3X. trit.

I

Iodatum
For gonorrhoea and gonoreal urethritis.
Dose— Lower potencies.

Imperatoria
For any affections of stomach.
Dose — ø, teaspoonful every two hours.

Influenzinum
Is a specific for catarrh, colds and influenza.
Potency — 30-th, every 3 hourly.

Indium Metalicum
An unique remedy in backache, epistaxis, megrim and sore-throat.
Dose — 6X. trituration.

Iris Foetidissima
Of use in headache and hernia.
Dose — Tincture and high potencies.

Itu Resina
Has proved to be great beneficial in stiff-neck, toothache and vulvitis. Also cures earache when the least dampness sets in.
Potency — 30-th attenuation.

Irisin

Gives instant relief and cures sick headaches and cholera morbus.
Dose — 6X. trit.
Ichthyolum
Excelent in winter coughs of old people. It is strongly antiparasitic. Polyarthritis, chronic rheumatism.
Potency — 3X.
Indol
Persistent desire to sleep. Constant motion of fingers and feet.
Dose — 6-th attenuation.
Iris Versicolor
Valuable for sick headache. Burning of whole alimentary canal.
Dose — ø., to 30-th. Tincutre, 10 drops.
Iris Tenax
Pain in ileo-caecal region ; appendicitis.
Dose — 30-th and higher.
Iris Florentina
Of use in delirium, convulsions and paralysis.
Dose — Higher.
Iberis Amara
Possesses great efficacy in cardiac diseases. Cardiac dyspnoea. Darting pains through heart. White stools.
Dose — ø. and 1-st potency.
Ipomea
Kidney disorders with pain in back. Much abdominal flatulence.
Dose — Tincture to 6-th potency.
Indigo
Of undoubted benefit in the treatment of epilepsy. Neurasthenia and hysteria.
Dose—thirtieth. Pure powdered Indigo placed on the wound cures snake and spider poison. Use also 6X. trit.
Iduretted Potass. Iod.
Expels tapeworms dead.
Dose — 30 grains Potass. and 4 grains Iodine to 1 OZ of water, 10 drops thrice daily.
Iodothyrine
Affects metabolism, reducing weight. Hence use in obesity.
Potency— 6-th to 30-th.
Iodoformum
Use in the treatment of tubercular meningitis. Chronic diarrhoea of children.
Dose — 2-nd trit. 3 grains on the back of the tongue will relieve attack of asthematic breathing.
Ingluvin
Relieves vomiting of pregnancy, infantile vomiting and diarrhoea.
Dose — 3X trit.
Illecebrum
For fever with catarrhal symptoms, gastric and typhoid fever.
Dose —12-th attenuation.
Insulin

Use in the treatment of diabetes. Also in acne, carbuncles, erethema with itching eczema.
Potency — 30-th.

J

Jacaranda Gualandi
For painful erections of penis ; phimosis. Prepuce painful and swollen. Chancroid. Chordee. Itching pimples on glans and prepuce. Rheumatic pain in right knee.
Dose — Tincture, 15-20 drops. Also 3X.

Justicia Adhatoda
Highly efficacious medicine for acute catarrhal condition of the respiratory tract. Coryza with paroxysmal cough, larynx painful, horse. Whooping-cough.
Dose — ø., 3-rd and higher.

Jaborandi
Eye strain from whatever cause. White spots before eyes. Smarting pain in eyes. Near-sighted. Also of use in exophthalmic goitre. Thyroid infections. Night-sweats of consumptives.
Dose—3-rd potency.

Jalapa
Cures colic and diarrhoea.
Dose —12-th and higher.

Juniperus Communis
Catarrhal inflammation of kidneys. Dropsy, with suppression of urine. Chronic pyelitis.
Dose — ø., 10 drop doses.

Juniperus Virginianus
Dysuria, burning, cutting pain in urethra when urinating.
Dose —Tincture.

Jatropha Curcas
Is of use in cholera and diarrhoea. Forced discharge; loud noise in abdomen like gurgling of water coming out of a bung-hole.
Dose — 30-th.

Juncus Effusus
Dysuria, strangury and ischuria. Asthmatic symptoms in haemorrhoidal subjects.
Dose — ø., and 1-st potency.

Juglans Cinerea
Occipital headache, associated with liver disturbances. Itching and pricking when heated. Eczema, specially on lower extremities.
Dose — ø..

Jonosia Asoca
Of great use in delayed and irregulr menses ; menstrual colic; amenorrhoea, pain in overes before flow.
Potency — Tincture.

Jequirity
Purulent conjunctivitis, granular ophthalmia. Keratitis.
Dose — Internally use 3X. Locally, diluted mother tincture.

Jaglandin
For duodenal catarrh and bilious diarrhoea.

Dose — 6X. trit.
Juniperus Sabina
A good remedy for recto-vaginal fistula.
Potency — 30-th.
Jasminum Officinale
Very useful in convulsions and tetanus.
Dose — Tincture.

K

Kedron
For uterine fibraoid, small tumors on breasts.
Dose — Thirtieth.
Keratin
Relieves any types of pain.
Dose — 3X. trit., 10 grain doses.
Kamala
Is best known as a remedy for tapeworm.
Dose — ø, half dram doses.
Karaka
Of use in paralysis.
Potency — Tincture.
Kerosolenum
Acts like a magic in convulsions.
Dose — Use moderate potencies.
Kissingen
Marvellous results are obtained by this drug in diabetes, corns and warts. Also of use in gout and albuminuria.
Dose — 12-th and higher.
Kali Silicatum
Very marked lassitude, desire to lie down all the time, emaciation.
Dose — Higher potencies.
Kali Salicylicum
Useful for vomiting of pregnancy. Chronic rheumatism.
Dose — 30-th and higher.
Kali Oxalicum
For lumbago and convulsions
Potency — Higher.
Kousso
Nausea and vomiting, virtigo, precordial anxiety, slowing and irregular pulse.
Dose — Tincture.
Kaolin
A remedy for croup and bronchitis. Soreness of chest along trachea.
Potency — 3X and 6X. trit.
Kali Sulph. Chromico
Chronic colds. Sneezing, red, watery eyes, irrilation of mucous membrane.

Dose — 12-th potency.
Kali Nitricum
Of great value in sudden dropsical swellings over the whole body.
Dose — 30-th.
Kali Aceticum
Use in diabetes.
Dose — Higher.
Kali Picricum
For jaundice, with violent eructations.
Potency — 30-th.
Kali Telluricum
Is of use in swellen tongue.
Dose — Higher.
Kali Arsenicum
Intolerable itching, worse undressing. Chronic eczema. Psoriasis. Numerous small nodules under skin.
Dose — 30-th.
Kalagua
For tuberculosis
Dose — Higher.
Kali Hydroiodicum
Profuse watery, acrid coryza, associated with pain in frontal sinus. Syphilis, indicated in all stages.
Dose — 3-rd potency. Use 1X trit., 3 times a day, for fibroid
tumors, metritis, sub-involution, hypertrophy.
Kali Cyanatum
Cancer of tongue and agonizing neuralgia. Difficult speech.
LDose — 200-th. Also 6X trit.

L

Lueticum
For puny growth, nocturnal fright and deafness. Unilateral arrest of development of the body.
Dose — 200-th.
Lac Vac. Defloratum
One of the most valuable remedy for appendicitis, obesity, sciatica, leucorrhoea, and for defective lactation.
Potency — 5-th attenuation and higher.
Lactic Vaccini Flos.
Is a specific remedy for diphtheria, sore-throat, leucorrhoea and menorrhagia.
Dose — Use moderate dilutions.
Linum Catharticum
Acts like a magic in amenorrhoea, laryngitis, and haemorrhoids.
Potency — 3-rd attenuation and higher.
Lippspringe
is of great service in jaundice, leucorrhoea and worms.

Dose — 30-th.
Lithium Muriaticum
Specific for heartburn.
Potency— 12-th attenuation.
Lobelia Dortmanna
Of use in headache and indigestion.
Dose — Tincture.
Lysidinum
Very useful in gout, lithiasis, and oxaluria.
Potency — 6X. trit.
Lapis Alba
Affections of glands, goitre, pre-ulcernative stage of carcinoma. Burning pain in breast, stomach, and uterus. Uterine carcinoma.
Dose — 6X. trit., and higher in dilutions.
Lathyrus
Paralytic affections of lower extremities. Infantile paralysis. Burning pain in tip of tongue.
Potency — 3-rd and higher.
Latrodectus Mactans
The best specific for angina pectoris.
Dose — 30-th potency. Also 6X. trit.
Lemna Minor
Acts especially upon the nostrils, nasal polypi, swollen turbinates ; atrophic rhinitis.
Dose — 6-th to 30-th. Also of the q, 20 drops.
Levico
Chronic and dyscratic skin diseases, chorea minor and spasms in scrofulous and anaemic children. Favours assismilation and increases nutrition.
Dose — Ten drops in a glass of warm water, 3 times a day.
Liatris Spicata
Of use in dropsy. Suppressed urination is most favourably influnced. Disrrhoea, with violent urging and pain in lower part of back.
Dose — Tincture. Locally, applied to ulcers and unhealthy wounds.
Lolium Temulentum
Trembling of all limbs.
Dose — Sixth potency, and higher.
Lycopus Virginicus
Lowers the blood-pressure, reduces the rate of the heart. Haemoptysis due to valvular heart disease. Also of great use in exophthalmic goitre and haemorrhoidal bleeding.
Dose — 30-th. In toxic goitre, 5 drops of tincture.
Lithium Carbonicum
Chronic rheumatism connected with heart lesions. Headache ceases while eating.
Dose — Third trituration.
Lachnanthes Tinctoria
A remedy for torticollis, rheumatic symptoms about neck.
Potency —30-th Tincture, in phthisis, 3 drops every 4 hours.
Lobelia Erinus
For malignant growths, exrremely rapid eevelopment. Corkscrew-like pains in abdomen.

Dose — ø, to 30-th.

Lobelia Syphilitica
Sneezing influenza, involving the posterior nares and fauces. Pain and gas in bowels, followed by copious watery stools with tenesmus and soreness of anus.
Dose — 30-th.

Latrodectus Hesselti
For loss of memory. Arrests intense pain in pyaemia. Great oedema in neighbourhood of wound.
Dose — 6-th potency.

Lactis Vaccini Floc.
Is of use in diphthria, leucorrhoea, menorrhagia and dysphagia.
Dose — Highest potencies.

Lac Caninum
Is valuable in tonsillitis, sore throat and diptheria, symptoms change repeatedly from side to side. Breasts swollen painful before menses. Decided effect in drying up milk in women who cannot nurse the body.
Dose — 30-th and higher.

Lactic Acid
For morning sickness, diabetes, and rheumatic pain in joints and shoulders, wrists, knees. Trembling of whole body while walking.
Dose — 30-th. Ten drops of tincture in a glass of water in gastro-enteritis. Locally, in the tuberculous ulceration of vocal cords.

Lac Vaccinum
For headache, rheumatic pains and constipation.
Dose — 30-th.

Lac. Vaccinum Coagulatum
Relieves nausea of pregnancy.
Dose — Thirtieth and the highest potencies.

Lappa Major
Eruptions on the head, face, and neck ; pimples, acne. Stys and ulcerations on the edge of the eyelids. Crops of boils and styes.
Potency — ø, to 30-th.

Lupulin
Best in seminal emissions.
Dose — 6X. trit. Locally, in painful cancers.

Lupulus
Conditions of the nervous system attended with nausea, dizziness, headache following a night's debauch. Infantile jaundice.
Dose — ø, 15 to 25 drops.

Lecithin
Use in anaemia and convalescene, neurasthenia and insomnia.
Dose — 2 grains of crude and 12-th potency.

Lachesis Lanciolatus
For haemorrhages from every orifice of the body.
Potency — 30-th.

Lignum Vitae

Is especially adapted to the arthritic diathesis. Very valuable in acute rhematism. Acute tonsillitis, syphilitic sore throat.
Dose — Tincture.

Linaria Vulgaris
Enteric symptoms and great drowsiness very marked jaundice, with splenic and hepatic hypertrophy.
Dose — Sixth.

Lonicera Pericylamenum
For irritability of temper, with viotent outburst.
Dose — Sixth.

Laurocerasus
Spasmodic tickling cough, in cardiac patients is often magically influenced by this drug. Asphyxia neonatorum.
Dose — ø.

Lapsana Communis
useful in sore nipples and piles.
Dose — 3-rd attenuation. Locally, tincture in sore nipples.

Lithium Benzoicum
Deep-seated pains in loins ; in small of back. Gallstones.
Dose — Use 3X trit.

Lippia Medicana
Persistent dry, hard, bronchial cough—asthma and chronic bronchitis.
Dose — 200-th.

Leptandra
A liver remedy, with jaundice and black, tarry stools.
Dose — ø, 30 drops. Also 3X. trit.

Lapathum Acutum
Nosebleed and headache following pain in kidneys; Leucorrhoea.
Dose — 30-rd potency.

Lithium Lacticum
Rheumatism of shoulder, and small joints relieved by moving about.
Dose — 3X trit.

Leptandrin
For hydropericardium.
Potency — 3X. trit.

Libradol
Is an excellent local application for any types of pain. Also apply to the spine for cerebro-spinal meningitis and for pain in abscess.
Dose — Tinctue.

Lactucarium
Cures impotence, sleeplessness and hydrothorax.
Potency — 1X. trit.

M
Madar

Is employed in the treatment of asthematic paroxysms.
Dose — 30 drops of tincture, once daily.

Meloe Majalis
For haemorrhages from any orifice of the body.
Potency — 30-th.

Melitagrinum
An unique remedy in varicocele and eczema of the glans and of the sulcus of the penis. Crusta lactea.
Dose — 200-th.

Morgan Pure (Paterson)
In indicated where there is a marked symptoms of skin eruptions, (e.g., itchy pustular eruptions on the face, scalp and neck ; Eczema on chin, forehead and ear passages; itchy eruptions behind ears ; Neuro-dermatitis on chin, forehead and scalp margins. Erysipelas face ; Acne on face.) or disturbance of the liver ; bilious headache, or actual pressure of gall-stones.
Potency — 202-th and 1002-th attenuation. Do not repeat this bowel nosode within 3 months.

Morgan Gaertner (Paterson)
Is employed in the treatment of skin, (e.g. Psoriasis — elbow; knees and ankles, legs or body. Eruptions, thigh; wrist. Herpetic eruptions on sole of foot. Papulo-pustular eruptions face, brow, scanlp,— crusty, scaling and cracked. Urticaria arms — large weals. Warts hands — large, flat or jagged. Shingles) and liver affections, but it is likely to be more useful where there is evidence of acute inflammatory attack, such as that found in cholecystitis. An effective remedy of renal colic. It is also of value in treatment in any case which has a 4-8 p.m. modality.
Dose — 202-th and 1002-th attenuation.

Malaria Officinalis
Has evident power to cause the disappearance of the plasmodium of malaria. Malaria cachexia. Functional hepatic diseases.
Dose — 6-th and higher.

Macrotin
Especially for lumbago.
Dose — 3-rd attenuation and 30-th.

Malandrinum
A very effectual protection against small-pox. Ill effects of vaccination.
Dose — 30-th and highest.

Myrica Cirifera
Marked action on the liver, with jaundice and persistent sleeplessness.
Dose — Tincture, 10 to 20 drops.

Mullein Oil
Has a pronunced action on the ear. Also for teasing cough at night or lying down. Enuresis.
Dose— Internally, q and lower potencies. Enuresis, 5 drop doses night and morning. Locally, for earache and dry. Scally condition of meatus. Also for teasing cough.

Myristica Sebifera
A remedy of great antiseptic powers. Inflammation of skin, cellular tissue and periosteum. Specific action in panaritium. Pain in the finger nails with swelling of the phalanges. Hastens suppuration and shortens its duration. Inflammation of middle ear, suppurative stage, Fistula in ano. Acts more powerfully often than Hepar or Silcea.
Dose — 3-rd to 30-th. dilutions.

Magnesia Boro Citrate
The best remedy for calculus in the bladder.
Dose —Dissolve 15 grains in one ounce of water and give a teaspoonful once a day. Use also 30-th attenuation.
Magnetis Polus Arcticus
Disturbed sleep, somnambulism, and for toothache.
Dose — 12-th and higher.
Magnetis Polus Australis
For ingrowing toenails.
Potency — Higher.
Mygale
Chorea is the principal therapeutic field of this drug. Constant motion of whole body. Uncontrollable movements of arms and legs.
Dose — 30-th.
Myosotis
Chronic bronchitis and phthisis. Cough with profuse muco-purulent expectoration, gagging and vomiting during cough.
Dose — ø, 2 to 5 drops.
Mercurius Iodatus Flavus
Right-sided throat affections, with greatly swollen glands. Mammary tumors.
Potency — Third trituration.
Mercurius Iodatus Ruber
Diphtheria and ulcerated sore-throat, especially on left side, with much glandular swelling. Early stages of cold, especially in children.
Potency — Third trituration.
Marum Verum
A remedy of first importance in chronic nasal catarrh with atrophy ; large, offensive crusts and clinkers. Polypi. Ozaena. Loss of sense of smell. Also of use in itching of anus, and constant irritation in the evening in bed. Ascarides, crawling in rectum after stool.
Potency — 6-th locally for polupi, dry powder.
Manganum Aceticum
Cellulitis, subacute stage, promotes suppuration and hastens regeneration. Involuntary laughter and involuntary weeping and walking backwards.
Dose — 30-th.
Manganese Colloidal
Is of great use in boils and other staphylococcal infections.
Dose — 3-rd potency.
Manganum Mur.
For bone-pains.
Dose — Higher.
Manganum Oxydat.
Pain in tibia, dysmenorrhoea, occasional uncontrollable laughter.
Potency — Use 3X.
Madura Album
A grand remedy for leprosy.
Dose — 6-th potency.

Metico
For difficult, dry, winter cough.
Dose — ø.

Methylene Blue
A remedy for neuralgia, neurasthenia, malaria, typhoid.
Dose — 3X attenuation. Locally 2% sol., in chronic otitis with foul smelling discharge.

Mentha Viridis
Scanty urine with frequent desire.
Dose — 30-th potency. Also of the mother tincture, 20 drops.

Mentha Piperita
Useful is gastrodynia.
Dose — Tincure. Locally, in pruritus vaginae.

Mutabile (Bach)
Is indicated where skin eruption atternates with asthmatic symptoms.
Potency — 32-nd, 202-th and 1002-th.

Manganise Dioxide
Very efficacious in amenorrhoea.
Dose — Mother trituration, 1 grain 4 times a day.

Momordica Cherentia
High temperature due to measles. Watery discharges from eyes and nose with constipation or diarrhoea.
Dose — ø, 5 drops every 4 hourly.

Morbillinum
Has been used as a prophylactic against measles.
Potency — 30-th, thrice daily.

Manganum Oxydatum Nativum
Acts like a magic in pain in tibia. Diarrhoea with colic.
Dose — 1X. trit.

Matthiola Graeca
Has cures abscesses, cancer.
Potency — ø, and higher.

Melastoma
Cures diarrhoea, pains in perinaeum and prostatic affections.
Dose — 30-th.

Mercurius Praecipitatus Albus
For dwarfism and eczema feciei.
Dose — 3X. trit.

Mercurius Sulphocyanatus
A good remedy for diphtheria and stricture of oesophagus.
Potency — 3X. trituration.

Moschus
A remedy for hysteria and nervous paroxysms, fainting fits and convulsions, catalepsy etc.
Potency — 3X.

Mephitis Mephitica
A great medicine for whooping-cough ; suffocative feeling, asthmatic paroxysms, spasmodic cough.

Dose — Use 30-th.
Mepato
The rectal symptoms are most important, with fissures of anus, with great constriction, buring like fire. Cures pterygium. Violent hiccough. Cracked nipples. Pin worms.
Dose — 30-th. Locally, the Cerate has proved invaluable in many rectal complaints.
Mercurius Auratus
For brain tumor ; swelling of testicles.
Dose — 6X. trit and higher in dilutions.
Mercurius Acet.
Eyes inflamed, burn and itch.
Dose — 2-nd to 30-th.
Millefolium
Use in continued high temperature. A valuable remedy for various types of haemorrhages.
Dose — ø, to 3-rd potency.
Myrtus Cheken
Chronic bronchitis with dense, yellowish sputum, copious expectoration keeps patient distressed and coughing.
Potency— Third.
Magnetis Poli Ambo.
burning lancinations throughout the body. Tendency of old wounds to bleed afresh.
Potency— Higher.
Menispermin
Specially indicated for leucocythemia.
Potency — 2X. trit., 2 grains 4 times a day.
Myricin
Of use in jaundice.
Dose — 1X. trit.
Menthol
Has proved curative in acute nasal catarrah ; in chronic eustachian catarrah, pharyngitis, laryngitis ; neuralgias, etc. Itching, especially pruritus vulvae.
Dose — Sixth. Externally for itching, use 1% sol.
Mercur. Cum Kali
For acute facial paralysis.
Dose — 30-th.
Mangifera Indica
One of the best general remedies for passive haemorrhages, uterine, renal, gastric, pulmonary and intestinal. Varicose veins.
Dose — Tincture.

N

Natrum Murbit
Cures headache, stinging pains in liver and spleen.
Dose —Tincture.
Narcotinum
Of great use in paralysis of bladder.

Potency — 30-th.

Natrum Hypochlorosum
This remedy is indicated for haematuria, priapism, scurvy, and toothache.
Dose — 30-th potency.

Nectrianin
A successful remedy for carcinoma, and epitheloima.
Potency — Lower triturations.

Nitrogenum Oxygenatum
Is employed in the treatment of enuresis, hysteria and congestion of lungs.
Dose — High potencies.

Nux Juglans
Cures ringworm, acne, flaulence, and pain in spleen.
Dose — 12-th and higher.

Niccolum Bromidum
Is of service in periodical haeaches of the congestive and neuralgic types.
Dose — 6X. trit.

Nitro-Muriatic Acid
Hepatitis and early cirrhosis of liver.
Dose — Well diluted, 10-drop doses.

Natrum Cacodyl.
Use in foul breath and mouth with bad odor.
Dose — 6-th potency.

Natrum Choleinicum
For constipation, diabetes, ascites.
Potency — 12-th trit.

Natrum Hyposulph.
For liver-spots.
Dose — 6-th trituration. Use also locally.

Natrum Lacticum
Rheumatism and gout ; gouty concretions, rheumatism with diabetes.
Dose — Thirtieth.

Natrum Salicylicum
One of the best remedies for the prostrating after-effects of influenza.
Dose — Third potency.

Natrum Silico-Fluoricum
A cancer remedy.
Potency — Twelfth trituration. Use carefully.

Natrum Selenicum
Horseness of singers, expectorate small lumps of mucus with frequent clearing of throat.
Dose— 30-th.

Natrum Succinate
Is of use in catarrhal jaundice.
Dose — 3-rd trit. 5 gr. every 3 hours.

Naphthaline
Emphysema in the aged wth spasmodic asthama. Whooping-cough, long and continued paroxysms of coughing. Phthisis pulmonalis. Opacity of the cornea.

Dose — Third trituration. For worms, and especially pin-worms, one-gramme dose. Externally in skin diseases, 5% ointment.

Narcissus Poeticus
Symptoms of nausea followed by violent vomiting and diarrhoea.
Dose — 1-st attenuation.

Negundium Americanum
Marked action on engorgements of rectum and piles with great pain.
Dose — Tincture, 10 drops every 2 hours. Also 30-th.

Niccolum Sulphuricum
Who suffer from periodic headache. Neuralgias of malarial origin. Useful in climacteric disturbances.
Dose — 2-nd trit.

Nyctanthes
Bilious and obstinate remittent fever ; sciatica ; rheumatism. Constipation of children.
Dose — ø, drop doses.

Nicotinum
Alternate tonic and clonic spasms, followed by general relaxation and trembling ; and speedy collapse; head drawn back, contraction of eyelids and masseter muscles; muscles of neck and back rigid; hissing respiration from spasm of laryngeal and bronchial muscles.
Dose — 30-th and higher. Use also 6X. trit.

Nabalus Serpentaria
For chronic diarrhoea, worse after eating, nights and towards morning. Dyspepsia, with acid burning eructations. Leucorrhoea with throbbing in uterus.
Potency — ø.

Nymphaea Odorata
Curative in ulcerative sore-throat.
Dose — Tincture and 3X.

Nuphar Luteum
Complete absence of sexual desire ; parts relaxed, penis retracted. Impotency, with involuntary emissions during stool, when urinating. Spermatorrhoea. Pain in testicles.
Dose — 6-th. Also 1 drop of tincture.

Nectranda Amare
For watery diarrhoea, dry tongue and colic.
Dose — First potency.

O

Ovyry
For proper development of fiminine characters.
Dose — 3X.

Oenanthe Crocata
Skin affections, especially lepra and itchthyosis. Epileptiform convulsions; worse, dyring menstuation and pregnancy. Puerperal eclampsia ; uraemic convulsions. Convulsive facial twitching.
Potency — 30-th, and higher.

Onosmodium Virg.

A remedy for migraine. Headache from eyestrain and sexual weakness. Use in sexual neurasthenia.

Dose — 30-th attenuation. Also of the q, 30 drops.

Origanum Majarona
Is effective in masturbation and excessively aroused sexual impulses. Lascivious ideas and dreams.

Dose — Third potency.

Oxytropis Lamberti
Patient walks backwards. Sphincter of rectum relaxed, stools slip from anus.

Potency — 30-th.

Ova Tosta
Leucorrhoea and backache. Pain of cancer. Warts.

Dose — Use lower potencies.

Oleum Jecoris Asellie
Atrophy of infants. Restless and feverish at night.

Dose— 3-rd trit. Locally, in ringworm, and nightly rubbing for dwarfish, emaciated babies.

Ovary Extract
For severe climateric flushings and for post-climacteric dyspepsia.

Dose — 3X. trit., 5 grain doses of ovarian gland thrice daily.

Oldenlandia Herbacea
It is very efficacious in acute and chronic malaria.

Dose — Tincture, 10 drops three times a day.

Oleum Ricini
Vary useful for epilepsy, haemoptysis, strangury and toothache.

Potency — ø, and 30-th.

Oxygenium
This remedy is indicated for cancer, diabetes, influenza and whooping-cough.

Dose — 30-th and upwards.

Oleum Succinum
For Hiccough.

Dose — Second potency.

Oxalis Acetosella
To remove cancerous growth of the lips.

Dose — The inspissated juice use as a cautery.

Ozonum
Use in sacral pain.   Dose — 200-th.

Ocinum Canum
Cramps in kidneys. Pain in ureters. Red sand inurine. Uric acid diathesis. Renal colic, renal calculus.

Dose — 30-th potency.

Oleander
Is of use in violent itching eruption, bleeding. Want of perspiration. Pruritus, especially of scalp.

Dose —3-rd to 30-th.

Oophorinum
Cutaneous disorders and acne rosacea. Climacteric disturbances. Ovarian cysts.

Dose — Lower trit. and also higher dilutions.
Orchitinum
Use after overiotomy, sexual weakness, senile decay.
Dose — 30-th.
Ostrya Virginica
Of great value in anaemia from malaria. Bilious conditions and intermittent fever.
Potency — 3-rd.
Ornithogalum
In chronic gastric and other abdominal indurations, cancer of intestinal tract, especially of stomach and caecum.
Dose — ø.
Orobanche
A remedy for sick, neurasthenic, and nervous headaches.
Dose — 30-th potency.

P

Persicaria Urens
For lichen urticarus, worse in the wormth of bed.
Potency — 30-th and higher.
Pond's Extract
Is externally applied for hurts and sprains. Chronic bleeding piles with prolapse of the rectum.
Dose — Pure pond's extract, and tincture.
Proteus (Bach)
Of great use in angio-neurotic oedema, herpetic eruptions at the mucocutaneous margins. Very useful in emotional hysteria, anginal attacks due to spasm of the coronary capillaries; Raynaud's and Meniere's disease. Cures epileptiform seizures and meningismus in children during febrile attacks.
Potency — 32-th, 202-th and 1002-th attenuation.
Pas Avena
Instantly relieves any kinds of pain or colic. It is very useful in headache, neuralgia, sciatica, hysteria, convulsions and insomnia.
Dose — ø, 1 teaspoonful in an ounce of hot water every 30 minutes for pains. Thrice daily for other cases.
Passiflora Compound
Is one of the best nerevous sedative. Invaluable in insomnia, convulsions, epilepsy, tetanus, chorea, paralysis agitans, locomotor ataxia, in spasmodic and non-spasmodic asthma.
Potency — ø, 25 drops thrice daily.
Phaseolus
Use in diabetes.
Potency — Sixth and higher.
Plantanus Occidentalis
For tarsal tumors.
Dose — Apply the tincture.
Pothos Foetidus
Is of use in asthmatic complaints.

Dose — ø, 30-50 drops.
Primula Obconica
Skin symptoms accompanied by febrile symptoms. Great itching, worse at night. Urticaria-like eruptions on the face, between fingers.
Dose — 12-th and higher.
Pyrus
Neuralgic and gouty pains. Spasmodic pains in uterus and bladder.
Dose — 6-th potency. the left side.
Pancreatinum
Indicated in intestinal indigestion ; pain an hour or more after eating. Lienteric diarrhoea.
Dose — 3X. 5 grains.
Paraffine
Valuable in constipation. Chronic constipation, with haemorrhoids and continual urging to stool. Obstinate constipation in children.
Dose — 3X trit. and 30-th potency.
Parthenium
A remedy for fevers, especially malarial.
Potency — Higher.
Passiflora Incarnata
Insomnia of infants and aged. Convulsions of children. Whooping-cough. Tetanus. Hysteria ; puerperal convulsions. Painful diarrhoea. Asthma.
Dose — Thirtieth potency.
Plantago Major
In the treatment of earache, toothache, and enuresis. Pyrrohoea alveolaris. Neuralgic earache, pain goes from one ear to the other through the head.
Dose — Tincture. Locally, use in toothache in hollow teeth, otorrhoea, pruritus and incised wounds.
Ptelea Trifoliata
Frontal headache. The aching and heaviness in the region of the liver is greatly aggravated by lying on.
Dose — Large doses of tincture, 30 drops, repeated several times. For asthma, 20 gtt. every 10 minutes for a few doses. Locally, in erysipelas.
Penthorum Sedoides
Very marked action in coryza, with rawness and wet feeling in nose. Itching of anus and burning in rectum.
Dose — Lower potencies. use also q, 30 drops.
Pilocarpinum Nitricum
Has most pronounced effects in alopecia, mumps, deafness and nausea of pregnancy.
Potency — 3-rd trit.
Primula Vulgaris
Cures any types of dropsy.
Dose — 30-th and higher.
Prinos Verticillatus
Very useful in diarrhoea and fever.
Potency— Thirteeth.
Pyrethrum Parthenium

Has gained high reputation in curing dysentery, fever and rheumatism.
Dose — Tincture.
Parotidinum
Is of great use in mumps, meningitis, orchitis.
Potency — 30-th and onwards.
Papaya Vulgaris
This remedy is indicated in gastrodynia and enteralgia and cures atonic dyspepsia and gastric catarrh. Is of service in the gastric derangements of pregnancy.
Dose — ø, and 30-th.
Parathyroid
Has benefited puerperal convulsions and epilepsy ; should be remembered in tetany, paralysis agitans.
Potency — 32-th attenuation.
Plumbum Aceticum
In servere pain and muscular cramps in gastric ulcer.
Dose — 3-rd potency. Locally as a application in moist eczema.
Piscidia
Pains of irregular menstruation ; regulates the flow. Insomnia, due to worry, nervous excitement, spasmodic coughs.
Dose — Use tincture, in rather material doses.
Piperazinum
For constant backache, with rheumatic arthritis.
Dose — Give 1 grain of first desimal trit., thrice daily.
Pulmo Vulpis
Persistent shortness of breath causing a paroxysm of asthma, with sonorous bubbling rales.
Potency — 6X trit.
Phenazone
Headache under ears with earache. Dark blotches on skin of penis, sometimes with oedema.
Dose — 2-nd decimal potency.
Prunus Spinosa
Of great use in ciliary neuralgia.
Potency — 6-th.
Prunus Virginiana
Used as a heart tonic. Cough, worse at night on lying down.
Dose — Third.
Pecten
Asthma preceded by coryza and burning in throat and chest. Attacks end with copious expectoration of tough, frothy mucus. Worse at night.
Dose — ø.
Pituitrin
Used chiefly for controlling over the growth and development of the sexual organs, stimulates muscular activity and checks bleeding after delivery. Also use in high blood pressure, prostatitis.
Dose — 30-th potency.
Pix Liquida

A great cough medicine. Muco-purulent sputum in chronic bronchitis. Scally eruptions, with intolerable itching, Alopecia.

Dose — 1-st to 6-th.

Phloridzin

Is of use in diabetes.

Dose — Second trituration. Daily doses, 15 grains.

Pinus Lambertina

For delayed and painful menstruation.

Potency — Third Potency.

Protargol

Externally apply in gonorrhoea after acute stage ; syphilitic mucous patches, chancres and chancroids.

Dose — 5% solution applied twice a day.

Planifolia

Is used as an emmenagogue and aphrodisiac.

Dose — 30-th.

Polygonum Aviculare

Found efficacious in phthisis pulmonalis and intermittent fever.   Dose — 3X. dilution and higher.

Phellandrium Aquaticum

Pain in milk ducts ; intolerable between nursing. Good for the offensive expectoration and cough in phithisis, bronchitis, and emphysema.

Dose — ø, to 6-th. In phthisis, use high potency.

Plumbum Iodat

Indurations of mammary glands, especially when a tendecy to become inflamed, sore, painful.

Potency — 30-th. Also use 3X.

Platinum Muriaticum

A remedy for violent occipital headaches, dysphagia, and syphillitic throat and bone affections.

Dose — Sixth trituration.

Plat. Mur. Nat.

Is of use in polyuria and salivation.

Dose — 30-th.

Prenanthes Serpentaria

Chronic diarrhoea, with pain in abdomen and rectum. Dyspepsia, with acid burning eructation.

Potency — ø.

Pediculus Capitis

Itching eruptions on dorsum of hands, feet, neck.

Dose — 200-th.

Psoralea Cor.

Very important in treating pain of cancer, ulcers. Foetid leucorrhoea. Pruritus, Uterine tumors.

Dose —3-rd potency.

Polyporus Pinicolus

Has a remarkable power over intermittent, remittent and bilious fevers, with headache, yellow tongue, constant nausea, faintness at epigastrium, and constipation.

Dose — Thirtieth.

Populus Candicans
A remedy for acute colds, especially when accompanied by a deep, horse voice, or even aphonia. Instantaneous voice-producer.
Dose — ø.

Pelletierinum
An anthelminitic, especially for tapwrorm.
Dose — 6X. trituration.

Paullinia Sorbilis
Used as a remedy for certain forms of sick headache.
Dose — 20 grains of the powder, must be given in material doses.

Pepsinum
Inperfect digestion with pain in gastric region. Diarrhoea due to indesgestion. Marasmus of children who are fed on artificial foods.   Dose— 3-rd trit.

Placenta
Helps increased secretion of milk of the nurning mother.
Potency — 3X.

Pilocarpus Microphyllus
A valuable remedy in limiting the duration of mumps. Exophthalmic goitre. Eye strain from whatever cause.
Dose — Third potency.

Plumbum Phosph.
Loss of sexual power. Locomotor ataxia.
Dose — 30-th.

Potass. Xantate
For loss of memory.
Dose — 1-st attenuation.

Pertussin
For the treatment of whooping-cough and other spasmodic coughs.
Dose — 30-th potency and higher.

Pareira Brava
Dribbling after micturition. Violent pain in glans penis.
Dose — 3-rd potency. Use also 10 drops of tincture.

Pneumococcin
Use in pneumococcus.
Potency — 200-th. 202 and 1002 are also available potencies.

Picrotoxin
Is indicated in epilepsy, locomotor ataxia.
Dose — 30-th. Use also 6X. trit.

Potash Acetate
For chronic eczema.
Dose — ø, 30 drops thrice a day.

Podophyllin
Of great use in diarrhoea, gall-stone colic and hydropericardium.
Potency — 3X. trit.

Phytolaccin

Cures chronic rheumatism, sore-throat, quinsy, syphilitic bone pains, tetanus and opisthotonos. Also very useful in fistula and haemorrhoids.

Potency — 4-th trituration, 6 grains at bed-time.

Polygonum Persicaria
Of use in renal colic and calculi. Gangrene.

Dose — Tincture.

Prerero Brena
It is very efficacious in renal colic, difficult micturition, violent pain in bladder and back, red sand or brick-dust in the urine.

Dose — Tincture, 30 drops in 2 ounce of hot water every half an hour.

Phytoline
Reduces fat, makes the muscles thiner, more firm and stronger. Cures rheumatism and gout associated with obesity, also removes sterility in obase subjects.

Dose — ø, 2 drops in an ounce of hot water, 4 times a day.

Pelargonium Reniforme
Used in dysentery.   Dose — ø.

Phenacetinum
Of great service in typhoid fever, uraemia and eruptions on face.

Dose — 30-th and above.

Phosphorus Muriaticus
Is found useful in asthma, coryza and ophthalmia.

Dose — Use moderate potencies.

Polygonum Sagittatum
For pains of nephritic colic, lancinating pains along spine. Burning inner side of right foot and ankle.

Dose — Use 2X.

Q
Quininum
Is a valuable remedy for intermittent and remittent fevers, cancerous ulcers, pruritus vulvae. Also of use in dysmenorrhoea, haematuria, and rheumatism.

Potency — 3X. trit., and also 30-th attenuation.

Quassin
One of the best remedies for atonic dyspepsia, with gas and acidity ; heartburn and gastralgia, regurgitation of food.

Dose — 3X. trit.

Quercus Glandium Spiritus
Is of use for chronic spleen affections. Takes away craving for alcoholics. Useful in gout, old malarial cases, with flatulence.

Potency — 3X. trit.

Quillaya Saponaria
Most effective in the beginning of coryza, frequently checking its further development. Cures symptoms of acute catarrh, sneezing and sore-throat.

Dose — q.

R

Ranuculus Ficaria
Is chiefly useful in haemorrhoids.
Dose — ø, and higher.

Rhodium Oxydatum Nitricum
This remedy is indicated in burning in and itching of anus, constipation, pains in ears, and impotence.
Potency — 3X. trit.

Rosa Canina
for affections of bladder, dysuria.
Dose —30-th and above.

Russula
Used in scrofula ; cough caused by tickling in throat.
Dose — 1X. trit.

Rumex Acetosa
For violent pains in the bowels. Also used in cancer.
Dose — 3-rd potency.

Rumex Obtusifolius
Nosebleed and headache following ; pain in kidneys leucorrhoea.
Potency — Sixth.

Rhus Aromatica
Renal and urinary affections, especially in diabetes. Enuresis due to vesical atony ; senile incontinence. Insures radical cure in blindness, chorea, convulsions, and enuresis.
Potency — Higher.

Rumin
Haematuria and cystitis. Severe pain at begenning or before urination. Constant dribbling.
Dose — ø, in rather material doses.

Rhus Glabra
Cures epistaxis and occipital headache. Foetid flatus. Ulceration of mouth. Dreams of flying through the air.
Dose — 1-st potency. Tincture, locally, to soft, spongy gums, aphthae, pharyngitis.

Rhodium
Fleeting neuralgic pains in head, over eyes, in ear, both sides of nose, teeth. Itching in arms, palms and face. Loose stools with griping in abdomen.
Potency — 200-th.

Rhamnus Californica
Of frequent use in rheumatism and muscular pains. Pleurodynia, lumbago, gastralgia. Inflammatory rheumatism, joints swollen, painful; tendency to metastasis. Vesical tenesmus ; dysmenorrhoea of myalgic origin ; pain in head, neck, and face.
Dose — Tincture, in 15-drop doses every four hours.

Rosa Damascena
Useful in the beginning of allergic rhinitis, with eustachian catarrh.
Dose — Tincture, 30 drops. Use also 3X.

Resorcin
For summer complaint with vomiting.

Dose — 3-rd trit.
Rhus Venenata
Erythema nodosum, with nightly itching and pains in long bones. Itching, > by hot water. Vescles. Erysipelas, skin dark red.
Potency — 6-th to 30-th.
Radium Bromide
Found effective in the treatment of rheumatism and gout, in skin affections generally, acne rosacea, naevi, moles, ulcers and cancers. Chronic rheumatic arthiritis. Severe aching pains all over, with resthessness, better moving about. Ithing all over body, burning of skin.
Dose — 12-th trit and thirtieth.
Rhamnus Frangula
Chronic diarrhoea with colic.
Dose — ø.
Rhamnus Purshiana
Palliative in constipation, as an intestinal tonic, and dyspepsia dependent theron.
Dose — 10 drops of tincture.
Rosmarinus Officinalis
Marked action on dificient memory. Menses too early ; violent pains followed by uterine haemorrhage.
Potency — 30-th.
Ricinus Communis
Increases the quantity of milk in nursing women. Anorexia with burning in stomack, pyrosis, nausea, profuse vomiting and incessant diarrhoea with purging.
Dose — Third potency. Tincture, 5 drops every four hours for increasing flow of milk.
Ranunculus Acris
Pain in lumber muscles and joints by bending and turning body.
Dose — 30-th.
Ranunculus Sceleratus
Cures vesicular eruptions, with tendency to form large blisters. Acrid exudation, which makes surrounding parts sore. Pemphigus.
Dose — 6-th potency.
Rhus Radicans
For occipital headache.
Potency — 6-th.
Rhus Diversiloba
In much swelling of face, hands and genitals. Violent skin symptoms, with frightful ithing. Eczema and erysipelas.
Dose — 30-th.
Rubia Tinctorum
A remedy for affections of spleen. Chlorosis andamenorrhoea. Tuberculosis.
Dose — ø, 10 drop doses.
Rubus Villosus
Diarrhoea of infancy ; stools watery and clay coloured.
Dose — 3-rd to 30-th attnuation. Also of the q, 20 drops.

S

Scutellarin
For many distresssing nerve symptoms, which are due to after-effects of two attacks of influenza
Dose — 1X. trit.

Sarza
Multiple hard tumours of breast, prolapsus uteri.
Dose — ø.

Scarlatininum
Small tumour of left breast and lymphomatous tumours of neck. Also for nephritis and sore-throat.
Potency — 32-th, 202-th and 1002-th attenuation.

Sodium Urate
Of great use in gout.
Potency — 3X. trit.

Sodium Bromide
For ovarian tumours.
Dose — 3X. trit., 8 grains at bed-time.

Sodium Silicate
For fistula proctalgia.
Dose — ø, 5 drops in water night and morning.

Sycotic Compound
The key-note of the nosode Sycotic Co. (Paterson) is 'irritability' of any system and has special action on mucous and synovial membrane.
Potency — 32-th and 1002-th attenuation.

Succus Amogara
Is a marvelleous remedy in all stages of syphilis, for boils, carbuncles, abscesses, diththeria and typhoid conditions. Also purifies blood. Dose — ø, 30 drops, every 4 hourly.

Sium
It controls convulsions and titanic spasms.
Dose — 30-th and upwards.

Sol.
A great remedy for cancer. Also indicated in headache, lupus, premature menses, paralysis and sunstroke.
Potency — 200-th.

Solanin
For paralysis of lungs.
Potency — 6X. trit.

Solaninum Aceticum
Is a specific for tetanus.
Potency — Lower trit., and also 30-th.

Salanum Arrebenta
Most important remedy of universal fame in curing swelling of and pain in breasts ; apoplexy, boils, urticaria and vertigo.
Dose — 30-th and higher.

Sperminum

Is chiefly useful in climacteric sufferings, and sexual weakness.
Dose — 3X. trit.
Stachys Betonica
has proved to be great beneficial in headache, vertigo and paralysis of diaphragm.
Dose — ø, and 30-th.
Sabbatia Angularis
For wounds and to establish the menstrual flow ; is indicated in periodic fevers, and dyspepsia.
Potency — Of the mother tincture, 40 drops.
Saururus Cernuus
Painful and difficult micturation.
Dose— 6-th potency.
Scolopendra
Terrible pains in back and loins, extending down limbs ; return periodically. Angina pectoris. Inflammation, pain and gangrene. Pustules and abscesses.
Potency — Thirtieth.
Scutellaria Lateriflora
Twitching of muscles. Spasms of children, during dentition.
Dose — ø, 30 to 60 drops.
Sepsin
A great remedy for septic states, with intense restlessness. In septic fevers, especially puerperal and also influenza and typhoid symptoms. All discharges are horribly offensive — menstrual, lochial, diarrhoea, vomit sweat, breath etc.
Dose — Use higher potencies. Should not be repeated too frequently.
Sisyrinchium Ang.
Of use in rattlesnake bites.
Dose — ø, in 15 drop doses. Also use 30-th.
Skookum-Chuck
Profuse, ichorus, cadaverously smelling discharge in otitis media. Eczema. Hay-fever, profuse coryza and constant sneezing.   Dose — 3-rd trit.
Solanum Carolinense
Convulsions and epilepsy, where the disease has begun beyond age of childhood. Use also in whooping-cough.
Dose — 25 drop doses of tincture.
Symphoricarpus Racemosa
Is highly recommended for the persistent vomiting of pregnancy. Gastric disturbances, fickle appetite, nausea, water brash, bitter taste. Constipation. Nausea, during menses. Nausea, worse any motion.
Dose — Lower and 200-th.
Sabal Serrulata
For general and sexual debility. Promotes nutrition and tissue building. Of great value in prostatic enlargement, epididymitis, and urinary difficulties. Valuable for undeveloped mammary glands.
Potency — Mother tincture, 20 drop doses.
Saccharin
Used in dyspepsia, loss of appetite, diarrhoea.
Dose — 30-th.

Saccharum Lactis
Has most suitable application towards the end of the labor en there is no mechanical obstruction and delay is due to uterine inertia.
Dose — 25 grammes dissolved in water, several times every half hour.

Saccharum Officinale
Acts as a nutrient and tonic, increasing weight and power. Acidity and anal itching.
Dose — 3—th and higher. Locally, in gangrene.

Strychninum
Spasms of muscles and tetanic convulsions with opisthotonos. The pains and sensations come suddenly and return at intervals. Potency — 30-th. Use also 3X.

Stannum Iodatum
Persistent inclination to cough. Trachial and bronchial irritation of smokers.
Dose — 6X. trituration.

Saponin
Much pain before the menstrual flow ; severe sore-throat, tonsils swollen. Sharp burning taste and violent sneezing. Very good for migraine. Pain in left temple, eye, photophobia, hot stitches deep in eye.
Dose — Lower potencies.

Santalum Album
Useful for aching in kidneys.
Potency — 30-th.

Sulphurous Acid
Has briliant results in ulcerative stomatitis, acne rosacea and pityriasis versicolor.
Dose — 3-rd attenuation. Use as a spray in tonsillitis. Relives pyrosis and prevent fermentation and flatulence, if taken 15 drops before each meal. It also removes thrush.

Strychinia Phosphorica
An excellent remedy in anaemia of spinal cord ; paralysis ; burning, aching and weakness of spine ; pain extends to front of chest. Hands and axillae covered with clammy perspiration. Acts upon muscles, causing twitching, stiffness, weakness and loss of power ; also acts upon circulation producing irregularity of pulse, and upon the mind, producing lack of control, uncontrollable desire to laugh. Used in chorea, hysteria, acute asthenia after acute fevers.
Dose — Third trituration.

Strychnin Nit.
Use for two weeks, to remove craving for alcohol.
Potency — 6X. trit.

Salix Alba
This remedy is employed in intermittent fever, when there is weakness of the digestive organs, passive haemorrhages and convalescence is slow.
Dose — Of the tincture, 25 drops. Also use 30-th upwards.

Spiritus Aetheris Nitrosi
Is indicated in low fevers of childhood, nausea and flatulence.
Dose — Of the spirit, from a fraction of a drop, well diluted.

Strychine Hypophos.
A special remedy for dipsomania, helps the vomitingand strengthen the nerves.
Dose — 1X. trit., 1 grian once daily.

Soda Sulpho Carbolate

For chronic Catarrh.
Potency — Dissolve one-half teaspoonful in a pint of warm water twice daily. Use ½ as a gargle.

Senecin
For functional amenorrhoea of young girls with backache. Also of great service in cirrhosis of liver.
Dose — 6X. trit.

Stillingin
Has a specific action in jaundice and constipation. Cures chronic periosteal rheumatism.
Potency — 30-th attenuation, and onwards.

Scrophulin
Use in scrofulous swellings and painful hamorrhoids.
Potency — 30-th.

Strychnos Tiente
A valuable remedy for tonic spasms, tetanus and asphyxia. Pain in eyes and orbits, with conjuntivitis. Dull backache, after excessive coitus. Hangnails inflamed ; itching and redness of roots of nails.
Dose — 6-th potency.

Sulphur Hydrogenisatum
A highly efficacious remedy in delirium.
Potency — 200-th and upward, and not too frequent doses.

Sulphur Terebinthinatum
For chronic rheumatic arthiritis ; chorea.
Dose — Use 1M and higher.

Sulfonal
Checks loss of control of sphincter. Mascular incordination. Vertigo of cerebral origin, cerebellar disease, ataxic symptoms, and chorea.
Dose — Third trit. Use as a hypnotic, 20 grains in hot water. It takes about two hours to act.

Sumbul
Is of use in insomnia of delirium tremens.
Dose — Tincture. For arterio-sclerosis, advise 2X every 4 hours.

Sal Marinum
Indicated in chronic enlargements of glands, especially cervical and auxiliary. Also very useful in constipation.
Potency — 200-th and higher.

Sarcolactic Acid
Of great value inthe most violent form of epidemic influenza, espicially with violent retching and greatest prostration.

Sodii Bicarbonas
n vomiting of pregnancy, with acetonuria.
Dose — 30 grains in water.

Spigelia Marylandica
Maniacal exitement, paroxysmal laughing and crying, loud, disconnected talking, vertigo, deliated pupils congestions.
Potency — 30-th and higher.

Spiraea Ulmaria

Used for elcampsia, epilepsy, and hydrophobia. Checks gleet and prostatorrhoea. Bites of mad animals.
Dose — ø.
Sarracenia Purpurea
Black objects move with the eyes.
Dose — 6-th potency.
Saraca Indica
Acts powerfully on abdominal pain, amenorrhoea, and menorrhagia.
Dose — Tincture.
Salol
Rheumatic pain in joints, with soreness and stiffness, headache over eyes ; urine violet-smelling.
Dose — 3-rd decimal trit.
Sambucus Canadensis
Great value in dropsies.
Dose — ø, 1 teaspoonful thrice daily.
Sanguinaria Nitrica
Is of use in polypus of the nose. Acute and chronic catarrh. Acute phryngitis. influenza. Chronic follicular phazryngitis. Nose feels obstructed. Profuse, watery mucus, with burning pain. Sneezing. Rawness and soreness in posterior nares.
Potency — 3-rd trit.
Sanguinaria Tartaricum
A remedy of mydriasis, dim vision.
Dose — 3X trit.
Sanguisuga
Haemorrhages, especially bleeding from anus.
Dose — Use 6X.
Saponaria Officinalis
Of great use in the treatment of acute colds, coryza, sore throat.
Dose —Thirtieth.
Solanum Tuberosum Aegrotans
For prolapse of the rectum, tumors of rectum look like decayed potato. Offensive odor of whole body.
Potency — 3-rd to 30-th.
Solidago Virga
For repeated colds of tuberculosis.
Dose — Use 2X. Oil of solidago, 1 ounce to 8 ounce alchohol, 15 drop doses to promote expectoration in bronchitis and bronchial asthma in old people.
Staphylococcin
Very efficacious in acne, abscess, furuncle ; empyema, endocarditis, etc.   Dose - 30-th and higher
Stellaria Media
Sharp, shifting, rheumatic pains in all parts. Chronic rheumatism, stiffness of joints ; parts sore to touch ; worse, motion.
Dose — 2X potency. Tincture, externally.
Stigmata Maydis

Has marked urinary symptoms, and has been used with success in organic heart disease, with much oedema of lower extremities and scanty urination. Enlarged prostate and retention of urint. Suppression and retention. Dysuria. Renal lithiasis; nephritic colic ; blood and red sand in urine. Tenesmus after urinating. Vesical catarrh. Gonorrhoea. Cystitis.

Potency — Tincture, 30 drop doses.

Succinic Acid
Hay-fever. Paroxysmal sneezing, dropping of watery mucus from nostrils. Inflammation through respiratory tract ; causing asthma, chest pains, etc. Itching of eyelids and canthi and nose worse drafts.

Dose— 6-th to 30-th.

Sulphur Iodatum
Obstinate skin affections, notably in barber's itch and acne. Popular eruptions on face. Weeping eczema.

Dose — 3-rd trit.

Soda Cocodyl.
For any type of tumors.

Dose — 12-th trit.

Sodium Chloraurate
Has more power over uterine tumors than any other remedy. Leucorrhoea, with spasmodic contraction of vagina. For high blood pressure due to disturbed function of nervous mechanism.

Dose — Second and third trit.

Soda Taurocholate
Fruitful against certain forms of hypoglobular anaemia, hypertrophy of the spleen and ganglia. Use in cases of dyspnoea, Cheyne-Stokes rhythm, acute pulmonary oedema, and intense exaggeration of the cardiac pulsations.

Potency — 3-rd trit.

Scopolamine Hydrobromide
A remedy for shock. Paralysis agitans; tremors of disseminated sclerosis. Dry cough in phthisis.

Dose — Third decimal trituration. Use in physiological dosage (50 grains) for mania and chorea ; insomnia.

Silphion Cyrenaicum
Phthisis pulmonum, with incessant cough, profuse night- sweats, emaciation.

Dose — 3-rd potency.

Simaruba Ferroginea
Is particularly useful in malarial affections, Has powers of antidoting snake-bites and stings of insects. Whole body seems numb with headache. Severe pain in eye-ball, with radiating pains around eye, shooting into nose. Scalding lachrymation and periodic supra-orbital neuralgia.

Dose — Lower attenuations.

Strychnin. Sulph.
A remedy of unquestioned benifit in gastric atony.

Dose — 12-th potency. Also 6X. trit.

Strychnin. Valarin.
Exhaustion of brain-power ; women of high nervous erethism.

Potency — 30-th.

Strych. et Ferr. cit.

Marked action in chlorotic and paralytic conditions ; dyspepsia, with vomiting of ingesta.
Dose — 3X trit.
Strychnin. Ars.
Paresis in the aged, relaxed musculature, prostration. Psoriasis ; chronic diarrhoea with paralytic symptoms ; compensatory hypertrophy of heart with begining fatty degeneration ;' marked dyspnoea when lying down ; oedema of lower extremities, urine scanty, high specific gravity. heavily loaded with glucose. Diabetes.
Potency — 6X trituration.
Succinum
Cures affections of spleen. Asthma, incipient phthisis, chronic bronchitis, pains in chest. Whooping-cough.
Dose — Third trit. Use also 200-th.
Strychonos Gautheriana
Used in exhaustion with vertigo ; numbness and tingling in hands and feet ; involuntary action of lower jaw. Pustules and boils; tertiary syphilis and paralysis, eczema, prerigo, old ulcers, leprosy, cancer of glandular structures, and bites of serpents. Removes fetor and haemorrhage in cancer, relives the healing process.
Dose — ø, in 10 drop doses.
Salicinum
One of the best remedies for deafness, tinnitus, influenza and Meniere's disease.
Potency — 6X. trit. and 30-th.
Salix Mollissima
Used with success in rheumatic affections and for scitica.
Dose — Thirtieth and onwards.
Salix Purpurea
Is indicated for diarrhoea, fever, parotitis and vertigo.
Potency— 30-th.
Sanguinarin
Specific for croup.
Dose — 3-rd trituration.
Scammonium
For diarrhoea and gastro-entritis.
Potency — Lower trit.
Schinus Molle
Acts like a magic in diarrhoea and vomiting ; griping pain in liver, drawing pain in spinal cord.
Dose — Tincture.
Scilla Maritima
Is very efficacious in diabetes, bronchitis, measles, whooping-cough and worms. Also of use in hydrothorax and pneumonia.
Potency — 200-th.
Septicaemin
An unique remedy in camp diarrhoea, dysentery and typhoid fever.   Dose — 30-th attenuation.
Scirrhinum
Cancerous diathesis ; enlarged glands ; cancer of breast ; worms.
Dose — Best in high potencies.

Sinapis Nigra
Is of use in hay-fever, coryza, and pharyngitis. Dry nares and pharynx, with thick, lumpy secretion. Nostrils alternately stopped.
Dose — 3-rd potency.

Streptococcin
Has anti-febrile action ; septic symptoms in infectious diseases. Rapid in its action, especially in its effect on temperature.   Potency— 30-th.

Selaginella
For bites snakes and spiders.
Dose — Use locally, macerating in milk.

Salicylic Acid
Acute articular rheumatism, worse, touch and motion. Sciatica. Knees swollen and painful. Also used in fermentative dyspepsia and Meniere's disease; tinnitus aurium and deafness.
Dose — 3-rd trit. In acute articular rheumatism, 5 grains every 4 hours.

Santoninum
Is of unquestioned value in the treatment of worm diseases, as gastro-intentinal irritation, itching of nose, restless sleep, twitching of muscles. Ascaris lumbricoides, and thread worms.
Dose — 3-rd trit.

Salix Nigra
Has marked action on the generative organs of both sexes. Libidinous thoughts and lascivious dreams. Satyriasis and erotomania. In acute gonorrhoea, with much erotic troubles, chordee. After musturbation; spermatorrhoea. Nymphomania.
Dose — ø, 20 drop doses.

Salvia Officinalis
Controls excessive colliquative perspiration when circulation is enfeebled.
Dose — ø, in 20 drop doses.

Sedum Repens
Cancer, specific action on abdominal organs.
Dose — 6-th potency.

Strontium Bromatum
Is an anti-fermentative and neutralizes excessive acidity. Relieves vomiting of pregnancy and nervous dyspepsia.
Dose — 30-th.

T

Thymus Gland Extract
Is of great use in arthritis deformans ; metabolic osteo-arthritis. High potencies very efficient in expthalmic goitre.
Dose —1X. trit., 5 grains 3 times daily.

Tuberculinum Testium
Very useful for alopecia areata, spinal curvature ; puny growth, ringworm of shoulder and chronic insomnia. Nocturnal enuresis, left-sided pluro-dynia.
Dose - 30-th.

Tathelin
It promotes quick development and growth of the body.

Dose — Give 1X. trit., 2 grains thrice a day.
Tanghinia
Acts like a magic in vomiting and paralysis.
Potency— 2-nd trit.
Tannin
Gives instant relief and cures constipation.
Dose — 3X. trit.
Teplitz
One of the most valuable remedies for tumours in breasts, eifficult speech and paralysis of tongue. Also of use in metrorrhagia, erysipelas, toothache and flatulence.
Dose — High potencies.
Thebainum
Used in tetanus.
Dose — 30-th.
Tanacetum Vulgare
Said to be a specific against effects of poison ivy. Of use in chorea and reflex spasms.
Dose — Lower potencies.
Terpin Hydrate
For whooping-cough, hay asthma and bronchial affections.
Dose — 3X, 2 grain doses.
Titanium
Is found efficacious in sexual weakness, with too early ejaculation of semen in coitus.
Dose — 6-th potency.
Teucrium Scorodonia
In tuberculosis with muco-purulent expectoration; dropsy ' orchitis and tuberculous epididymitis, especially in young individuals with tuberculosis of lungs, glands; bones and urogenitals.
Potency — Use 3-rd potency.
Trional
Insomnia associated with physical excitement.
Dose — Third trit and 30-th.
Tetradymite
Of use in coccygodynia, ulceration of nails; pains in hands, ankles, heels, and tendo-Achilles. Dose — 30-th.
Triosteum Perfoliatum
Is a very valuable remedy in diarrhoea attended with colicky pains and nausea, numbness of lower limbs after stool.
Dose — 6-th potency.
Thlaspi Bursa Pastoris
Excellent in chronic neuralgia. Ulrine haemorrhage, with cramps and expulsion of clots. Sore pain in womb on rising. Chronic cystitis, dysuria and spasmodic retention. Haematuria, brick-dust sediment. Renal colic, accumulation of gravel.
Dose — 6-th potency. Also of the mother tincture, 50 drops.
Thymus Serpyllum
Respiratory infections of children ; dry nervous asthma, whooping-cough, severe spasms but little sputum. Burning in pharynx, sore-throat worse empty swallowing.

Dose — Tincture.
Trichosanthes Dioica
For diarrhoea, pain in liver and dizziness after every stool.
Dose — 6-th and higher.
Turnera
Said to be of use in sexual neurasthenia ; impotency. Incontinence of old people. Chronic prostatic discharge. Frigidity of females. Aids the establishment of normal menstrual flow in young girls.
Potency — ø, 30 drop doses.
Taxus Baccata
Large flat itching pustules and badly smelling night. Sweats. Also of use in gout and chronic rheumatism.
Dose — 3-rd potency. Also of the q, 20 drops.
Typha Latifolia
Has curative action on diarrhoea and dysentery, summer complaint of children.
Dose — Tincture.
Terentula Cubensis
As a curative and preventive remedy of bubonic plague especially during the period of invasion. Pruritus especially about genitals. A great remedy for pain of death ; soother the last struggles.
Dose — 30-th and higher.
Tela Aranea
Nervous agitation in febrile states. Obstinate intermittents and continued chilliness. Dry asthma, with harrassing coughs; periodic headaches with extreme nervous erethism.
Dose — Thirtieth. Also use 3X.
Thallium
Valuable in paralysis of lower limbs. Relieves the violent pains in locomotor ataxia. Alopecia, following acute exhausting diseases.
Potency — Lower triturations and also thirtieth.
Thiosinaminum
For disolving scar tissue, tumors, enlarged glands. A remedy for Tabes Dorsalis, improving the lightning pains.
Dose — 30-th. In stricture of rectum, use 1X, 3 grains twice daily.
Turpethum Minerale
For watery stool, with burning in anus. Oedema of legs. Sneezing from direct rays of sun.
Dose — 1X.

U
Urkalkgneiss
Is employed in the treatment of hard painful tumours of breast.
Potency — 4X. trit.
Upas Artiar
Cures clonic spasms with vomiting, diarrhoea and prostration.
Dose — 6X. trit.
Uva Ursi

Cystitis, with bloody urine. Frequent urging, with severe spasms of bladder ; burning and tearing pain. Urine contains blood, pus and much tenacious mucus. Painful dysuria. Pyelitis.
Dose — ø

Urinum
Useful in acne, boils, scurvy, dropsy.
Potency — Lower triturations.

Uric Acid
Most curative in gout, gouty eczema, rheumatism, and lipoma.
Dose — Lower trit.

Usnea Barbata
Is a remedy in some forms of congestive headache; sunstroke.
Dose — Tincture and also 30-th.

Ustilago Maydis
Menorrhagia at climaxis. Cervix bleed easily. Emissions, with irresistible tendency to masturbation. Sprematorrhoea, with erotic fancies and amorous dreams.
Potency — 30-th and higher.

Uranium Nitricum
Is known to cure nephritis, diabetes, degenaration of the liver, high blood pressure and tendency to ascites and general dropsy.
Dose — Third trit.

Urtica Urens
A remedy for agalactia and lithiasis. Antidotes ill-effects of eating shellfish. Rheumatism associated with urticaria-like eruptions. Urticaria, burning heat, with formication, voilent itching.
Dose — ø, and lower potencies.

V

Vanad Ammon
Marked action on piles, perineal abscesses and fistula.
Potency — 12-th attenuation.

Veratrum Nigrum
Has gained high reputation in curing headache, tinnitus aurium and protracted menses.
Dose — Tincture, and higher.

Viburnum Tinus
Is amazyingly curative for deafness, pain in ovary and hypochondriasis.
Dose — 30-th and upwards.

Vichy.
Has proved to be great beneficial in gall-stones. diabetes and gout. Also of use in indigestion, stiff-neck and affections of uterus.
Potency — 6x. trituration and higher dilutions.

Voeslau
Is chiefly useful in seminal emissions, urticaria and vertigo.
Dose — Lower attenuations.

Veratrin
A successful remedy for collapse, vomiting, purging, and cramps in extremities.
Dose — 3-rd trituration.

Viburnin
It prevents miscarriage, cures spasmodic and membranous dysmenorrhoea. Also a general remedy for cramps.
Dose — 3X. trit.

Vaccininum
For indegestion with great flatulent distension. Pimples and blotches. Eruptions like variola.
Potency — 200-th. Use also 4X. trit.

Vaccinum Myrtillus
Said to be a specific in dysentery and typhoid.
Dose — 30-th.

Vinca Minor
A remedy for skin affections, eczema and especially plica polonica. Spots on scalp, oozing moisture, matting hair together. Corrosive itching of scalp. Dose — Third potency.

Viola Odorata
has a specific action on deafness, otorrhoea and deep stitches beneath ears. Ear affections with pain in eyeballs.
Dose — 6-th.

Vitex Trifolia
Sprains and pains, headache in temples, pain in joints ; pain in abdomen ; pain in testicles.
Potency — Thirtieth.

Viburnum Opulus
Often prevents miscarriage. A general remedy for cramps. Colicky pains in pelvic organs. Menses too late, scanty, lasting a few hours, offensive in odor. Spasmodic and membranous dysmenorrhoea. Leucorrhoea, excoriating and itching of genitals.
Dose — ø, and lower potencies.

Vanadium
Acts as a tonic to digestive functions.
Dose — 30-th.

Variolinum
To be efficacious in protecting against and aiding in the cure of small-pox. Also of use in excruciating backache.
Dose — 30-th.

Verbena
Allays pain in bruises and promotes the absorption of blood. Vesicular erysipelas. Epilepsy. insomnia and nervous depression.
Dose — ø, 30 drops.

Viscum Album
Lowered blood pressure. Rheumatism with tearing pains. Sciatica. Of use in epilepsy, chorea and metrorrhagia.
Dose — Tincture and lower potencies.

Vaccinium Myrtillus
Is found useful in diarrhoea and dysentery.
Potency — ø.

W

Wiesbaden
Most important remedy of universal fame in curing amenorrhoea, whillow, inguinal hernia and glaucoma. Also of use in falling of hair, excessive ear-wax and corns.
Potency — 6X. trit.
Wildbad
Is employed in the treatment of pains in bones, spinal paralysis.
Dose — Lower dilutions.
Wyethia Helenioides
Has been proved an excellent remedy in pharyngitis, follicular. Irritable throat of singers and public speakers. Used also in haemorrhoids, hay-fever symptoms ; itching in posterior nares.
Potency — 30-th.

X
X-Ray
Has the property of stimulating cellular metabolism. Pain in muscles of neck when lifting head from pillow. Itching eczema. Warty growths. Psoriasis.
Potency — 30-th and higher.
Xanthium Spinosum
Said to be specific for hydrophobia and is also recommended for chronic cystitis in women.
Dose — Thirtieth.
Xanthoxylum Frax.
For neuralgic dysmenorrhoea, hemiplegia and indigestion from over-eating.
Dose — 6-th.
Xerophyllum Tenax
Used in eczematous conditions and early stage of typhoid.
Dose — Use high potencies.
Xanthoxylin
Is chiefly useful in hemiplegia, painful haemorrhoids, neuralgic dysmenorrhoea and insomnia.
Dose — 3-rd trituration.

Y
Yoloxochitl
Use in pleurodynia, rheumatism when there is a general weakness and a stiffness upon the slightest exposure to a draft of damp air. Relieves erratic pains in the chest.
Dose — ø, in 5 drop doses.
Yohimbinum
Acts as a sexual stimulant. Causes hyperaemia of the milk glands and stimulates the function of lactation.
Dose — 3-rd potency.
Yerba Buena
Cures colic and relieves flantulence. Dose — ø

Z

Zinc. Phos.
Neuralgia of head and face; lightning-like pains in lomotor ataxia, brain-fag and vertigo; sexual excitement and sleeplessness. Herpes zoster.   Potency — 3X. trit.

Zea Italica
Possess curative properties in psoriasis and eczema rubrum. Mania for bathing. Pyrosis, nausea, vomiting, better drinking water.   Dose — 3-rd potency.

Zincum Oxydatum
Nausea and sour taste, vomiting of bile and diarrhoea. Flatulent abdomen, watery stools with tenesmus.

Dose — 1X. Is also used locally as an astringent to unhealthy ulcers, fissures, intertrigo, burns etc.

Zinc. Bromatum
Of great use in hydrocephalus.
Dose — 3X. trit.

Zinc. Cyanatum
A remedy for meningitis, and cerebro-spinal meningitis, paralysis agitans, chorea and hysteria.
Potency — 2X. trit.

Zincum Picricum
For facial paralysis ; brain-fag, headache in Bright's disease; seminal emissions ; loss of memory and energy.

Dose — 6X. trit.

Zinc. Iodatum
One of the best remedies for constipation, cough and phthisis.
Potency — 2X. trit.

THERAPEUTIC INDEX OF RARE MEDICINES

A

Abortion — Alnuin, Faecalis (Bach).
Abscess — Aqua Silicata.
Acetonuria — Sodii Bicarbonas.
Acne — Arctium Lappa, Nux Juglans.
Acidity — Ferrum Sulphurium, Insulin, Strontium Bromatum.
Agalactia — Urtica Urens.
Albuminuria — Eel Serum, Kissingen.
Allergic Rhinitis — Rosa Damascena.
Alopecia — Burgamont Oil, Pilocarpinum Nitricum, Pix Liquida.
Amblyopia — Cichorium.
Amenorrhoea — Ferri Et Strychniae Citras, Gastein, Jonosia Asoca, Linum Catharticum, Manganise

Dioxide, Rubia Tinctorum, Wiesbaden.
Anaemia — Ferrum Protoxalatum.
Anasarca —Apocynin.
Angina Pectoris — Haematoxylon Campechianum, Haematin, Latrodectus Mactans.
Angio-neurotic Oedema — Proteus (Bach).
Anuria — Eel Serum.
Aphthous Ulcer — Acid Nitro-hydrochloricum.
Apoplexy — Solanum Arrebenta.
Appendicitis — Iris Tenax, Lac. Vac. Defloratum.
Arthritis — Fraxinus Excelsior.
Ascites — Apocynin, Natrum Choleinicum.
Asphyxia Neonatorum— Laurocerasus.
Asthma — Aspidosperimin, Euphorbia Pilulifera, Egg Vaccine, Ferrum Aceticum, Lipppia Mecana, Madar, Pothos Foetidus, Pulmo Vulpis.

B

Backache — Calcarea Ovorum, Indium Metalicum, Ova Tosta, Piperazinum, Variolinum.
Barber's Itch — Sulphur Iodatum.
Basilar Meningitis — Cuprum Cyanatum.
Biliary Calculi — Fel Tauri.
Bilious Headache — Morgan Pure (Paterson).
Beri-beri — Boerrhavia Rep.
Blindness — Hura Crepitans, Russula.
Blood-poisoning — Gun-powder, Hemidesmus Indica.
Boils — Ferrum Iodatum, Manganese Colloidal, Urinum.
Bone-pain — Euphorbin, Manganum Mur., Wildbad.
Borborygmi — Digitalin.
Brain-fag — Anhalonium Lewinii, Zinc. Phos.
Brain-tumor — Mercurius Auratus
Breast Cancer — Scirrhinum.
Bright's Disease — Cainca, Zincum Picricum.
Bronchitis — Bolsamum Tolutanum, Glanderine, Kaolin, Pix Liquida.
Bronchitis (Chronic) — Lippia Mexicana, Myosotis, Myrtus Cheken,
Burbonic Plague — Tarentula Cubensis.

C

Cancer — Matthiola Graeca, Natrum Silico-Fluroricum, Oxygenium, Rumex Acetosa, Sedum Repens.
Cancer-pain — Calcarea Acetica, Euphorbia Heterodoxa, Ova Tosta.
Carbancles — Insulin, Succus Amogara.,
Carcinoma — Lapis Alba, Nectrianin.
Catarrh — Hepatica Triloba.

Catalepsy — Moschus.
Cataract — Cineraria Maritima Succus.
Chancroid — Jacaranda Gualandi.
Chilblain — Calcarea Lactica Natronata, Fragaria Vesca,
Chlorosis — Ferrum Citricum, Ferri Et Strychinae Citras.
Cholera — Ampelopsin, Coffea Mocha, Irisin.
Chorea — Morphinum Aceticum, Mygale, Passiflora
Cholecystitis — Morgan Gaertner (Paterson).Compound, Zinc. Cyanatum.
Chordee — Jacaranda Gualandi.
Cirrhosis (of Liver) — Nitro-Muriatic Acid, Senecin.
Clonic Spasm — Upas Artiar.
Coccygodynia — Tetradymite.
Collapse — Homeria, Veratrin.
Colic — Dioscorin, Jalapa, Yerba Buena.
Convulsion — Datura Metel, Hedera Helix,
Kerosolenum, Pas Avena,
Congenital Pyloric Stenosis — Dys. Co. (Bach).
Constipation — Augopora, Franzensbad, Musa Sapientum,
Natrum Choleinicum, Paraffine, Stillingin.
       — (of Children) — Collinsonin.
Coryza— Asparagin.
Corneal Opacities— Cineraria Maritima Succus, Naphthaline.
Conjunctivitis — Ferrum Phos. Hydricum, Jequirity, Strychonos Tiente.
Corn — Ferrum Picricum, Kissingen, Wiesbaden.
Cough — Mephitis Mephitica.
Croup — Kaolin, Sanguinarin.
Crusta Lactea — Melitagrinum.
Cystitis — Camphoric Acid, Fluid Cerefolius, Fabiana, Imbricata, Musa Sapientum, Xanthium Spinosum.
       — (Chronic) — Epigaea Repens.

D
Dandruff — Badiaga.
Deafness — Cheiranthus Cheiri., Lueticum, Viburnum Tinus.
Delirium Tremens — Coriaria Ruscifolia.
Diabetes — Arsenicum Bromatum, Insulin, Kissingen,
Natrum Choleinicum, Oxygenium, Phaseolus,
Phloridyin, Uranium NitricumDeafness — Cheiranthus Cheiri., Lueticum, Viburnum Tinus.
Delirium Tremens — Coriaria Ruscifolia.
Diabetes — Arsenicum Bromatum, Insulin, Kissingen, Natrum Choleinicum, Oxygenium, Phaseolus, Phloridyin, Uranium Nitricum.
Diarrhoea — Acid Sulphuricum Aromaticum,
Jalapa,Jatropha Curcas, Melastoma, Prinos Verticillatus,
Rubus Villosus.
Dipsomania — Strychnine Hypophos.

Diphtheria — Diphtheria Antitoxin, Lactis Vaccini Flos., Mercurius Sulphocyanatus.
Displacement (of Uterus) — Fluor. Aurant. Amar.
Dropsy — Kali Nitricum, Liatris Spicata, Primula Vulgaris, Urinum.
Duodenal Ulcer — Dys. Co. (Bach).
Dwarfism— Mercurius Praecipitatus Albus.
Dysentry— Chenomorha Anti-dysenterica, Pyrethrum, Parthenium, Typha Latifolia.
Dyspepsia — Franzensbad, Ferrum Citricum, Nabalus Serpentaria.
    — (Climacteric) — Ovary Extract.
Dyspnoea — Iberis Amara.
Dysuria — Juniperus Virginianus, Rosa Canina, Uva Ursi.
Dysphagia — Lactis Vaccini Floc., Platinum Muriaticum.
Dysmenorrhoea— Apiol, Gastein, Heliotropium Peru, Manganum Oxydat., Viburnin.

E

Earache — Itu Resina, Mullein Oil.
Ear-wax — Wiesbaden.
Eclampsia — Spiraea Ulmaria.
Eczema — Bixa Orellana, Fuligo Ligni, Plumbum Aceticum.
    — (Rubrum)— Zea Italica.
Elephantiasis — Bixa Orellana.
Emmenagogue — Gossypium Herb., Gossypin, Planifolia.
Emphysema — Antimonium Arsenicosum, Naphthaline.
Empyema — Staphylococcin.
Enuresis — Mullein Oil, Nitrogenum Oxygenatum.
Enteralgia — Papaya Vulgaris.
Epididymitis — Sabal Serrulata.
Epilepsy — Ferrum Cyanatum, Passiflora Compound, Picrotoxin.
Epithelioma — Nectrianin.
Epistaxis — Helianthus Annus, Hydrastin. Hydrochlorate, Indium Metalicum.
Erysipelas — Euphorbia Lathyris, Euphorbia Cyparissias.
Eructation— Aconitum Neomontanum.
Exophthalmic Goitre— Ephedrin, Lycopus Virginicus.
Exostosis— Helka Lava.

F

Fever — Canchalagua, Eucalyptus Globulus, Illecebrum, Prinos Verticillatus.
Fibroma — Hydrastininum Muriaticum.
Fistula — Aurum Foliatum, Helianthus Annus, Hydrastin, Juniperus Sabina, Myristica Sebifera, Vanad Ammon.

Flatulence — Ipomea, Nux Juglans, Yerba Buena.
Frontal Headache — Digitalin.

G
Gallstone — Bilirubin, Lithium Benzoicum, Vichy.
Gangrene — Polygonum Persicaria.
Gastrodynia— Bismuth Trisnitrate, Mentha Piperata.
Gastritis— Euphorbia Ipecacuanhae.
Gastro-enteritis— Geartner (Bach), Henchera.
Gastralgia— Gaultheria Oil.
Gastric Ulcer— Plumbum Aceticum.
Glaucoma— Wiesbaden.
Gleet — Spiraea Ulmaria.
Globus Hystericus— Agnilegia.
Goitre — Fucus Vesiculosus.
Gonorrhoea — Fabiana Imbricata.
Gonorrhoeal Urethiritis — Cynosbati, Iodatum.
Gout — Aether, Colchicin, Formica Rufa, Formic Acid, Fraxinus Excelsior, Gichtwasser, Natrum Lacticum, Sodium Urate.

H
Haematuria — Ficus Religiosa, Natrum Hypochlorosum.
Haemorrhage — Erechites Hieracifolia, Lachesis Lanciolatus, Meloe Majalis, Millefolium.
Haematemesis — Ficus Religiosa, Hydrastin. Hydrochlorate.
Haemoptysis — Ficus Religiosa, Helix Tosta, Oleum Ricini.
Haemorrhoids — Aloin, Galvanismus, Gastein, Hamamelin, Lycopus Virginicus, Mucuna Urens, Pond's Extract.
Hay Fever — Calcarea Lactica Natronata, Sinapis Nigra.
Headache — Asclepin, Fagus Sylvatica, Iris Foetidissima, Lobelia Dortmanna, Natrum Murbit, Veratrum Nigrum.
Heartburn — Lithium Muriaticum, Quassin.
Helminthiasis — Areca.
Hemiplegia — Coniinum, Xanthoxylum Frax.
Hepatic Cirrhosis — Acid Nitro-hydrochloricum.
Hepatitis — Cornin, Nitro-muriatic Acid.
Hernia — Iris Foetidissima.
Herpes Zoster — Zinc Phos.
Hiccough — Amyl Nitrosum, Mapato, Oleum Succinum.
Hoarseness — Ampelopsin, Natrum Selenicum
Hydrocele — Ampelopsin.
Hydrothorax — Apocynin, Lactucarium.
Hydrocephalus — Galvanismus, Hedera Helix, Zinc Bromatum.

Hydropericardium — Leptandrin, Podophyllin.
Hydrophobia — Spirea Ulmaria, Xanthium Spinosum.
Hypochondriasis — Viburnum Tinus.
Hysteria — Aquilegia Canadensis, Ferri Valerianicum,
Zinc. Cyanatum.

I

Ichthyosis — Betala Alba, Borax Veneta.
Impotency — Lacttucarium, Nuphar Luteum.
Impetigo — Ferrum Arsenicum.
Indigestion — Lobelia Dortmanna, Pancreatinum.
Influenza — Gelsemin, Influenzinum, Oxygenium.
Inguinal Hernia — Wiesbaden.
Insomnia— Fagus Cup., Lecithin, Pas Avena, Passiflora
Compound, Piscidia, Xanthoxylin.
Ischuria— Juncus Effusus.
Itching — Ambrosia Artemisiaefolia, Anagallis Arvensis,
Bombyx, Dolchos Puriens, Primula Obconica.

J

Jaundice — Carduus Marianus, Fel Tauri, Leptandra, Myrica Cirifera, Myricin, Stillingin.
— (Infantile)— Lupulus.

K

Keratitis— Jequirity.

L

Labor-pain— Dictamnus Albus.
Lachrymation — Ambrosia Artemisiaefolia.
Laryngitis — Linum Catharticum.
Leprosy — Bixa Orellana, Gynocardia Odorata, Hygrophilla Spinosa, Madura Album.
Leucorrhoea — Aletrin, Calcarea Ovorum,
Ferrum Bromatum, Hedeoma Pulegioides,
Lippspringe, Ova Tosta, Rumex Obtusifolius
— (in little girls) — Cubeba Officinalis.
Leucaemia — Benzenum.
Leucocythemia — Menispermin.
Lichen Urticarus — Persicaria Urens.
Lipoma — Uric Acid.
Lithiasis — Lysidinum.

Locomotor Ataxia — Duboisin, Passiflora Compound, Zinc. Phos.
Loss of Memory — Coriaria Ruscifolia,
Latrodectus Hessetti, Potass. Xantate.
Lumbago — Ginseng, Hymosa, Kali Oxalicum, Macrotin, Rhamnus Californica.
Lupus — Sol.

M

Malaria— Alstonia Scholaris, Calcarea Arsenica.
Marasmus — Glycerinum, Pepsinum.
Masturbation — Origanum Majorona.
Measles — Gelsemin, Morbillinum.
Megrim — Anhalonium Lewinii, Calcarea Lacto-phosph.,
Indium Metalicum, Onosmodium Virg.
Menorrhagia — Calcarea Cloride, Epihysterin.
Menarche — Corpus Luteum.
Meningitis — Iodoformum, Parotidinum, Zinc. Cyanatum.
Meniere's Disease — Proteus (Bach), Salicinum.
Metritis — Sanguisorba Offcinalis.
Metrorrhagia — Erodium Cicutarium,
Hydrastininum Muriaticum, Viscum Album.
Micturation — Eryngium Aquaticum, Mentha Viridis.
Miscarriage — Viburnin.
Mumps — Pilicarpinum Nitricum, Parotidinum.
Myalgia — Formic Acid.

N

Naevi — Radium Bromide.
Nasal Polypi — Lemna Minor.
Nausea — Euphorbia Corollata, Narcissus Poeticus, Zea Italica.
Nephritis — Fluid Cerefolius, Scarlatininum, Uranium Nitricum.
Nervous Depression — Verbena.
Nettle-rash — Cancer Astacus.
Neuralgia — Croton Chloral, Pas Avena.
          — (Ciliary) — Hyoscyamin.
Neurasthenia — Lecithin, Methylene Blue.
Neuro-darmatitis — Morgan Pure (Paterson).
Nymphomania — Ferula Glauca.

O

Obesity — Esculentine, Fucus Vesiculosus, Iodothyrine
Occipital Headache — Cereus Bonplandii

Oliguria — Eel Serum
Opthalmia — Jequirity, Phosphorus Muriaticus
Opisthotonos — Phytolaccin, Strychninum
Orchitis — Parotidinum, Teucrium Scorodonia
Osteo-arthritis — Thymus Gland Extract
Otitis — Methylene Blue
Otorrhoea — Aethiops Antimonalis, Viola Odorata.
Ovarian Cyst — Oophorinum
Oxaluria — Acid Nitro-hydrochloricum, Aqua Regia, Lysidinum
Ozaena — Glanderine

P

Panaritium — Myristica Sebifera
Paraplegia — Anhalonium Lewinii
Paralysis — Gelsemin, Iris Florentina,
Passiflora Compound, Parathyroid, Strychnia Phosph., Zinc Cyanatum
    — (infantile) — Lathyrus
Parotitis — Salix purpurea
Pemphigus — Ranunculus Sceleratus
Pertussis — Diptrix Odorata, Formalin
Pharyngitis — Arum Dracontium, Wyethia Helenioides
Photophobia — Saponin
Phithisis — Formalin, Gallic Acid, Myosotis, Succinum, Zinc. Iodatum
Piles — Lapsana Communis, Vanad Ammon
Pleurodynia — Gaultheria Procumbens, Rhamnus Californica, Vyloxochitl.
Plica Polonica — Vinca Minor.
Pneumonia — Scilla Maritima.
Polyuria — Plat. Mur. Nat.
Poliomyelitis — Bungarus Krait.
Polyarthiritis — Eosin, Ichthyolum.
Post-partum Haemorrhage — Cinnamonum.
Presbyopia — Duboisin.
Priapism— Hydrophobinum.
Prolapsus Uteri— Sarza.
Prostatitis— Fabiana Imbricata, Pituitrin.
Prostatorrhoea — Spiraea Ulmaria.
Prostatomegally — Fluid Cerefolius.
Pruritus Senilis — Fagopyrum Esculetum.
Psoriasis — Kali Assenicum, Morgan Gaertner(Paterson), X-Ray.
Pterygium— Guarea Trichiloides, Mapato.
Puerperal Eclampsia — Oenanthe Crocata.
Pyelitis — Epigaea Repens, Juniperus Communis, Uva Ursi.
Pyorrhoea — Emetine Hydrochloride.
Pyrosis — Ricinus Communis, Zea Italica.

R

Rayneud's Disease — Proteus (Bach).
Remittent Fever — Narcissus Poeticus.
Renal Dropsis — Ampelopsin.
Renal Colic — Morgan Gaertner (Paterson).
Rheumatic Fever — Hymosa.
Rheumatism — Guaiacum, Gauttheria Procumbens, Lignum Vitae, Stellaria Media
—(Chronic) — Kali Salicylicum
Rhinitis — Glanderine, Lemna Minor.
Ringworm — Crysophanic Acid, Nux Juglans.

S

Salivation — Aqua Regia.
Scabies — Gynocardia Odorata.
Scarlet Fever — Aconitum Radix.
Sciatica — Cervus Brasilicus, Gnaphalium, Gaultheria Procumbens, Nyctanthes, Pas Avena, Salix Mollissima.
Scrofula — Rumin.
Scurvy — Carya Alba, Natrum Hypochlorosum, Urinum.
Seminal Emissions — Voeslau, Zincum Picricum.
Septicemia — Echafolta.
Sexual Weakness — Sperminum.
exual Neurasthenia — Damiana, Onosmodium Virg.
Shock — Hyoscin Hydrobrom.
Sleeplessness — Arenearum Tela, Hyoscyamin, Lactucarium, Myrica Cirifera.
Snake-bite — Eupatorium Ayapan, Selaginella.
Sneezing — Asparagin, Quillaya Saponaria.
Somnumbulism — Magnetis Polus Arcticus.
Sore-nipples— Lapsana Communis.
Sore-throat — Euphorbia Peplus, Helianthus Annus., Helleborus Viridis, Indium Metalicum, Nymphaea Odorata.
Spasm— Nicotinum.
Spinal Sclerosis — Hyoscyamin.
Splenitis — Ceanothus Amer.
Spermatorrhoea — Camphora Bromata, Nuphar Luteum, Ustilago Maydis.
Spinal Curvature — Tuberculinum Testium.
Spinal Paralysis — Wildbad.
Sprains — Pond's Extract, Vitex Trifolia,
Sterility — Phytoline.
Stiff-neck — Hura, Itu Resina.
Strangury — Apocynin, Juncus Effusus, Oleum Ricnini.
Strabismus — Morphinum Muriaticum.

Suppression of Urine — Apocynin.
Sunstroke — Sol., Usnea Barbata.
Syphilis — Gynocardia Odorata, Succus Amogara.

T
Tape-worm — Granatum, Hagenia Abyssinica, Ioduretted Potass. Iod.
Tetanus — Jasminum Officinale, Passiflora Compound.
Tinnitus— Salicinum, Vertrum Nigrum.
Tonsillitis— Lignum Vitae.
Toothache — Coccinella Septempunctata,
Ferrum Sulphuricum, Galvanismus, Itu Resina, Natrum Hypochlorosum, Oleum Ricini.
Torticolllis — Lachnanthes Tinctoria.
Tuberculosis — Guaiacolum, Rubia Tinctorum
Tumor — Ammonium Fluoridicum, Cancer
Fluviatilis, Carcinosin, Fraxinus Americana, Soda Cacodyl., Thiosinaminum.
Typhoid Fever— Baptisin, Septicaemin, Vaccinum. Myrtillus, Xerophyllum Tenax.

U
Ulcer — Fuligo Ligni, Gratiola Officinalis., Hygrophilla Spinosa.
Uraemia — Asclepias Cornuti, Phenacetinum.
Urticaria — Cancer Astacus, Gaertner, Hygrophilla Spinosa, Urtica Urens.
Uterine Prolapse — Aletrin.

V
Vaginismus— Cocaine Hydrochlorate.
Varicocele— Melitagrinum.
Varicose Veins — Mangifera Indica.
Vertigo — Ethylum Nitricum, Kousso, Morphinum Sulphuricum.
Vomiting — Amygadalus Persica, Agaricus Rhalloides, Cadmium Sulph., Elaterin.
 — (of pregnancy)— Aletrin, Ingluvin, Strontium Bromatum.

W
Warts — Aurum Mur., Calcarea Calcinata, Ferrum Magneticum, Ova Tosta, X-Ray.
Whittow — Wiesbaden.
Whooping-cough — Casein, Coqueluchinum, Fluroform, Oxygenium, Pertussin.
Worms — Chelone.
Wounds — Hamamelin.
Writer's Cramp — Brachyglottis, Ferrum Phos., Hydricum.

www.ingramcontent.com/pod-product-compliance
Lightning Source LLC
Chambersburg PA
CBHW050203230526
45470CB00001B/221